"On each page it becomes obvious that this book was written by two experienced trainers, who love what they teach and who know how to captivate their students."
—**Frank Staemmler**, *Psychologist and Gestalt therapist, Würzburg*

"The book will have a wide and receptive audience: Gestalt training institutes, graduate classes for mental health, masters and doctoral students, and practitioners from a variety of modalities. I highly recommend it."
—**Ruella Frank**, *Founder and Director of the Center for Somatic Studies, New York*

"I have great respect for this book, both for the huge amount of serious work that the authors have put in on it and for the didactic style that allows even non-specialists to understand what gestalt therapy is."
—**Margherita Spagnuolo Lobb**, *Director Istituto di Gestalt HCC, Italy*

Gestalt Therapy Practice

This essential new book gives the reader an introduction to the fundamental concepts of gestalt therapy in a stimulating and accessible style. It supports the study and practice of gestalt therapy for clinicians of all backgrounds, reflecting a practice-based pedagogy that emphasises experiential learning.

The content in this book builds on the curriculum taught at the Norwegian Gestalt Institute University College (NGI). The material is divided into four main sections. In the first section, the theoretical basis for gestalt therapy is presented with references to gestalt psychology, field theory, phenomenology, and existential philosophy. In the later parts, central theoretical terms and practical models are discussed, such as the paradoxical theory of change, creative adjustment, self, contact, contact forms, awareness, polarities, and process models. Clinical examples illustrate the therapy form's emphasis on the relational meeting between therapist and client.

Detailed description of gestalt therapy theory from the time of the gestalt psychologists to today, with abundant examples from clinical practice, distinguishes this book from other texts. It will be of great value to therapists, coaches, and students of gestalt therapy.

Gro Skottun, PhD, is one of the founders of the Norwegian Gestalt Institute University College (NGI), where she is currently Pro-Rector and Associate Professor. She has taught gestalt therapy internationally for many years, mostly in Prague and Budapest. She is a co-founder of the NGI's professional journal, *Norsk Gestalttidsskrift*, for which she is currently editor, and has published several articles on gestalt therapy.

Åshild Krüger cand. Polit, MSc in gestalt psychotherapy, former Assistant Professor at the Lillehammer University College and former Assistant Professor at the Norwegian Gestalt Institute University College (NGI). She is co-founder of the NGI's professional journal, *Norsk Gestalttidsskrift*, and has published widely on gestalt therapy.

Gestalt Therapy Book Series

The Istituto di Gestalt series of Gestalt therapy books emerges from the ground of a growing interest in theory, research and clinical practice in the Gestalt community. The members of the Scientific and Editorial Boards have been committed for many years to the process of supporting research and publications in our field: through this series we want to offer our colleagues internationally the richness of the current trends in Gestalt therapy theory and practice, underpinned by research. The goal of this series is to develop the original principles in hermeneutic terms: to articulate a relational perspective, namely a phenomenological, aesthetic, field-oriented approach to psychotherapy. It is also intended to help professions and to support a solid development and dialogue of Gestalt therapy with other psychotherapeutic methods.

The series includes original books specifically created for it, as well as translations of volumes originally published in other languages. We hope that our editorial effort will support the growth of the Gestalt therapy community; a dialogue with other modalities and disciplines; and new developments in research, clinics and other fields where Gestalt therapy theory can be applied (e.g., organizations, education, political and social critique and movements).

We would like to dedicate this Gestalt Therapy Book Series to all our masters and colleagues who have sown fruitful seeds in our minds and hearts.

Coordinators
Jeff Allison and Stefania Benini

Editorial Assistant
Serena Iacono Isidoro

General Editor
Margherita Spagnuolo Lobb

Istituto di Gestalt

www.gestaltitaly.com   HCC Italy

Series Editor **Margherita Spagnuolo Lobb**

Gestalt Therapy Book Series

Series editor: Margherita Spagnuolo Lobb

For more information on the titles in this series, please visit www.routledge.com/ Gestalt-Therapy/book-series/GESTHE and www.gestaltitaly.com

Gestalt Therapy Practice

Theory and Experiential Learning

Gro Skottun and Åshild Krüger

Routledge
Taylor & Francis Group
LONDON AND NEW YORK

First published in English 2022
by Routledge
2 Park Square, Milton Park, Abingdon, Oxon OX14 4RN

and by Routledge
605 Third Avenue, New York, NY 10158

Routledge is an imprint of the Taylor & Francis Group, an informa business

© 2022 Gro Skottun and Åshild Krüger

Translated by Ann Kunish.

This book was originally published in Norwegian as *Gestaltterapi: Lærebok i teori og praksis* (Gyldendal Akademisk, 2017)

The right of Gro Skottun and Åshild Krüger to be identified as authors of this work has been asserted by them in accordance with sections 77 and 78 of the Copyright, Designs and Patents Act 1988.

British Library Cataloguing-in-Publication Data
A catalogue record for this book is available from the British Library

Library of Congress Cataloging-in-Publication Data
A catalog record for this book has been requested

ISBN: 978-0-367-72204-3 (hbk)
ISBN: 978-0-367-72205-0 (pbk)
ISBN: 978-1-003-15385-6 (ebk)

DOI: 10.4324/9781003153856

Typeset in Times New Roman
by Apex CoVantage, LLC

Contents

Preface to the English edition

As gestalt training programmes become more and more international, and gestalt therapists and coaches meet in international fora with increasing frequency, the usefulness of textbooks in a common language becomes apparent. While resources in English and a very few other widely understood languages have been available for decades, the perspectives found in countries where other languages are spoken are generally only accessible to speakers of those languages. Making our pedagogical texts available to each other in this manner is therefore a way to share our various perspectives on the teaching, theory, and practice of our profession.

The first edition of *Gestalt therapy: Textbook in theory and practice* was published in Norway in 2017. When we revisited the material prior to translation in 2019, we once again found ourselves discussing the nuances of how we choose to present the material. It also gave us an opportunity to correct discrepancies that had managed to sneak into the Norwegian text prior to publication.

As part of the process of creating an English edition of this book, a peer review was done based on selected chapters, the Norwegian introduction, and the table of contents. The feedback from this review was invaluable and has resulted in the inclusion of several new perspectives on the historical development and theoretical basis of gestalt therapy. We are grateful to our reviewers for their thoughtful input.

During the translation process it has been inspiring to see how a Norwegian text is recreated in English and becomes a book, chapter by chapter. It has been rewarding to discuss terms and concepts with our translator Ann Kunish as we have explored how best to present our ideas in English. Ann's expertise as both translator and gestalt therapist, combined with her attention to detail, has resulted in an English edition that we believe readers will enjoy and find useful.

As a result of this work, the reader will notice a few slight differences when compared to the first Norwegian edition. These changes will be incorporated into the second Norwegian edition. Our perspective on gestalt theory and the Norwegian practice-based pedagogy remains however the same.

It is our hope that this English edition will contribute to the constructive discussion and debate that exist in the international gestalt milieu.

Introduction

This book targets a broad group of readers.[1] The founder of gestalt therapy, Fritz Perls, himself emphasised the importance of spreading his therapy form to a broad audience. He clarified that gestalt therapy is pragmatic and applicable to more than just therapy. In this textbook, we accept his invitation and apply examples from areas other than therapy, such as coaching, counselling, and organisational development. This is a natural extension of the target audience, because the Norwegian Gestalt Institute University College (NGI) offers study programmes in all these areas.

Every textbook is closely related to a study programme and teaching, and we find it natural to say a few words about the function of this textbook in the experience-based teaching form at NGI. The educational foundation of our teaching builds on the philosopher John Dewey's (1859–1952) principle of *learning by doing*.[2] Our method enables experience-based learning processes, which can be described in three phases. The first begins with facilitated practical exercises. These are followed up with reflection, before the knowledge-based concept is finally presented theoretically and discussed with the teacher. The benefit of this teaching form is that the student is able to make the concepts her own. Concepts are integrated into the body, emotions, and thoughts. In other words, this is a practical pedagogy that is well suited for training therapists. It is personal and intimate. Kjeldahl (2012) points out that the final phase of learning, when a concept is presented in light of content and theory, has a tendency to be the weakest phase in this form of learning. We hope and believe that the book's systemised presentation of concepts will help strengthen this final stage of the learning process.

The content in this book builds on the curriculum taught at NGI. It lays the foundation for our teaching theory and is intended to be a support for clinical practice. The material is divided into four main sections, each of which is divided into chapters.

Part 1: the basis of gestalt therapy

In Chapters 1 and 2, the theoretical basis for gestalt therapy is presented, and we examine the roots of the therapy form in Europe in the early nineteenth century. Chapter 1 discusses gestalt psychology and Kurt Lewin's understanding of a person and her environment. This theme is examined further in Chapter 2, in light

DOI: 10.4324/9781003153856-1

of phenomenology's philosophical basic principle of being in the world here and now. In Chapter 3, we examine Laura and Fritz Perls' importance in gestalt therapy, where the development of this form of therapy is illustrated by a discussion of changing trends and by the presentation of central actors. The chapter concludes with a description of how gestalt therapy has evolved.

Part 2: Fundamental terminology and concepts

Chapters 4 through 11 mark the transition to a more pragmatic, practice-relevant approach. In Chapter 4, the relationship between field theory and gestalt therapy's relational approach is highlighted. We influence and are influenced by others, and our diverse and often conflicting needs affect our lives. Chapter 5 describes the gestalt therapy perspective of change and how this change can take place in the therapy room. The concept of creative adjustment is described in Chapter 6, and includes how people develop and adapt to their surroundings at any given time. People's understanding of who they are, how they can behave in different ways in different situations, and how impulses and needs lead to action are described in Chapter 7—the theory of self in gestalt therapy.

Chapter 8 describes concepts such as awareness. These are the basics the therapist uses in order to learn more about herself and her clients, not only during the course of therapy, but throughout life. Contact, described in Chapter 9, was the term Fritz Perls described as the most basic in gestalt therapy. Several of the theoretical models and techniques gestalt therapists employ are based on being in contact. Chapter 10 describes polarities as contradictions in and between people, and we discuss how these contradictions are related to conflicting needs the therapist can explore with the client in the therapy room. Chapter 11 discusses the gestalt 'therapeutic experiment'. This pragmatic term describes how the therapist creates situations where the client can experiment, verbally and nonverbally, with unknown and new forms of expression and behaviour that can increase the client's attention and create new experiences.

Part 3: contact forms

As the word suggests, the term 'contact form' describes the ways in which we humans are in relationships with others. There are many forms of contact, and these vary from situation to situation. There are six forms of contact in gestalt therapy. Perls et al. (1951) described five contact forms: confluence, introjection, projection, retroflexion, and egotism. The sixth, deflection, is described by Polster and Polster (1974). The contact forms are discussed in Chapters 12 through 17.

Part 4: Process models

Gestalt therapy is concerned with processes in the here and now, and the three gestalt process models support the therapist's attention to how therapy progresses. The three gestalt process models—often referred to as cycles—are the process of contact, the process of experience, and the process of change. These models are based on Fritz Perls' understanding of change and creative adjustment and are discussed in Chapters 18 through 20.

The examples given in this book are fictional but are based on the authors' experience from years of clinical practice.

Notes

1 In this book we have chosen to write *gestalt* rather than *Gestalt*. In his book *Gestalt Therapy* (2010), published by Routledge, David Mann argues for the use of a lowercase g, which he uses throughout his book. In his argumentation, Mann refers to Bloom, Spagnuolo Lobb, as well as Staemmler's (2008) Notes on Nomenclature. *Studies in Gestalt Therapy. Psychotherapy and Social Change: Dialogical Bridges*, *2*(1).

These examples are part of an ongoing discussion in the professional discourse about whether to capitalise the name of our method of therapy. We contemplated the various arguments for and against when making a choice for this book before ultimately deciding on *gestalt*.
2 This learning model as used by NGI is presented and discussed in Kjeldahl (2012), Krüger (2005), and Grendstad (1986).

References

Clarkson, P., & Mackewn, J. (1993). *Fritz perls*. London: Sage

Grendstad, N. M. (1986). *Å lære er å oppdage* [To learn is to discover]. Oslo: Didakta Norsk Forlag AS.

Kjeldahl, M. (2012). *"Det blir så veldig en del av en selv": En studie av læring i gestalt-terapeutisk perspektiv: Masteroppgave i pedagogikk*. ["It becomes so very much a part of oneself": A study of learning in a gestalt therapeutic perspective: Master's thesis in pedagogy.]. (Master's thesis). Retrieved from DUO Research Archive, http://hdl.handle.net/10852/30642

Krüger, Å. (2005). Gestaltveiledning: Modell for oppdagende læring i kontekst [Gestalt supervision: A model for discovery in learning in context]. *Norsk Gestalttidskrift*, *2*(2), 102–107.

Perls, F. S., Hefferline, R. F., & Goodman, P. (1951). *Gestalt therapy: Excitement and growth in the human personality*. London: Souvenir Press.

Polster, E., & Polster, M. (1974). *Gestalt therapy integrated*. New York: Vintage Books.

Part 1

The basis of gestalt therapy

Chapter 1

Gestalt psychology and field theory

What exactly does the word 'gestalt' mean? This is the classic question gestalt therapists are often asked by friends, acquaintances, and clients. The word 'gestalt' is German, and can be translated as 'form, shape' or 'an organised whole that is perceived as more than the sum of its parts'. In the theatre world it is not uncommon to hear the phrase 'to gestalt a role' as a way to describe the process by which an actor brings form and substance to a character. In a therapeutic context, we can say that the client comes to therapy to explore difficult experiences. With the therapist's support, the client creates the possibility to give form and content to—to gestalt—those experiences.

In this chapter, we describe the psychological basis for gestalt therapy, namely gestalt psychology, with emphasis on perception, key gestalt principles, and field theory. We provide a historical overview of the development of gestalt psychology, describe its basic theories, and discuss the influences these have had on gestalt therapy.[1]

The roots of the term 'gestalt'

The history of the term 'gestalt' stretches back in time to the poet Johann Wolfgang von Goethe (1749–1832). Goethe was also a naturalist; he believed that totality was more important than individual parts. A forest, a plant, or for that matter a human being, is first and foremost a gestalt that cannot be picked apart.

The term 'gestalt' reappears in the German psychology of consciousness in the 1890s. For the proponents of this school of thought, however, consciousness was focused more on individual trees than on the forest, although it was also thought that the forest as a whole was more than a collection of trees. It is, however, the so-called gestalt psychologists from Berlin in the beginning of the twentieth century who have become known as the founders of what we today call gestalt psychology. The gestalt psychologists, or the Berlin School as they also were called, consisted of a group of scientists who set out to demonstrate scientifically how we structure what we sense, or, to use our terminology, how we perceive what we sense.

DOI: 10.4324/9781003153856-2

A historical retrospect

From the late 1800s, psychology was a new science in full swing with research on human thought and behaviour. In laboratories, questions were raised about how we understand human consciousness, and psychologists made great progress in research. They developed hypotheses and concluded that images on the retina are a direct result of neurological processes between external stimuli and brain activity.

The psychologist Wilhelm Wundt (1832–1920), whose professional life took place during the era of the psychology of consciousness in the 1890s, was considered by his contemporaries to be a founder of the 'new experimental psychology'. He established the first formal laboratory for psychological research in Leipzig in 1879. In his opinion, experimental psychology should study simple psychological phenomena such as sensation, perception, attention, associations, and simple emotions; that is, the basic, elementary aspects of consciousness.

The psychological analyses of this school of thought were based in a reductionist, one-to-one correspondence between external objects and internal images. The tree I see is the same as the real, living tree. Consciousness is composed of individual parts—a so-called atomistic way of thinking, advocated by Wilhelm Wundt.

In line with this reductionist way of understanding human behaviour emerged another type of psychological understanding. Psychologist Christian Freiherr von Ehrenfels (1859–1932) was one of the first to question whether there were other scientific ways to understand consciousness. In contrast to the reductionists, he claimed that our senses perceive more than individual parts. He believed that what we see is not the parts that make up a tree, but rather the tree in its entirety. Thus, atomism was replaced by holistic thinking.

Ehrenfels was thus the first to use the term 'gestalt' to describe the sensory process by which we see objects as whole entities. It was in his footsteps the first gestalt psychologists followed when they formed their hypotheses about how we gestalt experience. The first was one of Ehrenfels' students, the philosopher and psychologist Max Wertheimer (1880–1943). Wertheimer was followed by his likeminded colleagues Kurt Koffka (1886–1941) and Wolfgang Köhler (1887–1967).

It is not surprising that Wertheimer and his colleagues became involved in the holistic and phenomenological school of thought. They read and studied the natural philosophers Spinoza and Goethe, two thinkers who, in addition to phenomenology, are considered central to the idea of the importance of the senses and the holistic idea that everything is connected. Wertheimer, Koffka, and Köhler were interested in music and other art forms; these interests were also fertile ground for scientific challenge to atomistic thinking.

The discovery of the phi phenomenon (motion illusion)

The gestalt psychologists went one step further and argued that we first and foremost perceive the totality of an object or experience, and that the whole is thus more than the sum of its parts. Wertheimer claimed that when we hear, or rather sense, a piece of music, we perceive the overall quality or expression, a qualitative whole beyond its individual notes. Wertheimer called this phenomenon *phi*.

This claim was not, however, well received, and it took time before *phi* could be explained scientifically. The famous discovery came one autumn day in 1910 as Wertheimer sat on the train watching telephone poles go by along the railroad tracks. He was aware that the distance between the poles seemed to be less than it actually was as the train passed. The overall picture as it was perceived by the senses there and then, as the train was in motion, was an illusion. The whole that emerges is illusory: we perceive movement without the poles actually moving. The conclusion is, in Wertheimer's view, was that we sense not only the sum of the parts, in this case the telephone poles, but the qualitative totality: movement.

Perception of gestalts

Wertheimer eventually moved to Berlin, where he met Koffka and Köhler. Together, the three established an active and enthusiastic research group that became known in relation to gestalt psychology. After the discovery of the *phi* phenomenon, Wertheimer and Köhler continued work on the hypothesis of perception and creating wholes. Having ascertained *that* we perceive, they directed their attention to *how* our impressions of the whole of a situation are formed; in other words, how we gestalt and structure phenomena.

The gestalt psychologists gave many compelling arguments that illustrated how totalities occur spontaneously; in other words, how perceptual impressions organise themselves. On this basis, they came to the following conclusions, taken from Teigen (2004/2015):

- All perception is the perception of organised forms: even two dots are not just dots, but a pair. The *phi* phenomenon is not two sensations, but a movement.
- It is not coincidental which parts of a field of stimulus come together to form a whole.
- A gestalt's appearance is not coincidental.

The law of prägnanz

Using a series of experiments, gestalt psychologists found that organisation takes form in certain ways and by specific laws, and that the fundamental principle behind these laws is the law of *prägnanz*. Wertheimer and Köhler found that our perception tends to find the clearest and simplest form. For example, we have a tendency to perceive a figure as complete, even when parts of the whole are lacking. This is shown in Figures 1.1 and 1.2.

When you see these figures, your mind automatically fills in the missing information; Figure 1.1 becomes a complete circle, Figure 1.2 an entire rectangle.

The law of *prägnanz* says that when we perceive something, we tend to seek and identify the totality that we feel to be the simplest and most obvious. If we

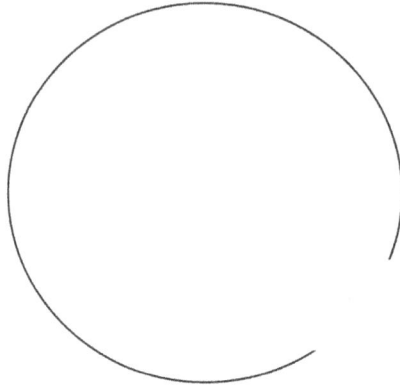

Figure 1.1

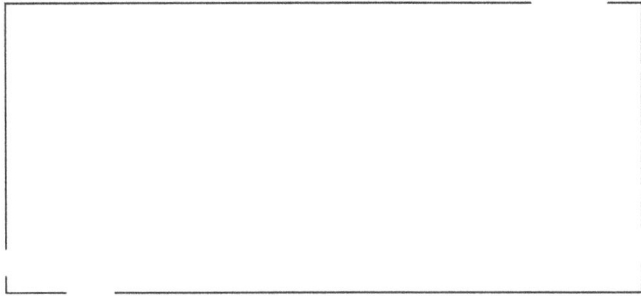

Figure 1.2

look at human behaviour in light of this law, we see that the simplest, most obvious and natural thing for people to do is often what they are accustomed to doing, or—as in Figures 1.1 and 1.2—to see what they are accustomed to seeing. This is an example of structures or gestalts that repeat. In the context of the therapy room, this means that the therapist sees the client's behaviour as the best, most obvious, and simplest way of being, even though it is not always the most appropriate for the client or the client's environment.

The principles of perceptual grouping were also called 'gestalt laws', 'gestalt factors', or 'gestalt qualities'. These principles describe which parts of the stimulus field are grouped together, and that these groups will also appear as the most regular and completed. We have certain ideals that we attempt to align with the world around us. This often succeeds, because on the whole, the world and perception follow the same laws.

The principle of figure-ground

The principle of figure-ground is also an example of an automatic organisation of sensory impressions that matches well with the way the world is actually organised. The organisation of figure-ground is perhaps the principle most often referred to by gestalt therapists. It was developed by the Danish psychologist Edgar Rubin (1886–1951), who began studying the phenomenon several months before Wertheimer began his investigations of *phi*.

Figure 1.3 is the well-known, characteristic example of how we tend to perceive something against the background of something else. This well-known image illustrates that when we focus on an idea or sensation, everything else disappears into the background. When we see the vase, the white area comes into the foreground and the black becomes a formless background. The opposite happens when the figure is perceived as two faces; the white area loses its contour and blends into the background while the profiles take shape and come to the foreground.

The 'aha' experience and problem-solving learning

Köhler was interested in how the process of gestalting occurred, and performed a series of experiments on chimpanzees to see how they solved specific tasks. Some of the most famous are the experiments done with the chimpanzee Sultan. Köhler placed Sultan in a cage and placed bananas out of reach. The chimpanzee was equipped with two bamboo poles, and the only way to reach the bananas was to put the poles together. Sultan was hungry and wanted the bananas. Initially, Köhler tried to help him by suggesting solutions. Interestingly, Sultan was not interested in the suggestions; instead, he concentrated on solving the problem himself. After much trial and error, he was angry and frustrated and gave up. He retreated to the back of the cage, showed no interest in his environment, and

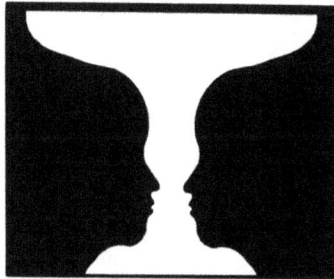

Figure 1.3

scratched his neck. Suddenly he stood up, walked over, and put the two poles together, bringing the bananas within reach. He was able to complete the task when he restructured the problem.

Köhler interpreted Sultan's behavior as an 'aha' experience (Madsen, 2016). With this and similar examples, Köhler demonstrated that solutions often happen in moments of insight, where the individual factors, all aspects of the problem, spontaneously organise themselves into a meaningful, comprehensive action in the situation. It was not possible to explain how Sultan had solved the problem by breaking down his action into individual factors (Neumann & Neumann, 2014). The result of Köhler's research and the theories he developed have had a great deal of influence on later theories of insight-based problem-solving and learning and are also fundamental to how gestalt theory views change and learning in the therapy room (see Chapter 4 on paradoxical change).

Summary of gestalt psychology and perception

The gestalt psychologists' conclusions about perceptions live on. After systematic testing of perception in the laboratory, they arrived at several basic principles. Although their methods were later criticised for not being thorough enough, there is no doubt that their work paved the way for later, more precise experimenting. Many of the gestalt psychologists' findings became part of the foundation of the theory of gestalt therapy, in particular the *phi* phenomenon, the law of *prägnanz* and related gestalt laws, and the principle of figure-ground. The gestalt view that the whole is greater than and not simply the sum of its parts; that phenomena such as experience, needs, and emotions are gestalted in a field; and the therapist's attitude that by following the law of *prägnanz* the client does the best she can in any given situation, all have their roots in gestalt psychology.

The attitude in gestalt therapy toward change and learning are influenced by Köhler's experiences with problem solving and learning via spontaneous insight. This means that the therapist can be present with the client in her frustration and attempts to find a solution, fully aware that as a therapist, she does not need to find a solution for the client.

Field theory

Gordon Wheeler (1998) discusses the importance of the first gestalt psychologists in the gestalt therapeutic context. He points out that a typical feature of the so-called Wertheimer models is that, despite persistent attempts to mark the distinction between the Wertheimer models and Wundt's reductionism, the classic gestalt psychologists nevertheless conducted their experiments in closed laboratories and under the rules of scientific control. The results were therefore limited and not applicable to clinical practice. Wheeler calls their research 'figure limiting', with no reference to anything other than the closed space for examination.

The big change that clearly marks a scientific epoch change, a historical milestone, and a paradigm shift, came with the groundbreaking thinking of the two gestalt psychologists Kurt Goldstein (1878–1965) and Kurt Lewin (1890–1947). Both belonged to the Berlin School and were of crucial importance in moving gestalt thinking, and thus studies of perception, out of the laboratory and into real life.

The organism and its environment

In the 1930s, the neuropsychologist Kurt Goldstein developed a theory of the 'structure of the organism', in which he saw all needs as special cases of a fundamental tendency toward completion or realisation, and which he called *self-actualisation*. This was a continuation of the gestalt psychologists' view of perception based on the principle of finality, where a situation that is unfinished or incomplete *requires* that it be completed or supplemented. The term 'self-actualisation' was used by Aristotle (384–322 BCE) and Carl Gustav Jung (1875–1961). It later became a key concept in the humanistic theories of personality. For Goldstein, however, it was the organism and its relationship to the environment that was the overarching gestalt. This gestalt strives for harmony and balance and has had a considerable influence on gestalt therapy theory.

The field

The founders of gestalt psychology used the field concept in a broad variety of contexts, ranging from problems of understanding brain processes and their relationship to phenomenal processes (for example Wolfgang Köhler) to the investigation of human perception and behaviour (for example Kurt Lewin). In a recent article, Stemberger (2019) has described three definitions in which the field concept is addressed in gestalt psychology: the phenomenal field, the psychic field, and the psychophysical field. In this book, we focus on Lewin's understanding of the field concept which includes the phenomenal and the psychic field.

Lewin was interested in examining perception in real life without the limitations of a laboratory. Based in gestalt theoretic principles, he aimed to develop a personality theory rooted in a dynamic, realistic life situation here and now. He wanted to change the focus from individual linear studies of man to the study of lived life experience. This opposition to the early gestalt psychologists is summarised by Wheeler (1998):

That is to say, the perceptual gestalten in the 'real life' situation do not merely rise and fade and succeed each other in a linear (or Associationist) fashion, as

> in the lab setting, but actually persist, coexist, and interact in a dynamic and mutually structured way . . . it is not such that gestalting of sensations in the field only come and go in a linear fashion, but that they are persistent and that they interact in a dynamically and mutually structured manner.
>
> (p. 28)

In the development of his field theory, Lewin (1936) was strongly influenced by his knowledge of gestalt psychology, physics, and phenomenology, which were under rapid development both before and during his lifetime. Lewin believed that the complex force of physics was a good metaphor for the tension that is created when people meet and influence each other, and used the term 'psychodynamic field' (Dyrkorn, 2014; van Baalen, 2002/2008b). Lewin (1951) understood that there was a big difference between a physical field and a psychological field between people. Field theory is as much about behaviour as about experience, but also behaviour was in Lewin's opinion a result of the total psychological field: the life-space that surrounds the individual. This life-space consists of the individual and the surrounding psychological world as it exists for him, and is not necessarily the same as a psychodynamic field. Analogously, the psychological field theory of Lewin (1951) originates from

> the basic statements . . . that (a) behavior has to be derived from a totality of coexisting facts, (b) these coexisting facts have the character of a 'dynamic field' in so far as the state of any part of this field depends on every other part of the field.
>
> (Lewin in Staemmler, 2006, p. 25)

Lewin argued that life-space has a structure that consists of subjective, more or less restricted and more or less accessible *regions*, which arise when the regions have different *valence*, that is, are more or less alluring or repulsive. A person's needs and the psychological conditions in his environment influence her equally. They contribute to the tension in her and the living-space she is part of (Staemmler, 2006). It is in this dynamic touch with what is around us, in this life-space of mutually influencing forces, that we develop, are shaped, and gestalt our lives.

Lewin's description and explanation of an individual's living-space is at times complex and difficult to understand; we have chosen not to delve into it further in this text. Instead, we examine the basic ideas in his field theory, which are used by gestalt therapists in clinical practice. We choose to define 'field' as follows: a field may be considered to be the sum of the reciprocal influencing forces in a limited area and for a given time (see Yontef, 1993, p. 297; Parlett, 2005, p. 47). On the basis of this definition, we will now discuss three characteristics of field theory. The first is *the principle of the interdependence of field forces*, the second is *the here and now*, and the third is *the importance of needs in regulation*.

The principle of the interdependence of field forces

In our discussion of field theory's fundamental principles, we give an example from everyday life, and therefore take a trip to the sandbox:

> Little Harry, four years old, is playing together with his three friends. They make roads and build houses in the sand with a great deal of enthusiasm. Harry's mother turns up in the middle of their activity; she has come to take him home for dinner. Suddenly, the mood changes—the children protest loudly. None of them wants to go home. Anger and tears ensue in the sandbox. Harry is the most vocal; his experience is that his mother soothes him if his protests are loud and persistent enough.

This short story illustrates how the dynamics between individuals in a field change—around them, between them, and in them. We can see that the interaction in the sandbox has its own dynamic; the way Harry, his friends, and mother interact is characterised by a mutual and inherent interdependence. When Harry thinks, feels, and acts, he affects not only the others, but also himself.

When his mother enters the scene, the picture changes dramatically. The children's quiet, normal interaction changes character—the energy rises and the dynamic quality changes form. It is no longer just about the children's activity, but also about the mother's intrusive intervention. A change occurs. When the field is changed by the mother's entrance, the dynamic between the children and between the mother and children is affected.

Regardless of what happens in a field, it affects the interaction in one way or another for each individual and between the participants in the unfolding field. This complex reciprocal interaction in the field is what Lewin called the principle of the interdependence of field forces, where all parts of a system are connected, and a change in one part changes all parts.

The field is in other words a hyper-complex system with a multitude of opportunities for something to take shape and find its structure. In gestalt terminology, we say that the figure in the field emerges from a complex background (see p. 11 on figure-ground). The processes are by no means simple and linear, as if one occurs as a result of another; rather, the field implies an inherent interdependence. Harry's version of the story in our example is admittedly different from that of his mother, yet the stories are related. In this way, their common story is created on the basis of each of their stories and the field they form together in the moment.

Before we move on to the next principle, we stop to examine the consequences field theory has on our understanding of what happens in the therapy room. When the therapist and client meet, they form a field together—a field in which both contribute to the gestalting of experiences and the process by which the experiences acquire meaning. It is important to take seriously the fact that both therapist and client are participants who affect the dynamic of the field, and that both contribute to the client's experience and action. Seen in light of phenomenology, this is about creating a situation where the information in the relational field is available here and now (Wollants, 2012). This leads us to the next characteristic of the field.

Here and now in the field

> Harry's mother recognises his vocal protests from previous occasions. Every time she arrives to fetch him, he screams in protest.

It can of course be useful to recognise behaviour patterns that repeat. In therapy, we also place great importance on experience as it shows itself in the current situation. In order to mark a distinction between past and present, gestalt therapists often use the phrase 'bringing past experience to the here and now'. This clarifies the distinction between what was and what is.

> Harry's mother sighs as usual in this situation, and states: 'Typical—here he goes again!'

When his mother sighs and comments on Harry's behaviour here and now, the situation is moved to the present: she becomes part of the field. She is part of the pattern that unfolds in the sandbox, and as she realises this, the possibility arises that not only Harry, but also she and the others—the entire situation—have the opportunity to change.

The subjective experience is influenced by what the individual senses, supposes, thinks, feels, and perceives together with the others, here and now. The individual's understanding is gestalted—that is, given meaning—in her interaction with the environment there and then.

Applied to the therapy room, we can say that the client's relational experiences show themselves here and now in the relationship with the therapist. The therapist supports the client in recreating past experiences so they can be explored in the moment. In this way, the client can recognise and discover what it is that prevents her development. In the field, the experiences of both therapist and client can figure. These experiences have shaped their wants, needs, expectations, fears, habits, and feelings of safety.

Lewin (1936) emphasises that only the present can influence what happens here and now. He points out that dynamic movement is only created between simultaneous events in the present. Even though the client brings up experiences from her past, these experiences acquire meaning in the context that exists here and now, while the future is brought in in the form of wishes, hopes, and expectations.

The importance of needs for regulation in the field

> We return to the sandbox. His mother's arrival arouses anger, frustration, and conflicting needs in Harry. On the one hand, he very much wants to continue to play, but on the other hand, he is hungry and wants to go home to eat. The more his mother nags, the more desperate he becomes.

This example tells us something about experiencing the tension that can exists between competing needs. Harry is torn between his mother's nagging and his own desire to continue playing with the others. In addition, his stomach is rumbling, and his need for food increases. In the midst of all this his frustration level increases. What should he choose? What is his most pressing need? What doesn't he need? These questions do not occur as conscious reflections on Harry's part; rather, they reflect his unclear needs and desires. Because of this, we can describe this field as one with inner tension.

Lewin argues that it is precisely this tension between competing needs that helps to regulate the field. In Harry's case, the excitement is almost unbearable. Fortunately, his mother intervenes and makes a clear choice: 'We're going home!' After a few more protestations, Harry calms down and is able to say goodbye to the other children. His mother's intervention regulates the field, and another way of being together takes shape.

Lewin used comparisons from physics to explain how the field is regulated. When positive and negative forces oppose each other, tension builds. As the tension builds, the system being charged is set in motion. Lewin believed that similar tensions arise in the social field between people, and that the degree of tension is determined by our needs. The degree to which the needs are charged, or their *valence*, as he referred to it, is determined by the extent to which the needs in the field are being met. A need that is met to only a slight degree, for example hunger when we have eaten too little, has negative valence, and positive valence when we have eaten too much. The needs, in this case hunger, regulate the field.

An example of mutually influencing forces is the tension generated when we have uncompleted tasks. Tension is created between the need to complete the task and the resistance that occurs because the task is difficult to complete.

The Zeigarnik effect

The gestalt psychologists showed us that we organise what we sense, in wholes. This urge to give shape and meaning was explored further by Lewin's Russian student, the gestalt psychologist Bluma Zeigarnik (1901–1988). She noticed that the waiters at the café remembered the customer's order in detail, but when the customer had received what he ordered, all details were forgotten. Waiters did not need to remember the orders at that point; the task was completed. Zeigarnik decided to investigate the phenomenon further in the laboratory in Berlin. She gave the participants puzzles to solve; half of the participants were interrupted before they were finished. When asked to repeat the tasks, they were able to remember most of the interrupted tasks. They had literally not finished. This phenomenon has since been called the Zeigarnik effect.

Zeigarnik's colleague Maria Rickers-Ovsiankina (1898–1993) examined the phenomenon further and was able to show that uncompleted tasks also have an impact on our behaviour. If we leave a task unfinished, it continues to gnaw at us until we have completed it. This experiment drew attention to emotions and behaviour, and to the fact that we humans have an urge to complete unfinished tasks.

We structure that which we perceive. According to field theory, these structures or patterns are formed based on the needs that arise in the field in which we find ourselves at any given time. Further, as we have seen, the perceiving subject gives these patterns a form that is the most useful there and then.

According to Lewin, the change in how we perceive the field is the most important way out of the deadlocked structures or patterns we develop in our interactions with the outside world—in the field. It is about clarifying these deadlocked structures and facilitating the development of new and more flexible forms. The key is to develop attention and be aware of the different ways in which the interaction happens. We will show examples of this in later chapters.

Lewin believed that imagination and creativity are essential for thawing frozen structures or patterns and bringing about change and movement in the field. Here, too, we find a clear relationship between gestalt therapy and its methodical use of experimentation. Use of colour, movement, imagination, and metaphor make it possible for clients to explore their own patterns or ways of being in contact with themselves and their surroundings.

Field theory summarised

Lewin's field theory has shown itself to be important for the development of psychology's understanding of man as a social being. Not only did Lewin make his mark and lay the foundation for social psychology as an independent science, but he also influenced the understanding of man as a social being in general. Lewin did not only challenge the beliefs of his colleagues, but also the development of psychology at the time.

In Chapter 4, we emphasise the connection between field theory and gestalt therapy's relational approach. Lewin's theories are fundamental gestalt terms that describe how we as gestalt therapists view the interaction between us and our clients and between our clients and their surroundings.

Note

1 Where no other sources are quoted, information in this chapter is taken from Kendler (1987) and Teigen (2004/2015).

References

Dyrkorn, R. (2014). *Lederen og teamet—Gestaltbasert coaching og teamutvikling* [The leader and the team—Gestalt-based coaching and team development]. Oslo: Gestaltforlaget.

Kendler, H. (1987). *Historical foundations of modern psychology*. California: The Dorsey.

Lewin, K. (1936). *A dynamic theory of personality*. New York: McGraw-Hill.

Lewin, K. (1951). *Field theory in social science: Selected theoretical papers* (D. Cartwright, Ed.). New York: Harper & Brothers.

Madsen, K. B. (2016). "Aha-opplevelse" ["Aha experience"]. In *Den Store Danske* [The great Danish encyclopedia]. A. Nygaard, D. A. Andersen, E. Both, J. H. Pedersen, K. Englev, L. Vistrup, P. Trier & U. Fugmann (Eds.). Retrieved from http://denstoredanske.dk/index.php?sideId=34308

Neuman, C. B., & Neumann, I. B. (2014). *Forskeren i forskningsprosessen* [The researcher in the research process]. Oslo: Cappelen Damm Akademisk.

Parlett, M. (2005). Contemporary gestalt therapy: Field theory. In A. L. Woldt & S. M. Toman (Eds.), *Gestalt therapy: History, theory, and practice*. Chapter 3. London: Sage.

Staemmler, F. M. (2006). A Babylonian confusion?: On the uses and meanings of the term "field". *British Gestalt Journal, 15*(2), 64–83.

Stemberger, G. (2019). Some remarks on the field concept in gestalt psychology. Extract from the article: Trombini, G., Corazza, A., & Stemberger, G. (2019). Manifest dream/association comparison: A criterion to monitor the psychotherapeutic field. *Gestalt Theory: An International Multidisciplinary Journal, 41*(1), 61–78. https://doi.org/10.2478/gth-2019-0005

Teigen, K. H. (2004/2015). *En psykologihistorie* [A history of psychology]. Bergen: Fagbokforlaget.

van Baalen, D. (2002/2008). Awareness er ikke nok [Awareness is not enough]. In S. Jørstad & Å. Krüger (Eds.), *Den flyvende hollender* [The flying Dutchman] (pp. 70–77). Oslo: NGI.

Wheeler, G. (1998). *Gestalt Reconsidered* (2nd ed.). Cambridge, MA: CIGPress.

Wollants, G. (2012). *Gestalt therapy: Therapy of the situation*. London: Sage.

Yontef, G. M. (1993). *Awareness, dialogue & process*. New York: The Gestalt Journal Press.

Chapter 2

Phenomenology and existentialism

We have seen that gestalt therapy's theoretical foundation is based on gestalt psychology. Now we will look at its philosophical points of departure, namely phenomenology and its offspring, existential phenomenology and French existentialism. The philosophy of phenomena is also the basis of the gestalt method, and the fundamental values of gestalt therapy have their historical roots in both German and French phenomenology and philosophy.

The word 'phenomenon' comes from the Greek *phainomenon*, which can be translated as 'that which appears or is seen'. Let us look at an example: imagine a light. Which images occur to you first? Perhaps you see a candle; maybe you see a light in the dark, maybe something else. Regardless, whatever comes to your mind is associated with light. Further, does what you see have a colour? Is it large or small? You are now in the process of describing the phenomenon of light from your perspective, as you see and perceive it right now. If someone else sees the same light, she sees it in her own way and from her subjective perspective. Your description of the light will therefore be as it emerges as a phenomenon for just you.

To perceive and form an understanding of something is always done from a subjective perspective, and that perspective is always formed in a field. According to field theory, all experience is influenced by the field (Lewin, 1951). We can summarise by saying that phenomenology is the study of the fact that—and how—we humans give shape and meaning to our experiences in the field.

This chapter is about the philosophical foundations of gestalt therapy. We begin by examining phenomenology as a methodological foundation in gestalt therapy and ethics as a foundation for the therapeutic attitude. In the last part of the chapter, we examine the importance of existentialist thinking in the gestalt-therapeutic form of therapy.[1]

From phenomenology

The fact that phenomenology is the philosophical basis for gestalt therapy has certain implications; this philosophy describes the ethical basis for our therapy form. In the following, we take a closer look at the tradition in which therapy is based. First, some history.

DOI: 10.4324/9781003153856-3

A historical retrospect

We return to the first part of the nineteenth century. In the presentation of gestalt psychology in Chapter 1, we saw that this period was marked by innovation in the natural sciences, including psychology. In the enthusiasm for new methods in the scientific approach, it was thought that human beings must be understood in the same way as everything else in nature and that behaviour could thus be explained by general principles. It therefore followed that by studying human behaviour in light of the unbiased principles of natural sciences, it would be possible to explain why we behave as we do.

At the same time, however, it was suggested that human behaviour could be explained with a basis in phenomenology. In our ensuing discussion, we therefore follow the same timeline as in our review of gestalt psychology. Here, however, we examine how this philosophical tradition has left its mark on gestalt therapy.

The philosopher and psychologist Franz Clemens Brentano (1838–1917) was among those who argued that human consciousness is neither static nor 'content' that can be observed in the way we do with the world around us. In his view, consciousness had to be described as a process.

With reference to Aristotle, Brentano believed that it is *how* knowledge comes into being that is important, not an analysis of why. He is credited with reviving the medieval construct of intentionality and using it in his concept of act psychology. Intentionality addresses the 'aboutness' of experience and refers to the idea that everything we feel, think, imagine, and perceive is about something. Each of these mental acts takes an intentional object. (Brownell, 2008).

Although Brentano initiated this school of thought, it was one of his students, Edmund Husserl (1859–1938), who systemised it and is considered the founder of phenomenology. His theories about phenomena were to be of great significance for our thinking today, not least in the social sciences, and thus also for the philosophical tradition on which gestalt therapy is based.

Like Brentano, Husserl believed that explanations obscure our spontaneous experiences, the information we perceive through our senses. He therefore felt that rather than attempting to explain our experiences, we should be open to immediate physical experience: what we see, taste, hear, and smell. It is namely via enhanced attention to the body's awareness of sensation that our consciousness clears, and we are able to understand and acknowledge our experiences.

Following this principle of the senses as the source of consciousness, phenomenological experiences happen here and now. This applies to past experiences that spontaneously occur here and now, or directly experienced sensation as it occurs and is lived in the moment. One of Husserl's and thus phenomenology's central theses was therefore that the road to recognition goes through the senses.

Exploring phenomena

Gestalt therapists are trained to use an open phenomenological approach in the therapy room. Emphasis is on supporting and encouraging the client to explore her subjective experiences through questions such as: 'What do you notice now?'

'How does it feel to . . . ?' 'What happens when you do more of . . . ?' 'What are you aware of when . . . ?' The client might say: 'I'm sad', and the therapist might respond: 'What does "sad" mean to you? How do you feel sad right now?' The therapist says this in order to support and encourage the client to describe the experience from her own perspective.

The psychologist Ernesto Spinelli (1989/2005) points out how this phenomenological approach is used in psychotherapy. His explanation is considered an exposition of basic principles for the practice of gestalt therapy. With reference to the fundamentals of phenomenology, he shows three ways of being that the therapist strives for in her process together with the client. These three ways of being are not only meant to be purely methodological, but also describe a therapeutic attitude.

The first is *to put aside* predetermined opinions about how something is—*to have an open rather than predetermined attitude*. We have probably all experienced how quickly we form opinions about how something or someone is. The man wearing a suit becomes synonymous with a businessman, whereas the man dressed in rags is a drug addict. Such preconceived notions and attitudes become prejudices, and can sometimes evolve into fixed opinions on how someone or something should be and therefore should be understood.

Prejudices and beliefs about others are often present in the meeting between therapist and client in the therapy room. When the client comes to the first session, we might form an impression of who and how the client is when we shake hands for the first time. We have a tendency to make up our minds about things quickly, and the phenomenologists challenge us to put aside our prejudices. We are encouraged to be open to the immediate experience and thus be open to what makes itself apparent here and now. The therapist's task is therefore to be aware of her own beliefs about the other, and to strive to meet the other with openness and impartiality.

The second phenomenological way of being is the therapist's focus on *description rather than explanation*. Description helps us to stay in the immediate experience. Contrary to explanation, description helps us to sense the true and most accurate experience. Explanation is often our default mode, and is indeed necessary—not least in our time, where we tend to abstract and theorise—to train our awareness and attention to what is actually being experienced here and now. To facilitate a descriptive way of being, it is of great help for the exploratory process to ask open-ended questions that begin with what or how, rather than why, which tends to close processes.

The third phenomenological way of being is *to consider all information to be equal*. This has to do with how the therapist relates to information she perceives and senses in the field. In this awareness of and attention to the process, the therapist is encouraged to follow the process without jumping to the conclusion that some sensory data is of greater importance. This attention is naturally of particular importance in phases where a phenomenon begins to take shape in the field. Spinelli (1989/2005) encourages the therapist to 'avoid making immediate, misleading hierarchically based judgements' (p. 21).

The challenge for the therapist is therefore to wait together with the client in the early stages of the process before choosing to focus on specific information. At this point, it is important to expand the sensory field and attention together with the client. Together and as individuals we pay attention to what is in the field: signals, as yet unspoken. We seek to give what we experience through our senses enough time and room for expression, so that the client can find her answer in the field.

The phenomenological method is in other words a guideline for the therapist's ethical stance in the meeting with the client. We will now extend this ethical perspective on therapeutic processes by turning to a philosophical direction that evolved on the basis of Husserl's phenomenology: existential phenomenology.

From existential phenomenology

It was the Dane Søren Kierkegaard (1813–1855) who first described man as an 'existing creature'. While the philosophers of his time were interested in the universal aspects of man, that is, man's essence, Kierkegaard believed that man is a self-determining, *existing* being (Stigen, 1986). It is these budding thoughts about existence that were developed further some decades later in the phenomenological research community that surrounded Husserl in Germany. His two assistants, Martin Heidegger (1889–1976) and Edith Stein (1891–1942), helped formulate, each in his or her own way, the content of the tradition that was eventually called existential phenomenology. In the following passage, we also refer to the two central and contemporary existence philosophers Maurice Merleau-Ponty (1908–1961) and Martin Buber (1878–1965).

Existence philosophy emphasises phenomenology's view of human existence in the world: that we are in the world with others and our existence requires a special attention to those with whom we are in the world. In psychotherapeutic work, the therapist has a particular ethical responsibility to meet the other. We will now examine these elements from two perspectives: the body's sense of the other and the welcoming attitude in the meeting with the other.

The body's sensation of the other

Edith Stein (1989) was interested in how the senses, the body's sensations, are the cornerstone of all human encounters. She expressed her question in a concrete and recognisable way:

> Let us take an example to illustrate the nature of the act of empathy. A friend tells me that he has lost his brother and I become aware of his pain. What kind of awareness is this? I am not concerned here with going into the basis on which I infer pain. Perhaps his face is pale and disturbed his voice toneless and strained. Perhaps he also expresses his pain in words.
>
> (p. 6)

Stein pointed out that the perception of the other, 'I see you' and 'you see me', results in a bodily sensation resonance in us—a condensed experience that not only consists of thoughts and feelings, but also the body. With reference to Stein,

Staemmler (2012) quotes Abram (1997) as an example that it is this bodily sensation we feel when we for example see someone else fall off a bicycle:

> When I watch a stranger learning to ride a bicycle for the first time, my own body, although it is standing solidly on the ground, inadvertently experiences the uncertain balance of the rider, and when that bicycle teeters and falls I feel the harsh impact of the asphalt against my own leg and shoulder.
>
> (p. 139)

Merleau-Ponty (2005) is one of few Western philosophers who takes the perspective that our understanding of the world is based in our bodies' experience of our surroundings or situation. Together, the body and its surroundings are an existential inner relationship or structure where each reacts to the other. Merleau-Ponty uses the example of an organist who is about to play an organ that is new to him. He adapts so quickly to the new instrument's idiosyncrasies that it cannot be explained by muscle memory or adaptation. The organist creates an existential, intentional relationship to the instrument.

Merleau-Ponty claims that the body is perceptive:

> my body is not only an object among all other objects . . . but an object which is *sensitive to* all the rest, which reverberates to all sounds, vibrates to all colours, and provides words with their primordial significance through the way in which it receives them.
>
> (2005, p. 275)

It is the body that perceives and lays the foundation for the words that express the experience we have in the meeting the other. Staemmler (2012) summarises: 'It is precisely my body which perceives the body of another' (p. 132). This bodily awareness in the meeting with the other is thus the foundation for being able to put oneself in the other's place.

It is essential that the therapist is trained to be aware of such sensations when together with the client. The therapist's position as a professional implies that she also has a particular responsibility to facilitate the meeting with the client. By virtue of her profession, the therapist is also in a position of power (Crocker, 2005). Regardless of how accommodating the therapist is, there will always be an asymmetry of authority between therapist and client. It is therefore of fundamental importance that the therapist is aware of her ethical responsibility to meet the other.

Meeting the other

With this in mind, we turn to the existential phenomenologist Martin Buber and his philosophy about *the meeting between people*.

Buber (1923/2000) begins with the assertion that there are two basic ways in which we humans relate to each other. He describes these as the relational factors:

'I–it' and 'I–thou'. 'I–it' is characterised by relating to others in the same way we relate to things around us. An 'I–it' meeting is a situation in which people see each other more as objects; they distance themselves from and are objective in their meetings with each other. In such situations, taking care of the practical matters at hand becomes more interesting than the human relationships between them, and the others around them are simply a means by which they can achieve a goal. The usefulness of the other is central, and there can be a temptation to exploit the other's position.

The other relationship that is described is the 'I–thou' relationship. In this relationship, there exists a possibility other than exploitation: an ideal relationship between people based on a meeting of equals. The attitude and behaviour that characterises this relationship are composed of mutual recognition of each other's individuality. It is this type of meeting that is the goal. These meetings occur in the moment—as a gift, and in wonderment over our implicit acknowledgement in the mutual respect and trust that exists in the field. One example is the teacher who long believed that a pupil was inept, but who was able to set aside her prejudices in her meeting with the pupil, thereby recognising and being curious about experiences that are different to her own. In the context of the therapy room, we can see that Buber's concern was that the therapist should not see clients as objects that are used to help to solve their problems, but as subjects, and with respect for the individual and her uniqueness.

We emphasise that to strive for an 'I–thou' relationship does not mean that therapists will never find themselves in an 'I–it' relationship with their clients (Hycner & Jacobs, 1995). In some situations a client will require practical advice, or will be in a crisis situation where she is paralysed and might need someone to assist her in making contact with family, an employer, or the health care system. The therapist will also use her knowledge in practical matters, such as making agreements with clients that concern the therapy process or payment, as well as when choosing various forms of therapeutic approach.

From French existentialism

We are now at the philosophical core of gestalt therapy. The phenomenological explorations and ethical reflections of human encounters underlie the values of gestalt therapy.

The fundamental values of gestalt therapy

As with its methodology, gestalt therapy's values are rooted in phenomenology. Although the method is rooted in Husserl's description of how consciousness and meaning arise, the values and view of human nature are based in phenomenology's philosophical offshoot, existentialism.

Existential phenomenology arose in the twentieth century in two directions: religious and atheist (Stigen, 1986). If we follow the timeline of the history of gestalt therapy, we find traces of both. Here, we discuss French existentialism.

The existentialist tradition has fertile ground in the French philosopher Jean-Paul Sartre's (1905–1980) well-known texts from the middle of the twentieth century. He studied under Husserl in Germany, and his critical approach to Husserl's fundamental texts on phenomenology resulted in the foundation of existential philosophy. This influenced European thought in a broad range of areas, such as literature, theatre, psychology, psychotherapy, politics, and sociology.

Among other things, Sartre challenged Husserl's idea of how consciousness and meaning become direct perception. Sartre believed that the emphasis on how things become what they are—the very essence of sensation—stole attention from the real issue, namely the importance of experience and the fact that we exist. We are what we are as a function of 'being-in-the-world'. Existence is about how we seek to create meaning in our lives and the situation in which we find ourselves at any given time. There is no absolute truth; reality is subjective and unique to the individual, and it is up to us to deal with what we experience.

The consequence of this freedom is that we must constantly choose how we live our lives. Ultimately, we have the choice to accept that we live and that we will die. It is only when we realise that life comes to an end that we—paradoxically—have the option to choose whether to live fully. It is only when existence leads us to this shocking moment of realisation that we, naked and alone, have the chance to see and choose life openly and honestly.

The possibility inherent in change is in other words in our own hands. Man becomes that which he makes himself. Sometimes in life we are made uneasy by the way we choose to live our lives. Illness or other events cause us to question the circumstances of life, and the need for change arises. Sometimes it also becomes clear that the way we live our lives follows conventional patterns, which causes us to question the meaning of life. Our life situation there and then puts us face to face with pure existence: that something is as it is, and we therefore begin to wonder if life as we live it is basically meaningless.

Fundamental values in practice

It is precisely this issue of the need for change that is central to and indeed the point of the processes of psychotherapy, and thus also gestalt therapy. The client seeks a therapist because her life situation has reached a point where the need for change arises. The therapist's task is to meet the other with a supportive attitude, be willing to be present along with the other, and to facilitate in such a way that the client can openly investigate the difficulties in her life and thereby discover what she needs in the context of her life.

The French gestalt therapist Gonzaque Masquelier (2002) reminds us that the therapy room has in many ways been charged with existence. The lived life here and now is itself in focus. Open phenomenological exploration makes it possible for the client, together with the therapist, to discover new opportunities, even in the face of life's harsh realities. Both client and therapist hope that the process creates the possibility for something new to happen, and that through the process, a solution to the difficulties will make itself known.

In the therapy room, existence is brought into sharp relief. The therapy room magnifies life and life experiences, experiences that are often marked by the pain and confusion that unresolved issues cause. Life creates opportunities and imposes limitations. By virtue of being human, we live under *the paradoxical conditions of life*. Existence philosophy describes these paradoxes as the existential pressures that underlie all human life. We will now discuss Masquelier's review of four of these principal pressures: finality, solitude, responsibility, and imperfection.

Finality

To realise that we are going to die is to realise that we live. Life's paradox unfolds in the act of living and investing in life. To plant a tree and help it to grow is to realise that the tree's life will one day come to an end. Live, then die.

The fact that things come to an end is relevant for endings in life itself. A friendship ends, a pet dies, or a marriage ends in divorce. Such terminations can be limiting; they can depress us and make us despondent. The paradox is that that which ends seems to have in it the possibility of something new. In the limitations are also possibilities. In other words, when we realise that something is over, we also see opportunities for something new.

This life-and-death paradox also affects the processes of therapy. Perhaps it is here, in this room devoted to exploration of the challenges of life, that existence is made clear to us. We recognise that this life paradox becomes particularly clear in light of gestalt therapy's emphasis on the view that life is lived here and now (Kachel, 2014). To bring the client's story to the here and now is the core, says Masquelier (2002): 'That is to say, what are we going to decide to do, here and now, with our past, with our future, which we know to be limited? . . . by facing the unavoidable reality that is our finality, we can find multiple ways of positioning ourselves' (p. 81).

Solitude

To realise that something ends and thus is finite can create a feeling of loneliness. Masquelier discusses three forms of solitude: interpersonal, intrapersonal, and existential. All of these, understandably enough, come up in therapy.

Interpersonal solitude is about being alone and lonely, involuntarily. We can no doubt all feel solitude to a greater or lesser degree when we are together with others, either in the experience of being on the outside of our peer group or perhaps also in the most extreme sense of having no friends at all. We might recognise this social solitude when friendship becomes superficial and lacks good, meaningful conversation. This experience of interpersonal solitude is not unusual and is, not surprisingly, also the reason many seek therapy.

Many can no doubt also recognise experiences of *intrapersonal solitude*. As the wording implies, this solitude has to do with feeling a certain foreignness to oneself. Sometimes this form of solitude can occur when work becomes overwhelming and a feeling of being burned out arises. This inner solitude can create an experience of losing touch with oneself. Often it feels like being at a loss for something without being able to identify that something; floating through life without a sense of meaning and purpose. Clients in therapy need to rediscover the experience of who they are.

Unlike interpersonal and intrapersonal solitude, *existential solitude* is something we recognise without attempting to counteract it. To be human is lonely, and we ask ourselves: 'Do I have a predetermined place in the universe, or am I just a coincidental collection of atoms? Is there a God who gives meaning to life, or am I alone and ultimately left to my own devices?'

Unease and a fear of not belonging, whether in relationships or existential, are often topics in the therapy room. These topics touch our emotional selves and stir up unrest in both client and therapist because we are human beings. Despite the fact that these are important questions in our lives, it can naturally take time before the client brings existential themes into her conversations with the therapist. It is generally only when the therapeutic relationship feels safe and is well established that such issues arise. This applies especially to existential questions.

Responsibility

A third theme that existence philosophers were interested in was to realise one's own responsibility to be a participant in one's own life. The existential limitations we face when we take responsibility and stand up for ourselves bring with them anxiety and a desire to avoid responsibility by turning our backs on the limitations. Perls (1947/1969) was interested in the tendency we humans have to avoid and evade responsibility. He used a practical example from everyday life, pointing out the difference between the active statement 'I dropped the cup on the floor' and the passive 'the cup slipped out of my hands'. The passive form gives the impression that it is not I who is to blame for the cup falling; *I* am not responsible. The opposite is to realise that I am a participant in my own life, which entails the freedom to choose. The person who must and can choose is none other than myself.

Sometimes in life we are faced with choices that require more of us than the usual everyday decisions. Such situations stick out in our minds, and often become topics in therapy—and are of course familiar to the therapist as well. We can probably all recognise how easy it is to assign blame to others, for example in statements such as 'My colleagues are absolutely hopeless, I can't put up with them any longer!' In therapy we have the opportunity to explore the claims we make about others and situations, and therefore the possibility to discover that problems and challenges change when we assume our share of responsibility in our roles as colleagues.

Imperfection

Being accountable for one's actions also creates a sense of inadequacy and of not being able to fulfil requirements. To be human is to live in the existential pressure that exists between having to meet requirements and not being able to do so, thereby experiencing the fear of being imperfect. Masquelier (2002) reminds us how this feeling of inadequacy leads us to find ways to 'escape'. Making others the scapegoat is one such way to escape the feeling of imperfection.

Marie has sought therapy because she is struggling with her marriage and relationships with her husband. She is upset that he does not do more to contribute to their mutual happiness. She is also upset about his supervisor, who requires too much overtime. Both the husband and the supervisor are made scapegoats.

In therapy, she however realises that she also has a responsibility to make the marriage work. She learns to tolerate the fact that her husband is not perfect. In this way, she develops greater acceptance for the fact that she herself is not perfect.

In gestalt therapy, clients like Marie are challenged to rediscover their basic choices: 'What do you need?', 'What do you need to do to get where you want to be?' The therapist helps the client to understand her needs and set realistic boundaries, but also challenges her to go beyond these when they limit her.

The question of 'meaning' comes up at some point in all forms of therapy. Fritz Perls liked to challenge all established dogmas and categorical statements. To begin with, he would tend to ask the individual to think about existential questions: 'What is the meaning of life?' When the answer began to become clear, the next question would be: 'What is the meaning of life itself?'

Some last thoughts

In gestalt therapeutic thinking in recent decades there has been an increased interest in returning to the sources of gestalt theory—not least to the clear connection between the practice of gestalt therapy and phenomenology.

A clear red thread running through these texts is precisely the phenomenological description of awareness in the contact between people. Fritz Perls' descendants were interested in the exchange between people. Man is 'in the world', and the body's sensitivity is a source of empathy for others. The meeting between people is the focus.

In line with phenomenological thinking, to gestalt an experience is about *the fact that* and *how* something becomes meaningful and how we understand that meaning in the environment we find ourselves at a given point in time. This applies to both how the individual perceives and gives meaning to—gestalts—the tree in the forest or the cup on the table, and how certain events are understood and acquire meaning.

Gestalt therapy's phenomenological roots underline therefore the basic principle that the gestalting process takes shape in and is a function of the individual's exchange with her environment. The acquisition of meaning—the experiences we have now and over time—do not take place in isolation in the individual, separate from others. On the contrary, we understand something against the background of something else and, it is important to note, in the context and the environment in which we find ourselves here and now.

Note

1 Where no other sources are given, this chapter is based on Kendler (1987) and Teigen (2004/2015).

References

Abram, D. (1997). *The spell of the sensuous: Perception and language in a more-than-human world*. New York: Vintage Books.

Brownell, P. (Ed.) (2008). *Handbook of theory, research, and practice in gestalt therapy*. Newcastle: Cambridge Scholars Publishing.

Buber, M. (1923/2000). *I and thou*. New York: Scribner.

Crocker, S. (2005). Phenomenology, existentialism, and Eastern thought in gestalt therapy. In A. Woldt & S. Toman (Eds.), *Gestalt therapy*. London: SAGE.

Hycner, R., & Jacobs, L. (1995). *The healing relationship in gestalt therapy: A dialogic/self-psychology approach*. New York: The Gestalt Journal Press.

Kachel, C. B. (2014). Eksistensielt press i terapirommet [Existential pressure in the therapy room]. *Norsk Gestalttidsskrift, 11*(2), 68–78.

Kendler, H. (1987). *Historical foundations of modern psychology*. California: The Dorsey.

Lewin, K. (1951). *Field theory in social science: Selected theoretical papers*. D. Cartwright (Ed.). New York: Harper & Brothers.

Masquelier, G. (2002). *Gestalt therapy: Living creatively today* (K. Griffin & S. Reeder, Trans.). Paris: Author.

Merleau-Ponty, M. (2005). *The phenomenology of perception* (C. Smith, Trans.). London: Taylor & Francis e-Library. (Original work published 1945)

Perls, F. S. (1947/1969). *Ego, hunger and aggression*. London: Vintage Books.

Spinelli, E. (1989/2005). *The interpreted world: An introduction to phenomenological psychology* (2nd ed.). London: Sage.

Staemmler, F. M. (2012). *Empathy in psychotherapy: How therapists and clients understand each other*. New York. Springer.

Stein, E., Saint, 1891–1942. (1989). *The collected works of Edith Stein, Sister Teresa Benedicta of the Cross, discalced Carmelite* (Vol. 3). Washington, DC: ICS Publications.

Stigen, A. (1986). *Tenkningens historie* [The history of thought] (3rd ed.). Oslo: Gyldendal.

Teigen, K. H. (2004/2015). *En psykologihistorie* [A history of psychology]. Bergen: Fagbokforlaget.

Chapter 3

The founders of gestalt therapy

Despite solid roots in German theory and philosophy, gestalt as a form of therapy first saw the light of day in the post-war United States, on another continent and in a different time. The German-born Frederick Perls (who changed his name to Fritz when moving to the States) and his wife Lore (who changed her name to Laura) were fleeing a war-torn Europe, and eventually, in cooperation with the American anarchist Paul Goodman, developed the therapy form that was given the name gestalt therapy.[1]

In this chapter, we follow the Perlses, mainly Fritz, on the path that led to the creation of gestalt therapy in the United States in the 1960s. Our discussion begins with Fritz Perls' contacts in the professional psychoanalytic community. This is followed by a brief reunion with contemporary theory and philosophy, and finally a presentation of how the therapy form was established in the United States.

Personal and professional development

Let us start at the beginning—not in the United States, but in Germany in the late nineteenth century. Fritz Perls (1893–1970) grew up in a Jewish family with a caring mother and a strict, often absent father. After completing his basic education with distinction, he continued to study, this time psychiatry, specifically neuropsychiatry.

When World War I broke out he enlisted as a doctor, an experience that would make an indelible impression on him. History tells us that it was after these powerful experiences he could always be seen with cigarette in hand. In the following years he established a practice as a psychiatrist, and it was also during this period that he visited the gestalt psychologists' laboratories in Berlin. It was there he met his future wife, Laura (née Lore Posner, 1905–1990). Laura was a talented, intelligent, hardworking woman who came from a rich cultural Jewish family. She was a graduate student of gestalt psychology; had studied the development of existential ideas in the writings of Kierkegaard, Heidegger, Buber, and Tillich; and was familiar with work of the phenomenologists Husserl and Scher. Overall, Laura had a great influence upon the development of Fritz Perls' ideas from 1926 until the end of his life.

DOI: 10.4324/9781003153856-4

Fritz Perls was a respected psychiatrist and neurologist, but the underlying conflicts with his father persisted and troubled him, and the accumulated frustrations eventually led him to psychoanalysis.

His contact with the psychiatrist Karen Horney (1885–1952), known for her criticism of the contemporary traditional form of psychoanalysis, influenced him greatly. She would become one of his most important supporters throughout his life. The intimate and compassionate way in which she met Perls in the therapy room made a lasting impression on him. Horney was a vibrant presence, unlike in classic Freudian therapy where the therapist was neutral and distant. Fritz Perls and Karen Horney developed what they called a 'friendly-professional' relationship. Decades later they met again in the United States, and stayed in contact from that point throughout Perls' life.

Perls took these lessons from the close, personal relationship he experienced in therapy with him when he moved to Vienna, the mecca of psychoanalysis. He wanted to learn more and participated therefore in both analysis and professional supervision with several analysts. When some years later he moved back to the city of his birth, he established his own practice, although he was at this point still faithful to the traditional psychoanalytic form of the time. There can therefore be no doubt that Perls had a psychoanalytic understanding and way of thinking. Nevertheless, experience gained from Horney's close, personal, and unorthodox therapy form led him to a more unconventional way to practice analysis.

Here we introduce another key but very unpleasant experience that would come to influence Perls' further choices: his contact with the conservative analyst Eugen Harnik (1893–1931). Perls described Harnik's therapy as one of the worst he had experienced as a client. He struggled through months of talking on the couch without hearing a single response from the analyst. He experienced the silence as a nightmare, and it was at this point that Perls truly understood the importance of the relationship in the therapy room. The analyst's distance and exclusionary absence, and thus the patient's experience of total solitude, brought him to a realisation that would later become one of the core themes in gestalt as a form of therapy: the importance of the real, living contact in the relationship between therapist and client here and now.

After his desperate, lonely, and eerie experience with Harnik, Horney recommended that he consult the psychoanalyst Wilhelm Reich (1897–1957), whom she believed was the one who could offer Perls what he needed. She was correct—his work with Reich was the highlight of Perls' quest for a relational meeting in the therapy room. Reich did not distance himself by hiding behind his analysis notes; in the same way as Horney, he talked with the client. He was present, interested, and participated in the conversation.

In addition to challenging the traditional method of analysis, Reich was also interested in the psychological idea of 'body armour' and the organism's self-regulation (Bowman, 2005, p. 7). He pointed out that a person's typical way of thinking, feeling, and acting can often be understood as a defense and control mechanism aimed at one's own impulses and the demands of the environment.

Reich went even farther than Freud in relation to the role of sexuality, and developed theories of sexual life energy and orgone energy, which should be measured, accumulated, and released physically. He felt that people had problems because they did not allow energy in their bodies to move freely and that it was better not to repress sexual desires and fantasies. His therapy consisted therefore of attempting to 'loosen' individuals via muscle stimulation. He moved to Norway in 1934, both because he disagreed with the psychoanalytic association in Berlin and because of his political activity as a Marxist. In Norway he had a great deal of influence in the psychoanalytic community and created a stir with his theories about body armour, his ideas about sexual freedom, the nature of orgasm, and orgone therapy. Reich settled in the United States in 1939 where he discarded his original ideas about character and body armour and devoted himself to his theory of orgone energy. He was later jailed and prosecuted for his attempts to treat somatic illness, such as cancer, with orgone therapy. The wave of sexual freedom that washed over the United States after World War II was greatly influenced by Reich and his followers' free attitude towards sexuality and sexual relations.

Fritz Perls was inspired by Reich's way of thinking about man as organism and about how the body protects itself against unpleasant experiences. Perls continued Reich's thinking, which affected his understanding of man as an organic and sexual being. He agreed to Reich's ideas about 'the function of the orgasm' and the 'genital character' and was positive to a lived sexuality, which is illustrated by the several sexual relationships he had during the period he was in psychoanalysis with Reich (Bocian 2010).

Influences from contemporary currents

Fritz Perls could be both challenging and provocative and likely felt at home in the radical bohemian culture of the time, of which he became a part in the 1920s. The Berlin bohemians, with their 'anything goes' attitude, were known for their criticism of the status quo. Here, innovative writers, dancers, architects, poets, painters, leftist intellectuals, and others met, all of whom gave themselves over to the currents of a new era in a new century. Twenty-year-old Fritz Perls stood in the middle of this radical era as a newly qualified doctor and an atheist, with fresh memories of a frustrating adolescence. He prospered and thrived in this atmosphere and in the company of the people with whom he came in contact.

There he met the famous expressionist dancer Gret Palucca (neé Margarethe Paluka, 1902–1993), who, incidentally, was a student of the innovative choreographer Mary Wigman (1886–1973), later known as the founder of dance therapy. Fritz Perls was enthusiastic—both he and Laura were fascinated by dance and movement as a creative, spontaneous, and personal expression.

Fritz Perls also got to know and was a student of the contemporary director Max Reinhardt (1873–1943). It was through his association with Reinhardt that he learned how one could express feelings through vocal range and gestures in the theatre. Fritz Perls noted Reinhardt's belief that the way in which we humans express ourselves is of more importance than can be captured in words.

His contact with contemporary theatre and dance taught Fritz Perls about drama's form and techniques, which he developed further. These would become central to the design of gestalt therapy. His ability to facilitate when, how, and which themes in therapy can be played out, while simultaneously taking advantage of energy as it emerges, can be recognised in the partly theatre-like atmosphere that was often present in his demonstrations of gestalt therapy. He had a continuing desire to facilitate a stage where client and therapist could explore life's themes together in a defined space here and now.

Fritz Perls' desire to facilitate a stage reached its zenith when, after moving to the United States, he organised the first of what he later called his 'circuses'. He and the client conducted a therapy session on stage in the presence of a large audience. After one-to-one therapy was completed, he turned to the audience and spoke with them about what they had witnessed. Again, we see a Fritz Perls who broke new ground. The impression of him on stage in conversation with the audience provides a picture of a man who, despite his anti-social, self-centred, and individualistic behaviour, paradoxically sought community.

Some years later, Fritz Perls' interest in theatre was also influenced by the psychiatrist and theatre creator Jacob L. Moreno (1890–1974), who became the founder of the therapy form psychodrama. By the 1920s, Moreno had already developed forms of role-playing in which participants played out and dramatised scenes and people from their own lives in creative ways. Fritz Perls incorporated Moreno's ideas in his inspiration from theatre and dance, and developed them into his own type of role-play, which today can be recognised in gestalt therapy 'experiments'. Moreno was later a significant influence on the intellectual and radical community in New York in the 1950s, which Laura and Fritz Perls also became a part of when they settled in the United States.

Ideas from contemporary theory and philosophy

It was not only in the unorthodox psychoanalytic professional community that Fritz Perls found an understanding that we humans are formed and are (re)invented together with others, but also, as we have seen, in the contemporary rethinking of theory and philosophy.

Both Laura and Fritz Perls were well acquainted with the gestalt psychologists and their investigations of perception. From 1926 Fritz Perls worked for a period as an assistant at the gestalt psychologist Kurt Goldstein's (1878–1965) Institute for Research into the Consequences of Brain Injuries. At the same time, the young Kurt Lewin began his investigation of field theory and its application to real life outside the laboratory (see Chapter 1). As we have seen, this theory is central to the theoretical basis of modern gestalt therapy.

Psychology was not, however, the only discipline that generated interest at the time. Philosophy was also developing rapidly, and Fritz Perls now found himself in the enthusiastic phenomenological research community that existed in Germany at the time. It is appropriate here to note that Laura Perls was also one of Goldstein's assistants, and that she was particularly interested in the contemporary philosophy of human existence. Both Heidegger's *Mitsein* ('being-with') and Sartre's 'freedom, responsibility, anxiety' were concepts that later became key elements in the philosophical fundamental basis of gestalt therapy (see Chapter 2). It was Laura who became the greatest influence on the philosophical perspective in our therapy form. She was influenced by Merleau-Ponty and his theories about the phenomenology of perception, which became visible in her way of being assertive to bodily movements, gestures, and breathing. She was also captivated by the mystically oriented Martin Buber (p. 24) and the radical theologian Paul Tillich, and had many confidential conversations with both of them. She was of course also well acquainted with contemporary trends in French thinking and Sartre's ideas of existence. It also seems obvious that she discussed these philosophical ideas with Fritz—conversations that undoubtedly left lasting traces in the philosophical basis of gestalt therapy.

Fritz Perls was also familiar with the philosophers referenced above, but was more fascinated by the work of Salomo Friedlaender (1871–1946). Friedlaender was a philosopher and the author of widely read, wacky, grotesque stories written under the pseudonym Mynona. His basic philosophical themes of creative indifference and polar differentiation are in fact the starting points for Perls' therapy theory reflections (Frambach, 2003). For gestalt therapy, Friedlaender's philosophy contributed to a method of integrating polarities (see Chapter 10), the concept of the 'fertile void', and a more thorough understanding of the emergent gestalt.

In addition to the influence of existentialism and Friedlaender's ideas, it is important to mention that gestalt therapy was also influenced by Asian philosophy. In his later days, Fritz Perls also became interested in the meditative Zen Buddhism. During and after his trip to Japan in the 1950s, and with the help of his friend and Zen expert Paul Weisz, he worked hard to deepen gestalt therapy in light of this way of thinking. This applied particularly to the following areas: 'awareness in the moment' as compared to the Zen Buddhist term 'mindfulness', 'the paradox of change' in the context of the 'Zen Buddhist paradox', and finally the use of 'I will' rather than 'I should', equivalent to the emphasis in Zen Buddhism on the non-moralising attitude in relation to oneself and others.

Laura and Fritz took with them the lessons learned from contemporary trends and knowledge of key concepts in theory and philosophy when they were forced to flee in the 1930s from the growing Nazi threat in Fritz's native Germany.

Interlude in South Africa

The journey was long, and the Perlses ended in South Africa as guests of the prime minister and philosopher Jan Smuts. Despite the enforced flight and homesickness, they now had the time and space to work on writing and formulating theory.

At this point, Fritz Perls was still interested in contact with the Freudian psychiatry and wrote a scientific article that he would use as a basis for participation in a conference. The article was rejected, but he continued to work on the text, which—with important input from Laura—eventually became the book *Ego, Hunger and Aggression* in 1947 (Perls, 1947/1969).

Although at that time they had already gathered ideas and thoughts for a new form of therapy, *Ego, Hunger and Aggression* is primarily intended as a contribution to the psychoanalytic discourse. Strangely, despite the rejection of his article, Fritz Perls continued to want to be a part of this academic community. He believed that this book would be an alternative to the Freudian method. In a brave and bold opposition to the established professional milieu, he called the new form of analysis 'concentration therapy'. The book consisted of the ideas he had collected over a long period, including from the South African prime minister Jan Smuts' theories of holism, the German philosopher Salomo Friedlaender's theory of polarities, Kurt Goldstein's theory of holism and the organism and its environment, the gestalt psychologists' theory of perception and field theory, and phenomenological and existentialist philosophy.

To the United States

When Laura and Fritz moved to the United States and New York a few years later, it was natural for them to contact the psychoanalytic professional community and thus the alternative analytic form that was now in development. Here, Fritz met among others his good friend and therapist Karen Horney, as well as other key professionals such as Erich Fromm (1900–1980) and Harry Stuck Sullivan (1892–1949). At the time, everyone in this professional group was already familiar with research on Sullivan's term 'interpersonal psychoanalysis' (Sullivan, 1953) and thus also for the significance of relationships in therapy, a topic that later became central to gestalt therapy.

Fritz Perls flourished and grew in this academic community, both as a person and professionally. It was as if he had come home and found a resting place after a long journey—a place where he could digest his experiences and was able to further nuance the theory and method of this therapeutic method that had begun to take shape.

Gestalt therapy is born

Laura and Fritz eventually expanded their circle of acquaintances and came into contact with among others the politically radical anarchist Paul Goodman (1911–1972). He was a sociologist, writer, and poet. Though he was married and had three children, he was bisexual and lived a free sexual life. He was well versed in philosophy and brought Aristotelian ideas into early gestalt therapy (Bowman, 2005). Goodman was also influenced by Wilhelm Reich, with whom he went to psychoanalysis before he met Perls.

Goodman and Fritz Perls had rewarding and interesting professional discussions, which became the basis for a book they collaborated on about the new form of therapy they developed.

One of Fritz Perls' former clients, Ralph Hefferline (1910–1974), was invited to join them. He contributed to the book's first section with descriptions of the practical exercises, all of which facilitate the reader's development of awareness and attention. Perls contributed with his thoughts, but it was mainly Hefferline and Goodman who wrote the book, which was entitled *Gestalt Therapy: Excitement and Growth in Human Personality* (1951). In this book, most sections that deal with theory were written by Goodman. He brought to the writing his own synthesis of Aristotle's ethical and biological writings and the biological and problem-solving bent of the American pragmatists Dewey and James, as well as a number of Taoist and philosophical principles of nature (Crocker, 2005). In time, the book became the theoretical basis of the therapy form and is therefore naturally also the basis for the development of gestalt therapy in later generations.

Perls later wrote articles which mainly elaborated the therapy form's application in practice. Some of his texts were meant to emphasise the distinctiveness of gestalt therapy and were therefore partly or entirely written verbatim. After his death, some of the previously unpublished texts were printed in the gestalt therapy journal the *Gestalt Journal*.

Gestalt therapy in development: the pros and cons

Not long after the book *Gestalt Therapy* was published, Laura and Fritz, together with Paul Goodman, decided to establish what would become the first of many gestalt institutes in the United States, namely the New York Institute for Gestalt Therapy. Laura was reluctant to participate in establishing the institute because she was too busy with children, grandchildren, and her own practice, and did not want to take on more responsibility. But the first lecture by Fritz was so popular that Laura found herself taking on a group of twenty people for practicum, which turned out to be the beginning of a lifelong task. In her talk on the occasion of the New York Institute's twenty-fifth anniversary, she mentioned Fritz's involvement in the institute's beginnings:

> It is not easy to talk about Fritz's role in the development of the Institute . . . Fritz's genius was in his intuitive insights and uncanny hunches, which then had to be substantiated in more exact elaboration. Fritz very often did not have the patience for this detailed work. He was a generator, not a developer or an organizer. Without the constant support from his friends, and from me, without the constant encouragement and collaboration, Fritz would never have written a line, nor founded anything.
>
> (Perls, 1992, pp. 27–28)

Fritz was, however, restless in New York, and embarked on a tour of the United States to introduce the new therapy form. In both small and large arenas, with relatively large audiences present, he demonstrated how he worked as a gestalt therapist. His performances were very well received—they were so popular that many of the listeners were inspired to create their own gestalt institutes throughout the United States, in Cleveland, Miami, San Francisco, Los Angeles, California, as well as Vancouver Island in Canada.

While Fritz Perls was travelling and later when he lived at Esalen in California, Laura stayed in New York and took care of their two children. Fritz ignored them; he lived like a guru and often slept with his clients or trainees. Laura, together with Isadore From, later became central leaders of the New York Institute. From was a friend of Paul Goodman, and though he was not a writer, he had a considerable impact on the development of gestalt therapy through his training in New York and in other states.

Despite the success of Fritz Perls' travels, a challenge arose. He presented his work in an oral form, without proper use of references for theoretical concepts. This imprecision led to a situation in which the various institutes perceived his message differently and the audience was left with differing understandings of what gestalt therapy actually was. The lack of written documentation was to have consequences for how the therapy form was perceived. This lack of clarity followed the therapy form to the next generation of therapists, who revised the theory in the 1980s.

Toward the end of his tour in the United States, audience members began to see a change in Fritz Perls' presentation of gestalt therapy. In the 1960s he moved more and more away from both phenomenology's relational principles and the gestalt psychologist Lewin's field theory. He became markedly more individual-oriented, dogmatic, and assertive. This change is not only recognisable in his writing, but also in short film clips where he demonstrated therapy in a populist and simplistic way.

Both the content of what he said and the way he behaved appeared to be related to his attraction to current trends, such as the hippie movement's emphasis on individual freedom and the right to personal development. Fritz's enthusiasm for these modern ideas seemed to make him more egotistical. He now claimed that the most important thing for man is to think about himself and his own needs. These individual-oriented statements stood in sharp contrast to his earlier theories, such as gestalt therapy's basic premise that man grows and develops in relation to others. This way of being, which was foreign to both his family and his former followers, followed him to his death on 14 March 1970.

Laura Perls continued to work in New York, Canada, and Europe until she died in her hometown of Pforzheim in 1990. Laura's contribution to the development of gestalt therapy is often underestimated. Through her training, workshops, and lectures at the New York Institute as well as on her journeys in the United States and Canada, she shared and showed in practice her opinions and take on gestalt theory. She was critical to Fritz's way of promoting gestalt therapy in his last years, how he used techniques in his demonstrations, and his confrontative stance. She saw gestalt therapy more as an art form and stayed close to the original theories about field theory, the organism in its environment, creative adjustment, and contact. In her opinion, gestalt therapy was an existential, experiential, and experimental approach, and she explored what she called the obvious, that which was immediately accessible to the patient's or her own awareness. She worked with body awareness: breathing, posture, coordination, continuity, and fluidity in movement; with gestures, facial expressions, voice, and language (Perls, 1992).

Gestalt therapy has had a large sociocultural impact because of its anarchistic roots and its skepticism toward bureaucracy. Many of the early contributors to gestalt therapy, such as Martin Buber, Franz Koffka, Jan Smuts, and Paul Goodman, were engaged in the anarchistic movement (Bowman, 2005). This skepticism created friction between gestalt practitioners and the established systems in medicine and academia, and has given the impression of gestalt therapy as anti-academic, anti-intellectual, and anti-establishment.

Another important factor for the growth of gestalt therapy was the human potential movement that began in the 1960s, which focused on change and growth for 'normal' people without psychological problems. The movement was influenced by humanistic psychology and Abraham Maslow's theory of self-actualisation and concept of the hierarchy of needs. The Esalen Institute in California was founded in 1962 as a center for the study and development of human potential, and Fritz Perls had many of his large group demonstrations or 'circuses' there. He influenced many of the known practitioners in various fields of human potential, such as Alan Watts, Virginia Satir, Illana Rubenfeld, Ida Rolf, Will Schutz, and Sam Keen. These practitioners contributed in many different ways to gestalt therapy without carrying its banner. The humanistic movement was after some years strongly criticised for a lack of effectiveness as a serious agent of change after several outcome studies. The movement was also the subject of much scrutiny and was accused of being quasi-religious and narcissistic. This criticism was also directed at gestalt therapy as a consequence of the individualistic perspective taken by Fritz Perls in his later years (Bowman, 2005).

Gestalt therapy was spread by Laura and Fritz Perls and their colleagues and followers who travelled, demonstrated, and taught gestalt therapy. This led to the growth of institutes in the United States, Canada, South America, and Europe. Among the most important institutes in the United States are those in New York, Cleveland, San Diego, and Los Angeles.

A new day, a new paradigm

Many of those who met Laura and Fritz Perls in the 1960s were not acquainted with the theories and models of which they had spoken and written. For new generations of gestalt therapists, it has therefore been necessary to turn to the therapy form's basic thinking and thus not only recreate, but also further develop the theory of gestalt therapy as well as its philosophy and practical methods.

Parlett (2005) points out that today's relational stance marks a paradigm shift in gestalt therapy. As therapists, we are part of and organise the mutual reality or shared field, and in turn are created and organised by it.

Wollants (2012) argues that the gestalt therapy of our time is in a 'paradigm shift', that is a so-called fundamental and systematic shift in mindset.[2] This change is first and foremost an academic showdown with first-generation gestalt therapy, particularly with reference to the individual-oriented book written by Perls, Hefferline, and Goodman in 1951 and the tendency to explain the theory in an individualistic context.

The historic shift in the understanding of gestalt therapy came in the transition to the 1990s. A new generation of gestalt therapists now posed the necessary critical questions. Among these, Gordon Wheeler's book *Gestalt Reconsidered* (1998; first published 1991) was particularly important. The book's subtitle marked the transition to a new way of thinking: *A New Approach to Contact and Resistance*. A showdown with the older generation was thus a fact. This pioneering book inspired several of today's writers. Wollants (2012), for example, is sharp in his criticism of the older Fritz Perls' understanding of concepts. He criticises him for his unilateral individual-oriented perspective, and states that this individual orientation is tantamount to the dehumanisation of man, '*to treat him as less than human*' (p. 115). Yontef (1993) and Staemmler (2007) are also representative of this shift in gestalt therapy.

Gestalt therapy training and research

By the 1970s, the gestalt milieu in the United States and Europe was developing to the point that several gestalt institutes educated gestalt therapists, and training programmes that spanned two or three years came into being. In the beginning, this education was characterised by a combination of self-development and teaching of the basic gestalt-theoretic concepts and terms, and much teaching took place in the form of therapy demonstrations. The curriculum's content was influenced by the first teachers' sources of inspiration. Much of the teaching was influenced by Fritz Perls' confrontational style with its emphasis on the use of techniques, while other teaching was influenced by Laura Perls' supportive, body-oriented, and more empathetic style (Hostrup, 2010). Some institutes emphasised individual development, others had a more relational, contact- and field-oriented direction from Lewin. This created conflicts within and between institutes (Bowman, 2005).

Another challenge for the institutes was the continuing conflict between the need to be true to gestalt therapy's anarchistic roots and the need to adapt teaching to society's demands and expectations. Laura Perls (1992) was aware of this challenge and said the following in an interview with Daniel Rosenblatt in 1984: 'Any therapy, or anything one does in a concentrated way with people, is a political act. Starting with teaching' (p. 19). The rise of both national and international member organisations has especially led gestalt therapy in a more academic direction, with common criteria for teaching and an emphasis on supervision, ethics, and continuing education for therapists. The European Association for Gestalt Therapy (EAGT) puts forth this argument on their website:[3]

> The creation of minimum Training Standards for Gestalt therapy must be seen against the background of the professionalization of psychotherapy across Europe, specifically the recent dramatic increase in the number of local, national, and European organizations for psychotherapy concerned with establishing standards of training and ethical practice.
>
> The credibility of Gestalt therapy as a competent and ethical approach to the healing of human suffering and to personality development requires similar attention to be given to the establishment of high standards of training and ethical practice.

Over time, teaching in many institutes has become more and more organised, adapted to the criteria set by the EAGT, and in some countries adapted to criteria for colleges and universities, making it possible for institutes in those countries to offer programmes at the bachelor and master levels. Courses of study have been developed with their own curricula, criteria for and minimum hours of praxis, examinations, supervision, mandatory therapy for students, and participation in colloquia study groups. Institutes employ trainers and supervisors and have administrations that follow up students and ensure that national criteria for study programmes are met.

Gestalt therapy is both an art form and a craft (Zinker, 1977; Kolmannskog, 2019). At the same time, it is a therapy form that today has an academic foundation and is based on research (Brownell, 2016; Kolmannskog, 2019). Students are expected to understand the therapy form's theoretical basis and defend the choices they make in their role as therapists. This presupposes a high standard of teaching and a varied pedagogical approach. Trainers must be prepared to lead traditional lectures, group work, and therapeutic work; to be supervisors in a classroom setting; and to read and evaluate students' written work, including final qualifying exams.

The paradigm shift in the transition to the 1990s also laid the foundation for developing a tradition of research in gestalt therapy. Research is essential to establish the effectiveness of clinical practice. The peculiarity of psychotherapy is that the therapist usually sits unobserved with the client. One of the functions of research is to monitor the performance of psychotherapy, which in turn helps to build confidence in the therapy form and thereby increases its quality (Brownell, 2008).

Academic quality is thus closely linked to research. Researching practice reinforces reflection of the concepts the therapist uses in her work. In other words, research bridges the gap between practice and theory.

Roubal et al. (2016) point out that gestalt therapists often show great interest in clinical practice, but that this enthusiasm naturally leads to a one-sided emphasis on practice at the expense of developing the therapy form scientific and theoretically. This imbalance has resulted in it taking time before research in gestalt therapy was given the attention the subject needs and deserves. In recent decades, however, there has been increasing interest in developing good research instruments that are in line with the therapy form's basis and in accordance with phenomenology (Fogarty, 2015).

Research in gestalt therapy is relatively young, but the growing interest has resulted in several books focused entirely on research (Barber, 2006; Strümpfel, 2006; Brownell, 2008; Roubal et al., 2016). Many contributions have also been published in peer-reviewed journals such as the *Gestalt Journal*, the *Gestalt Review*, and the *British Gestalt Journal* (O'Leary, 2013). There are also articles in other journals and chapters in books all over the world presenting research or research projects. Gestalt therapists also take part in gestalt research conferences, where research methods and projects are presented. Brownell (2016), Evans (2016), and Spagnuolo Lobb (2016), among others, have described various research methods that might be relevant for gestalt therapists.

Kolmannskog (2019) claims that the gap between gestalt therapy and research is being bridged by research in both gestalt therapy and psychotherapy. Today, a multi-method approach enjoys a greater degree of acceptance, with a lesser degree of dominance from positivism and a greater appreciation for a pragmatic, practice-oriented approach where the therapist is also a researcher or actively participates in research: 'We have a knowledge-based practice—a practice that is informed by research—but also practice-based knowledge, research that emerges from practice' (p. 34). It is easier for gestalt therapists and students to do research when they can use their own or colleagues' practice as a point of departure for research in a dialogic or phenomenological approach. They can conduct qualitative studies with different methods of data collection, such as structured or unstructured interviews and participant observation. Kolmannskog argues that students can conduct research via case study in their final projects. In this way, students become accustomed to conducting research during their training, which can motivate them to conduct research as practicing therapists.

It is important to emphasise that there are already studies that show that in many cases, gestalt therapy is just as effective as other psychotherapeutic methods. This is particularly true in *The Heart and Soul of Change* (Duncan et al., 2010), which presents a summary of sixty years of research on psychotherapy. This summary shows that psychotherapy, including gestalt therapy, works, and that there are common factors shared by psychotherapeutic methods that create results.

In addition, there are currently two research projects, one in England (Stevens et al., 2011) and one in Italy (La Rosa et al., 2019), involving CORE-OM (Clinical Outcome Routine Evaluation Measure). These both show that clients experience positive effects in gestalt therapy.

In Norway, a research project is being conducted where the CORE-OM form is used concurrently with a gestalt diagnosis form in a therapeutic context, in order to determine whether there is a correlation between the two. The intention is to validate the gestalt diagnostic form so that therapists can use it in research (Mjelve et al., 2015). The gestalt diagnosis form measures four aspects of contact and is developed by Daan van Baalen (2002/2008, 2019).

Gestalt therapy today

Gestalt therapy has grown throughout the world, and today there are training institutes, membership organisations, research groups, and many types of conferences spread around the globe. Different kinds and branches of gestalt therapy, coaching, counselling, supervision, and organisational work are offered in private practice, psychiatry, community work, schools, in business, etc. There are training courses in gestalt therapy at the university level and as part of higher education systems in many countries. Gestalt therapy still struggles to be fully recognised by health care systems and insurance companies in several countries, and much work is being done nationally and internationally to lobby for recognition as an approved psychotherapeutic method on the same level as cognitive therapy or psychodynamic therapy. It is important in this work to show through research that gestalt therapy works in a clinical setting, through international interdisciplinary research.

Summary

Laura and Fritz Perls' legacy is alive and well. The emphasis new generations place on a profession's origin is central to all historical development, also for gestalt therapy. We have described how gestalt therapy took shape in the United States, with a background in Europe and in Fritz and Laura's knowledge of gestalt psychology and existential philosophy. Perls and Goodman's first book on gestalt therapy provided the first written foundation for the therapy form. Thanks to the meticulous efforts of new generations to pinpoint the therapy form's theoretical, philosophical, and scientific basis, gestalt therapy has recovered its roots and a foundation for further development has been laid.

Notes

1 This chapter is based on Clarkson and Mackewn (1993) where no other sources are mentioned.
2 The term 'paradigm shift' was defined by the science philosopher Thomas Kuhn (1962). In the history of a profession, it is inevitable that a fundamental new scientific way of thinking will occasionally take place. Established theories are discarded in favour of a more fruitful way of thinking about the profession's academic concepts. (See also Teigen 2004/2015, p. 347.).
3 https://www.eagt.org/joomla/index.php/2016-02-25-13-29-31/tranining-standards

References

Barber, P. (2006). *Becoming a practioner researcher: A gestalt approach to holistic inquiry*. London: Middlesex University Press.
Bocian, B. (2010). *Fritz Perls in Berlin 1893–1933*. Bergish Gladbach: Verlag Andreas Kohlage.
Bowman, C. E. (2005). The history and development of gestalt therapy. In A. L. Woldt & S. M. Toman (Eds.), *Gestalt therapy: History, theory, and practice* (pp. 3–20). London: SAGE.

Brownell, P. (Ed.). (2008). *Handbook of theory, research, and practice in gestalt therapy.* Newcastle: Cambridge Scholars Publishing.

Brownell, P. (2016). Warrant, research and the practice of gestalt therapy. In J. Roubal (Ed.), *Towards a research tradition in gestalt therapy* (pp. 18–34). Newcastle upon Tyne: Cambridge Scholars Publishing.

Clarkson, P., & Mackewn, J. (1993). *Fritz perls.* London: Sage

Crocker, S. (2005). Phenomenology, existentialism, and Eastern thought in gestalt therapy. In A. Woldt & S. Toman (Eds.), *Gestalt therapy: History, theory, and practice* (pp. 65–80). London: SAGE.

Duncan, B. L., Miller, S. D., Wampold, B. E., & Hubble, M. A. (2010). *The heart & soul of change: Delivering what works in therapy* (2nd ed.). Washington: American Psychological Association.

Evans, K. (2016). Research from a relational gestalt therapy perspective. In J. Roubal (Ed.), *Towards a research tradition in gestalt therapy* (pp. 64–78). Newcastle upon Tyne: Cambridge Scholars Publishing.

Fogarty, M. (2015). Creating a fidelity scale for gestalt therapy. *Gestalt Journal of Australia and New Zealand, 11*(2), 39–54.

Frambach, L. (2003). The weighty world of nothingness: Salomo Friedlaender's "Creative indifference". In M. Spagnuolo Lobb & N. Amendt-Lyon (Eds.), *Creative license: The art of gestalt therapy.* Wien: Springer Verlag.

Hostrup, H. (2010). *Gestalt therapy: An introduction to the basic concepts of gestalt therapy* (D. H. Silver, Trans.). Copenhagen: Hans Reitzlers Forlag. (Original work published 1999).

Kolmannskog, V. (2019). "Vi blir bedre håndverkere": En studie av den akademiske studentoppgaven ved Norsk Gestaltinstitutt Høyskole ["We become better craftspeople": A study of the academic student paper at the Norwegian Gestalt Institute University College]. *Norsk Gestalttidsskrift, 1*(1), 31–54.

La Rosa, R., Tosi, S., Settani, M., Spagnuolo Lobb, M., & Francetti, G. (2019). The outcome of research in gestalt therapy: The Italian CORE-OM research project. *British Gestalt Journal, 28*(2), 14–22.

Mjelve, L. H., Skottun, G., & van Baalen, D. (2015). Bruk av CORE-skjemaer i gestaltterapi [The use of CORE forms in gestalt therapy]. *Norsk Gestalttidsskrift, 11*(2), 8–29.

O'Leary, E. (2013). The present and future of international gestalt therapy. In E. O'Leary (Ed.), *Gestalt therapy around the world* (pp. 327–332). West Sussex: Wiley-Blackwell.

Parlett, M. (2005). Contemporary gestalt therapy: Field theory. In A. L. Woldt & S. M. Toman (Eds.), *Gestalt therapy: History, theory, and practice.* Chapter 3. London: Sage.

Perls, F. S. (1947/1969). *Ego, hunger and aggression.* USA, New York: Vintage Books.

Perls, F. S., Hefferline, R. F., & Goodman, P. (1951). *Gestalt therapy: Excitement and growth in the human personality.* London: Souvenir Press.

Perls, L. (1992). *Living at the boundary.* Gouldsboro, ME: The Gestalt Journal Press.

Roubal, J., Francetti, G., Brownell, P., Melnick, J., & Zeleskov-Djoric, J. (2016). Introduction: Bridging practice and research in gestalt therapy. In J. Roubal (Ed.), *Towards a research tradition in gestalt therapy* (pp. 1–15). Newcastle upon Tyne: Cambridge Scholars Publishing.

Spagnuolo Lobb, M. (2016). Research in gestalt therapy: A way of developing our model. In J. Roubal (Ed.), *Towards a research tradition in gestalt therapy* (pp. 35–44). Newcastle upon Tyne: Cambridge Scholars Publishing.

Staemmler, F. M. (2007). On Macaque monkeys, players, and clairvoyants: Some new ideas for a gestalt therapeutic concept of empathy. *Studies in Gestalt Therapy*, *1*(2), 43–63.

Stevens, C., Stringfellow, J., Wakelin, K., & Waring, J. (2011). The UK gestalt psychotherapy CORE research project: The findings. *British Gestalt Journal*, *20*(2), 22–27.

Strümpfel, U. (2006). *Therapie der Gefühle: Forschungsbefunde zur Gestalttherapie* [Therapy of feelings: Research findings on gestalt therapy]. Bergisch Gladbach: EHP.

Sullivan, H. S. (1953). *Interpersonal theory of psychiatry*. New York: Norton.

Teigen, K. H. (2004/2015). *En psykologihistorie* [A history of psychology]. Bergen: Fagbokforlaget.

van Baalen, D. (2002). Gestaltdiagnoser [Gestalt diagnoses]. In S. Jørstad and Å. Krüger (Eds.), *Den flyvende hollender* [The flying Dutchman] (pp. 15–46). Oslo: NGI.

van Baalen, D. (2019). Phenomenological research in organisations. In M. Spagnuolo Lobb & F. Meulmeester (Eds.), *Gestalt approaches with organisations* (pp. 129–141). Siracusa: Istituto di Gestalt HCC Italy.

Wheeler, G. (1998). *Gestalt reconsidered* (2nd ed.). Cambridge, MA: CIGPress.

Wollants, G. (2012). *Gestalt therapy: Therapy of the situation*. London: Sage.

Yontef, G. M. (1993). *Awareness, dialogue & process*. New York: The Gestalt Journal Press.

Zinker, J. (1977). *Creative process in gestalt therapy*. New York: Random House.

Part 2

Fundamental terminology and concepts

In the second part of this book we describe concepts that are fundamental to gestalt therapeutic work. These concepts primarily have their basis in gestalt psychology and existential phenomenology (Chapters 1 and 2) and were developed by Fritz Perls and his colleagues and successors. The first concept will be described in Chapter 4, 'The Field in Practice'. Lewin's field theory and Perls' and Goodman's understanding of this theory are the basis for this chapter. We emphasise the connection between field theory and gestalt therapy's relational approach: that we influence and are influenced by others, and how our diverse and often conflicting needs characterise our lives. Lewin's theories are fundamental gestalt terms that describe how we as gestalt therapists view the interaction between us and our clients and between our clients and their surroundings.

In Chapter 5, we discuss the gestalt view of change and how this change can take place in the therapy room. Gestalt therapists do not regard themselves as 'agents of change', but instead believe that change can occur spontaneously and paradoxically when clients become more aware of and attentive to themselves in their interactions with their surroundings. Paradoxical change is partly based on what are called 'aha' experiences or moments of spontaneous insight and is one of several ways in which people learn. The gestalt psychologists described this as being a result of insight-based learning.

The understanding of how gestalt therapy views the ways in which humans develop and adapt to their surroundings is described in Chapter 6. Fritz Perls called this 'creative adjustment'. Perls' point of departure for calling all human adjustment to the environment creative is based in his view that every situation and every moment is to be regarded as new; we can never repeat exactly what we have done in a similar situation—we always react in a new way. By increasing the client's attention to how she adjusts to challenging situations in life, the therapist can see the situation as 'new'. She becomes aware that there are several possible forms of creative adjustment in the given situation, and moreover that there are forms other than those the client has previously experienced.

Our understanding of who we are, how we can behave in different ways in different fields, and how impulses and needs lead to action are described in Chapter 7, in which we discuss the theory of self. The concept of 'self' is described as a

DOI: 10.4324/9781003153856-5

function of a situation and expresses how humans influence and are influenced, and that people become who they are together with others in a situation.

Concepts such as awareness and attention, which are described in Chapter 8, are in a sense what we strive to teach both ourselves and our clients during a course of therapy, and indeed during the course of an entire life. Increased awareness of who we are together in the therapy room can lead to a spontaneous recognition and paradoxical change, and to an awareness that we have more choices in a situation than we were aware of. At the same time, being aware and attentive are concepts we use continuously as therapists and are therefore described in this book as part of the conceptual basis of therapy. Awareness and attention are closely linked to phenomenology—to seeing phenomena as they are, with the least possible degree of interpretation.

The concept of contact, described in Chapter 9, was emphasised by Fritz Perls as being the most fundamental concept in gestalt therapy. Several of the theoretical models and techniques used in the gestalt method are based on being in contact. Views on contact—that is, how we understand the models that have been developed on the basis of Perls' view—are controversial and used in different ways in the therapy room. In this book, we present our theoretical thoughts about contact and how we use it as a model for the practice of therapy.

In Chapter 10, we discuss polarities, another of the important concepts in gestalt introduced by Fritz Perls, and which has its basis in, among other things, Lewin's view of the field and needs. The thinking surrounding polarities has led to many useful techniques and ways in which to practice gestalt therapy, which we illustrate in several theoretical models and practical examples.

In the therapeutic relationship, the therapist employs both dialogue and experimentation as 'methods' with which to help clients gain insight and a new understanding about themselves that can lead to change and growth. In Chapter 11, we address experiments. We show how the therapist can facilitate the client's ability to explore, both verbally and non-verbally, new and unknown forms of expression and behaviour that can increase attention and create new experiences. We present examples of types of experiments the therapist can use in different situations to help the client learn to become aware and mindful of bodily sensations, how she senses her surroundings, and the ideas she has about herself and the situation she brings into the therapy room.

Chapter 4

The field in practice

After reviewing the historical basis of gestalt therapy, we move on to how it is practiced, and the concepts from which therapists can draw support. The paradigm shift of the 1990s set the stage for today's understanding of gestalt therapy's place in a relational field perspective, where the therapeutic process is understood to be an *interactive* process that is formed by the here-and-now relationship between client and therapist. Earlier emphasis on therapeutic techniques and assessments are replaced by attention to the here and now that unfolds in the relationship. Rather than being an expert dispensing advice from on high, the therapist has a cooperative function in the field. Research on what works in psychotherapy has confirmed that in order for the client to benefit from therapy, it is crucial that the therapeutic approach be based on the relational interaction between therapist and client (Day, 2016).

Parlett (2005) discusses the therapist's function in this relational interaction, and describes four factors that are essential to therapeutic work in the field: the therapist's co-creative function in the field, how the therapist contributes to the organisation of the field, the therapist's attention to the here and now in the field, and how the therapist defines the parts of the field. These factors are intended to be guiding principles for therapeutic work, and are the background for the further description of the practice of gestalt therapy as explained throughout the rest of this book. In the course of this chapter, we illustrate our points with brief glimpses taken from the practice of gestalt therapy.

The therapist as co-creator in the field

Gestalt therapy's existential basis establishes that the therapist is part of and not an observer of the field that exists between therapist and client. The role of therapist is not to be an objective observer from the outside; rather, she actively contributes to the process together with the client, is present in the field with the client, and is personal and spontaneous. The therapist is not neutral, but can, like all living beings, influence and be influenced. Each theme that comes up in the therapeutic field, such as the client's sense of sadness, will somehow also affect the therapist, whether it stems from a feeling of sadness or sadness made explicit in words or

DOI: 10.4324/9781003153856-6

tears. Both client and therapist are influenced by what they sense and what happens in the field between them.

Therapist and client both contribute to how the phenomena emerge in the field; together, they create the process (Slagsvold, 2016). Parlett (2005) uses dance as a metaphor for this mutual process of creation:

> Two dancers create a dance together that is a product of each dancer's creativity and self-regulation in light of the other dancer's dance. At a particular time, the dance seems to 'take over'. The field itself, once organized and structured, begins to 'regulate the dancers'.
>
> (p. 48)

As we mentioned in our explanation of the philosophy of existence, interactive processes are also key in Buber's philosophy of dialogue (see Chapter 2). Dialogue is about meeting the other. The therapist is present with the client; she strives to be empathetic and place herself in the position of others. Existence philosopher Edith Stein expresses it thus: 'It is as if for a moment I leave myself, momentary switches to the other, taking part in the pain of others. In this immersion moment it is as if I lose myself in the other' (Stein, 1989). This ability to place oneself in the position of others is crucial when faced with people who seek help and support in difficult phases of life. In order to maintain and further develop this attitude to the other, the therapist participates in clinical supervision and meets with her own therapist.

In addition to emphasising the necessity of the therapist's empathic attitude, Hycner (1991) reminds us of another central concept from the work of Martin Buber: inclusion. While empathy is about entering completely into the pain of others, 'inclusion is . . . a turning of one's *entire* existence to the other and the concentrated attempt to experience the other person's experience *as well as* one's own' (p. 43). In other words, to perceive the pain of the other and immerse oneself in it as a shared experience while maintaining one's own perspective and experience. Therefore, the therapist strives to develop a dual skill: a presence where she is primarily is empathic, putting herself in the position of the other, but where she simultaneously incorporates the relational experience—both her own experience and that of the other. In other words, the therapist not only practices seeing from the other's perspective, but also includes herself in the relationship. The therapist develops and works on empathy and inclusion in clinical supervision and her own therapy.

We end this section with a glimpse from a cooperative process in the therapy room between the therapist and Susanne:

THERAPIST: 'When you describe the break with your boyfriend, I feel sad . . . '
SUSANNE: 'Yes, I'm sad . . . it hurts to think about him . . . '
THERAPIST: (sensing her own sadness and tears) 'Yes, sad . . . '
SUSANNE: 'It hurt so much when he went out the door for the last time . . . '

THERAPIST: (senses sadness and associations to parting) 'Do you see him now?'

SUSANNE: (tears) 'Yes . . . he goes . . . to the door and turns to me . . . '

THERAPIST: 'Yes, breaking up is sad . . . is there anything you want to say to him?'

SUSANNE: (quiet, tears) 'Harry, I'm sad that you're leaving, and I know it's over . . . ';

(quiet, hesitant . . . then says to Harry) 'I wish you all the best . . . '

The therapist contributes to the organisation of the field

We have pointed out that the tendency in gestalt therapy's early years was for the therapist to use certain set techniques. In the new paradigm, this predetermined approach is no longer relevant. Clarkson and Mackewn (1993) emphasise that 'Gestalt therapy is not, however, about techniques or quick catchy gimmicks: it's a process of working with phenomenological awareness, experimenting, creating and dialoguing' (p. 151). Today, the field and the relational process between therapist and client are the basis for our choice of interventions. The emphasis is on the therapist who uses her creativity and affects change on the basis of field experiences between herself and the client—in the relational meeting, there and then.

Affecting change is first and foremost a function of the therapist being present with awareness in the therapeutic field with the client. The therapist senses whether the time is right for change, and thus whether the timing is right to support the mobilisation of energy (see Chapter 20). If, on the other hand, the energy of the field drops, there may be a need for change in the tempo of the relational dance. In such tempo changes, the therapist is aware of the needs of the relationship here and now in this particular field with this particular client. She is aware of the client's past experiences and thus senses what the field between them can tolerate. She senses whether the time is right to suggest an experiment. In this way, the therapist allows body resonance to guide her in how she affects the field (Frank, 2016).

When the therapist is conscious about what she is aware of in the field together with the client, she can choose how to proceed based on what occurs in the field there and then. Her conscious awareness is something she feels, senses, and reflects on; it is not determined by rules or theoretical references. Conscious awareness becomes the basis for influencing change and reaction, like changing the pace in a spontaneous dance there and then.

PATRICIA: 'I'm still struggling with this conflict with my colleague'.

THERAPIST: 'You're going in circles . . .?'

PATRICIA: 'No! *He's* the one who's making things difficult . . . '

The therapist listens. This is not the first time Patricia has told her about this conflict. As she listens, an idea occurs to her. She is inspired to propose an exercise that she believes can help Patricia to sort out her relationship with her colleague. She is eager and mobilises energy and is on the verge of interrupting Patricia in order to suggest something, but a sense of unease holds her back. She continues to listen.

PATRICIA: 'He's always yelling at me . . . No matter what I do, it's always wrong . . . '

Again, the therapist notices that her urge to interrupt increases. Once again, she is on the verge of speaking. She inhales, thinking about what she is going to say, clears her throat.

Patricia suddenly becomes silent. The therapist waits . . . she feels her muscles tightening.

PATRICIA: ' . . . when I talk about him, I suddenly start thinking about my uncle . . . '

Patricia collapses in her chair, gasps . . . and the story of the assaults she has experienced comes out.

Here and now

The expression 'here and now' is one of the most well known in gestalt therapy. With field theory as a basis for our therapy form, bringing the now-perspective into therapy is justified. Lewin (1936) states the obvious: only in the now can anything be changed. It therefore seems obvious that the 'now' perspective is also part of the therapeutic process. Zinker (1987) follows up Lewin's definition by pointing out how the now opens up 'to being fully here with *all* of oneself, one's "body and soul"—open to all possibilities' (pp. 3–4). Likewise, Spagnuolo Lobb (2003) points out how life is embraced when the field is explored here and now, and thus the process of life itself is improvised there and then.

Being here and now is to live in life's continuous motion, moment by moment. This also applies to the here and now of the therapeutic process. The therapist senses both change and stability. When something becomes clear and thus a figure in the field, the stage is set for exploration here and now. The client is thus encouraged to bring her experiences to the present moment, and it is this 'now' that the therapist explores.

Wheeler (1998) points out, however, that gestalt therapists' emphasis on the here and how has a tendency to be too one-sided. He points out the danger of the therapist becoming suspended in the here and now at the expense of seeing the present in the light of past experiences. He reminds us that which makes itself known now is also based in the client's life experience, an experience that has been formed and given its meaning over time. It is therefore important to emphasise that gestalt therapy is also about taking the client's life experience seriously. In this way, the therapist is encouraged to be open to all time aspects in exploration together with the client. Therapist and client explore the client's 'there-and-then' past experiences as well as what is happening in the moment 'here and now'. Parlett (2005) calls for a flexible attitude by moving away from the one-sided 'here and now' to flexible shifts between, for example, 'there and then', 'here and then', and 'there and now'. It is not unusual that a topic that emerges as a figure in the field here and now can be traced to the past—the 'there and then'.

Defining the field

Parlett (2005) points out that the field perspective calls us to consider human behaviour and experience in a wider context where we are open to long-term patterns and persistent styles of self-organisation. This means that the therapist also is aware of themes brought up by the client from her past and considers her family, cultural, and socio-economic context. The attention to aspects of time in gestalt therapeutic practice leads us to another central theme in the therapist's awareness, namely the delimitation of the field. In the preceding paragraph, the therapist had already begun a delimitation of the field. When the process concerns what is happening here and now in the space between therapist and client, the therapist works in the delimitated here and now. In the next session, a memory from the client's childhood might be the theme. The field can then, for example, be limited to what happened there and then.

The delimitation of a field is primarily practical and useful for the therapist. Instead of having to deal with past, present, and future, the therapist chooses the one that feels most natural, often on the basis of what appears to be the figure here and now. Delimitation in the field helps the therapist to structure the processes that come and go. Other examples of delimitation could be when the figure in the field is about the client and her relationship with her husband, the client and her relationship with her mother during childhood, or simply the relationship between therapist and client:

> We can switch the emphasis from reality to role play, from experiencing something at a physical bodily level to visual fantasy, to searching for a metaphor, to telling the story. We can notice not just the immediate figure that is present but ongoing features, the structures and repetitive patternings arising in the field . . . the versatility and power of the therapist to engage fully and deeply with the client and his or her reality are often enhanced by 'movement in the field' as well as by 'reconfiguring the field'.
>
> (Parlett, 2005, pp. 51–52)

Field boundaries are particularly relevant in working with couples and groups, especially because the field may appear to be complex and chaotic. In both of these situations, delimiting the field becomes essential to and useful for managing the process. When working with groups, there are several possibilities, such as working with only one participant (the therapist–participant field), with the relationship between two or more participants, or with the group as a whole. Working with couples and groups is about working with fields and fields within the field. Such work also follows the principle that the smaller, inner field affects the group field as a whole (Dyrkorn, 2014).

This model is primarily intended to facilitate a clear and ordered structure for a process that includes multiple perspectives and that can otherwise often be confusing. Lewin points this out when he writes that the field is characterised by tensions, needs, and conflicting needs, force and counterforce. Defining the field can be a support to therapists as they observe and participate in the process.

Summary of key elements of the field in practice

- Note how the therapist and client affect each other.
- Be aware of the various fields: small and large fields can constantly change— the whole affects the parts, or smaller fields, and the parts affect the whole, or larger field.
- The therapist can choose which field she works in and with.
- There is a close relationship between gestalt psychology, the law of *prägnanz*, figure-ground formation, and creative adjustment.

The field in practice summarised

The model for therapy presented in this chapter is an example of how field theory gives therapists a practical tool with which to structure and keep track of therapeutic processes. Because additional fields can be active simultaneously, it is absolutely necessary for the therapist to be able to identify the separate fields. Good field delimitation is a method, a practical tool for keeping track of all the information that emerges when we are dealing with multiple fields simultaneously. A clear delimitation of the fields is crucial in order to see figures and how they are formed. Defining the field in this way is also highly applicable and useful in the therapeutic work done between a single client and therapist. Defining the fields facilitates overview and a good framework for here-and-now processes and is thus helpful for the therapist's awareness of the choices she has of the available fields, such as here and now or then and there.

Not least, field in practice is about the therapist's work with processes in the therapy room. There has been a growing awareness in parts of the gestalt milieu of the importance of the relationship between therapist and client for the therapeutic process. This development has led to increased attention on the significance of field theory for clinical practice, and not least to a greater understanding of the contribution of phenomenology to ethical reflections on clinical practice (Joyce & Sills, 2014). In recent decades, research on psychotherapy has shown that the quality of the relationship between client and therapist is essential to good therapy (Norcross, 2011). Field in practice is about how the therapist is aware and present, and cognisant of her influence and co-creative function in the here and now together with the client.

Field or situation?

There is a debate in the international gestalt-therapeutic scientific community as to whether Lewin's field concept should be expressed as *situation*, a term Lewin himself also uses on occasion. This has led to what Staemmler (2006) refers to as a 'Babylonian confusion' (p. 64). Wollants (2012) prefers to use the term 'situation' in place of field because he believes it is closer to everyday experience than the—in his opinion—unclear and ambiguous term 'field'. He is supported by Robine (2002), who believes that 'field' is too imprecise and can therefore easily be perceived as an overarching concept with imprecise content. The British authors Joyce and Sills (2014) use 'situation' a few times but seem to prefer 'field' in their many good examples taken from gestalt-therapeutic practice. A brilliant explanation of the field and its application in practice can be found in Parlett (2005). In the epilogue to Wollants' (2012) book about the situation, however, Parlett supports Wollants' argument that the concept of situation is more useful in an everyday setting than is the more ambiguous word 'field'. He summarises this diplomatically: 'the fundamental "unitary" message is the same' (p. 116). This last point of view is also supported by Staemmler (2010), who points out that 'situation' is far more pragmatic and useful for practice than 'field', which he considers a more abstract term.

References

Clarkson, P., & Mackewn, J. (1993). *Fritz Perls*. London: Sage Publications.

Day, E. (2016). Field attunement for a strong therapeutic alliance: A perspective from relational gestalt psychotherapy. *Journal of Humanistic Psychology, 56*(1), 77–94.

Dyrkorn, R. (2014). *Lederen og teamet: Gestaltbasert coaching og teamutvikling* [The leader and the team: Gestalt-based coaching and team development]. Oslo: Gestaltforlaget.

Frank, R. (2016). Self in motion. In *Self: A polyphony of contemporary gestalt therapists*. J.-M. Robine (Ed.), (pp. 371–386). France: L'Exprimerie.

Hycner, R. (1991). *Between person and person*. New York: Center of Gestalt Development.

Joyce, P., & Sills, C. (2014). *Skills in gestalt counselling & psychotherapy* (3rd ed.). London: Sage.

Lewin, K. (1936). *A dynamic theory of personality*. New York: McGraw-Hill.

Norcross, J. C. (2011). Foreword: The therapeutic relationship. In B. L. Duncan, S. D. Miller, B. E. Wampold, & M. A. Hubble (Eds.), *The heart and soul of change: Delivering what works in therapy*. Washington DC: American Psychological Association.

Parlett, M. (2005). Contemporary gestalt therapy: Field theory. In A. L. Woldt & S. M. Toman (Eds.), *Gestalt therapy: History, theory, and practice*. Chapter 3. London: SAGE.

Robine, J.-M. (2002). From field to situation. In J.-M. Robine (Ed.), *Contact and relationship in a field perspective*. Bordeaux: L'Exprimerie.

Slagsvold, M. (2016). *Jeg blir til i møte med deg* [I become me together with you]. Oslo: Cappelen Damm.

Spagnuolo Lobb, M. (2003). Therapeutic meeting as improvisational co-creation. In M. Spagnuolo Lobb & N. Amendt-Lyon (Eds.), *Creative license: The art of gestalt therapy* (pp. 1–10). New York: Springer.

Staemmler, F. M. (2006). A Babylonian confusion: On the uses and meanings of the term "field". *British Gestalt Journal*, *15*(2), 64–83.

Staemmler, F. M. (2010). *Continuity and change*. Keynote given at the conference of the Association for the Advancement of Gestalt Therapy in Philadelphia, USA, June 2010.

Stein, E., Saint, 1891–1942 (1989). *The collected works of Edith Stein, Sister Teresa Benedicta of the Cross, discalced Carmelite* (Vol. 3). Washington, DC: ICS Publications.

Wheeler, G. (1998). *Gestalt reconsidered* (2nd ed.). Cambridge, MA: CIGPress.

Wollants, G. (2012). *Gestalt therapy: Therapy of the situation*. London: Sage.

Zinker, J. (1987). Presence as evocative power in therapy. *Gestalt Review*, *1*(2), 3–4, 8.

Chapter 5

The theory of change

Most of us have periods in our lives in which we are not satisfied with ourselves and try to change our behaviour or our weaknesses. Often, we succeed. For example, we manage to lose weight, exercise, or eat healthier. This can give a good sense of accomplishment. Often, however, we are unable to change, despite the fact that we try our best. Clients who come to therapy often belong to this group. Some want to be kinder to their children, to be more patient, less irritable, and slower to anger. Some are struggling with anxiety, lack energy, are unhappy with themselves, or are incapable of making choices. Many have struggled for a long time and are looking for a solution to their problems when they seek out a therapist. This is the case with Mona in the following example.

Mona comes to therapy because she feels down and depressed. Her relationship with her boyfriend, with whom she lives, is not going well, and she is unhappy at work. In the first two sessions, she tells the therapist a little about herself, about her relationship with her partner Ben, how she is at work, and how lonely she feels. She has many explanations as to why she is having such a hard time and says that she has tried many things to make it better without feeling that it has helped.

After the session has begun, the therapist notices that Mona's upper body is slumped over, and that she does not look at the therapist as she speaks. Her words come fast in a monotonous and plaintive tone of voice. Mona says that she does not know if she will continue to live with Ben, and wonders what she should do to feel better at work. She does not feel that anyone at work cares about what she does, and she feels sad and lonely. The therapist notices that she herself is affected by Mona's depressed mood and is confused by her torrent of words and explanations. She thinks that it is time to interrupt Mona.

The therapist repeats what she has heard Mona say: 'Mona, I hear you say that you feel lonely, that you're not sure you'll continue to live with Ben, and that you don't know how to feel better at work. As you spoke, I noticed that you're sitting slumped in your chair and that you look sad'.

DOI: 10.4324/9781003153856-7

Mona looks up at the therapist: 'Yes, I feel sad and depressed, I don't know what to do. I care about Ben, but things are so bad between us, he doesn't understand me, and that's how it is at work, too, I don't know what I should do'. Mona begins to cry; the tears flow.

The therapist repeats again what she heard Mona say, pointing out that she sees that Mona is crying. Mona continues to cry, as she occasionally says more about how miserable she feels, how she feels that her life is hard, and that she is stuck without knowing what to do. After a while Mona stops crying, but she continues to sit slumped over without looking at the therapist.

The therapist repeats again: 'I hear you say that your life is hard, you're stuck and don't know what to do. Could you repeat what you said, and look at me while doing it?'

Here the therapist wants to make Mona aware of the content of what she says, and that she (the therapist) hears and sees her. When Mona sits slumped over without looking up, the therapist suspects that she is not aware of what is going on with herself and with the therapist. The therapist has a hypothesis that Mona can feel alone and depressed when she does not see others around her or is not aware that someone sees and hears her.

Mona nods and looks at the therapist as she says a bit hesitantly: 'My life is hard . . . I'm stuck . . . and I don't know what to do. It's a little weird for me to say that'.

The therapist repeats what Mona said, and asks her to repeat it again while she continues to look at her (the therapist).

Mona straightens up slightly in her chair, and says: 'My life is hard . . . I'm stuck . . . and I don't know what to do'. As she speaks, her voice grows louder. She sits up and looks directly at the therapist and says, a little surprised: 'Hmm, yes, it's true, that's strange. . . . My life is hard, I don't know what to do, and I'm stuck. It's as if I feel it differently inside me—as if I'm almost relieved when I know that I'm stuck. As if I agree in a way that I don't know what I want'.

Mona looks straight at the therapist, breathes, and smiles slightly. The therapist and Mona talk a bit about how this recognition of being stuck means that Mona feels she can look at the relationship with Ben and her job in a new way, without knowing what she will do in the future.

Instead of trying to solve Mona's problem, the therapist chose to interrupt Mona's explanations when she began to repeat herself and the therapist sensed that she was becoming depressed and confused herself. The therapist chose to focus on what she believed was the most important out of everything Mona had said, and they took turns repeating words verbatim. By repeating in this way, the therapist held Mona's focus and awareness in the challenging circumstances that she up to this point had tried to avoid feeling; namely, that she was stuck and did not know what to do.

When Mona repeated the sentence the first time, she felt the pain and discomfort and began to cry. She awoke to the truth of what she said and acquired new insight into the situations that she up to his point had tried to find solutions for. This recognition came spontaneously, and Mona felt an emotional and physical change.

Afterwards, Mona is able to think differently about her problems. She still has not found a solution to her difficulties, but the new insight has changed her understanding of her struggles. She feels lighter and less depressed, and it is as if she has a different perspective on herself, her relationship with Ben, and her job. In gestalt therapy we call this spontaneous insight and paradoxical change. Mona stops thinking that she should change and be different than she actually is. Often, this takes longer than in this example, but here we condense it to illustrate the steps in this type of process (see Chapter 20 on the process of change).

In this chapter, we provide a brief introduction to what is meant by spontaneous insight and paradoxical change, how gestalt psychology, Lewin's field theory (Chapter 1), phenomenology (Chapter 2), and Buddhism (Chapter 3) all have influenced the understanding of these concepts, and how this understanding is expressed in the therapist's attitudes and practices.

Spontaneous insight

In the example above, the therapist meets Mona with an accepting and friendly attitude. This therapeutic attitude is an important basis for Mona's new experiences.

The concept of spontaneous insight can be found in both gestalt psychology and Buddhist philosophy. The concept of paradoxical change is based on phenomenology but can also be found in Buddhism. First, we present the concept of spontaneous insight from gestalt psychology.

In the experiment described on pp. 11–12, Köhler showed how the chimpanzee suddenly solved a problem and had an 'aha' experience or spontaneous insight. The example with Mona also shows spontaneous insight. In retrospect, it cannot be explained precisely what it was that made her suddenly change her outlook on her life, beyond the fact that she allowed herself to feel her frustration, and that the therapist helped her to clarify some of the factors in her situation—that she was sad, stuck, and did not know what to do. In light of an increased attention on some parts of the whole, the whole was suddenly organised in a new way. This spontaneous insight led to a change in the way Mona looked at herself and her life.

The theories of Köhler and the other gestalt psychologists are the background for how Fritz Perls understood change. Perls saw fixed and inflexible behavioural patterns in the client as a result of an inadequate organisation between the client and her surroundings. His point of departure was in what the gestalt psychologists called the formation of figure-ground, which is an explanation of how people organise sensory impressions in such a way that something is in the foreground and the rest is background, where people choose that which is most important to them at the moment, and leave the rest in the background (Chapter 1 and p. 11). Perls argued that when this figure-ground formation is fixed, the therapist can work to increase the client's attention to herself and the surrounding environment, and that this can cause the client to see her situation in a new way (Clarkson & Mackewn, 1993). What previously was an unclear and fixed figure can become clearer and more interesting and meaningful. We can recognise this in how Mona felt stuck until she gained new insight and a new understanding of herself and her relationship to the environment. We call this paradoxical change.

Paradoxical change

The theory of paradoxical change was formulated by Arnold Beisser (1970/2006) as follows:

> *change occurs when one becomes what he is, not when he tries to become what he is not*. Change does not take place through a coercive attempt by the individual or by another person to change him, but it does take place if one takes the time and effort to be what he is—to be fully invested in his current positions.
>
> (p. 77, our italics)

Beisser's claim that change occurs when we become what we are, not when we try to become what we are not, refers to a central gestalt therapeutic method; namely, supporting the client's awareness of her own situation during the therapeutic process (see Chapter 8 on awareness). Beisser's characterisation of gestalt therapeutic change as a process in which someone becomes what she is means that the client can become conscious of all her feelings and experience her sensations, but not that she will necessarily act on them. This means that the client experiences her annoyance (and perhaps also her tendency to be violent) completely, and in this way becomes conscious that she is angry and possibly even becomes able to carry out aggressive actions. In this way, the client can discover who she is at any given time. This is a prerequisite for being able to behave differently in the future, if she should so wish (Staemmler, 2016).

We recognise in Beisser's statements the gestalt psychological basis that comes from Köhler's experimentation with figure-ground formation. Wheeler (1998) has summarised this as follows:

> Mere concentration of attention, by or with the subject, especially on some parts of the field that are characteristically out of awareness, will by definition

produce some reorganization of the field—and the potential, at least, for a corresponding behavioral change, of one kind or another.

(p. 39)

This summation also brings Kurt Lewin's field theory in as a clarification of the fact that a person's surroundings are always limited in time and space (see Chapters 1 and 4). Figure-ground formation always occurs in a field; the example of Mona illustrates this. The specific therapy session detailed above, composed of Mona and the therapist together in the therapy room, was the field in which Mona experienced a new understanding of her relationship with her partner and of her situation at work.

Seeing things as they are

In the phenomenological method it is fundamental that the therapist see phenomena as they present themselves in the moment, and not interpret or assign them subjective meaning (Chapter 2) (Krüger, 2002/2008). The phenomena that capture the therapist's interest can also be compared with that which figures and is of importance in the situation, that is, 'what is', which is always a subjective experience *for someone*. These phenomena can be impressions from the outside world and especially the therapist's *own* feelings, fantasies, thoughts, and bodily sensations. All this stems from experienced phenomena that are personal and are only available to the individual who has the experience. Put another way: 'that which is', in this context, does not objectively exist and cannot be identified. It cannot be investigated in the same way as a broken arm or an appendix. There is no universal truth, such as gravity, which is a universal reality, nor anything outside of ourselves that we can use as support, such as a tree or another human being. 'That which is' cannot be objectified; it must be understood metaphorically in the context in which it occurs (Staemmler, 2016). In the example of Mona, 'that which is' is her insight into the fact that she is stuck and does not know what to do.

The therapist's phenomenological attitude can also be found in Buddhist philosophy and other branches of therapy that recognise that a friendly attitude to oneself promotes change (Staemmler, 2016). In the example of Mona, we hear how depressed and alone she feels, and how helpful it is for her that the therapist has a different attitude toward her. In Buddhism, this is described as practice in attention. This means:

to bring consciousness back to the present moment, and to maintain this attention in all aspects of life, no matter how pleasant or unpleasant these situations are. Being attentive therefore also means not categorising or evaluating the content that emerges in consciousness, but rather simply observing it: an attentive attitude is characterised by being open to all experiences in the moment.

(Zwiebel, 2009, p. 1007, our translation)

Fritz Perls' understanding of paradoxical change and impasse

Perls was influenced by both phenomenology and Buddhism. He expressed himself in a slightly more nonchalant manner about change in one of his seminars.

> You never overcome *anything* by resisting it. You can only overcome something by going deeper into it. If you are spiteful, be *more* spiteful. If you are performing, increase the performance. Whatever it is, if you go deeply enough into it, then it will disappear; it will be assimilated. Any resistance is no good. You have to go full into it—swing with it. Swing with your pain, your restlessness, whatever is there.
>
> (Perls, 1969, p. 240)

This quotation from Perls reveals how he worked with clients. He held the client in what he called the 'impasse', where the client and the therapist are forced to acknowledge that they do not see solutions (Staemmler, 1994). Perls observed that the client sometimes played a role, assuming characteristics that were not part of her personality. He believed that when the client became aware of the fact that she did not know how to behave or that she had not been aware of her needs, something new could happen. Perls did not believe that the therapist should act as an agent of change. In this approach to therapy, he was ahead of his time (Beisser, 1970/2006). (See also Chapter 20 on the process of change.)

Beisser's and Perls' statements show the way in which we understand that *psychic change* is possible in psychotherapy, especially *in gestalt therapy* (Staemmler, 2016).

To accept what is: suffering, pain, and resistance

The view of suffering and pain is central to Buddhist thinking. In Buddhism, suffering is understood as man's basic condition, and pain is the reality we acknowledge in the moment. 'Life is not always the way we want it to be. Suffering comes into our lives as dissatisfaction, disappointment, frustration, and stress. The origin of suffering lies in ourselves, our minds, attitudes, and actions' (Braathen, 2011, p. 24, our translation). The suffering we experience depends on how much we resist acknowledging the pain. The more resistance we feel and express, the more we will suffer (Shapiro & Carlson, 2009). Take resistance away, there is no suffering, only pain. In a Buddhist perspective, this gives us the ability to control and even be freed from suffering when we acknowledge the pain that exists in the moment. This perspective is reflected in what we have written above about recognising 'what is' and paradoxical change. In gestalt therapy, the therapist works with just that: to explore and acknowledge resistance to pain and difficulty in the client's life.

These attitudes from phenomenology and Buddhism that were embraced by both Perls and Beisser have influenced the gestalt view of change, in that the therapist is more interested in *what* and *how* the client experiences a situation than in *why* the client behaves as she does. The therapist is not concerned with causal relationships or finding solutions, but rather in phenomena and experience. Beisser referred to the author Proust, who wrote: 'To heal a suffering one must experience it to the full' (Beisser, 1970/2006, p. 78). The therapist does not work within the medical paradigm where one looks for a diagnosis in order to find a treatment, but rather within a paradigm characterised by phenomenology and *seeing what is* (van Baalen, 2013).

Finding one's footing

Fundamental to all change is that *we know where we* are, so that we can orient ourselves and discover where we want to go, so as to follow our path. The first questions a foot orienteering athlete asks herself when she is given a map and compass are: 'Where am I?' and 'Where am I on the map?' She then checks the location of her next control point and determines how to get there. The same process occurs in therapy. Søren Kierkegaard (1998) formulated the importance of that the helper—in this case, the therapist—begins where the one who needs help is:

> If one is truly to succeed in leading a person to a specific place, one must first and foremost take care to find him where he is and begin there. This is the secret in the entire art of helping. Anyone who cannot do this is himself under a delusion if he thinks he is able to help someone else. In order truly to help someone else, I must understand more than he—but certainly first and foremost understand what he understands. If I do not do that, then my greater understanding does not help him at all.
>
> (p. 45)

It does not help to ask how the client wants to be, or about the direction she wants her life to take. She must first see and acknowledge where she is, no matter how uncomfortable and painful the acknowledgement can be. Beisser (1970/2006) also writes about this in his article:

> change can occur when the patient abandons, at least for the moment, what he would like to become and attempts to be what he is. The premise is that one must stand in one place in order to have firm footing to move and that it is difficult or impossible to move without that footing.
>
> (p. 77)

The client may experience getting such a foothold through her recognition of how and where she is. Staemmler (2009/2016) puts it this way:

> It is thus the foundation of their own psychological reality—and by that I do not mean a purely cognitive 'know thyself!', but a living experience. It is about first coming to oneself, then being able to grow beyond oneself.
>
> (p. 6, our translation)

Many clients who come to therapy, counselling, or coaching need help to see where they are in their lives and what is important to them. This is the case for Christine, who has been fired from her job.

> Christine was recently laid off from her job in a bank as a result of restructuring and downsizing. An advisor in HR suggests that she speak with a gestalt coach for help to find out what she can do next. Her life has been turned upside-down since learning that she is going to unemployed in just a few months. Much of her existence is based on her job; this will make it much more difficult financially, especially because she the breadwinner in a family with two children. She will lose colleagues and tasks she enjoys. When Christine comes to coaching, she is determined to find a new job as soon as possible.

CHRISTINE: 'I hope you can help me find a new job. I need a reliable income as soon as possible'.

COACH: 'I understand what you want and am happy to help. First, though, I wonder—did the layoff come as a surprise?'

CHRISTINE: 'Yes, absolutely. There had been a lot of talk about restructuring, and that it would mean that some of us would be let go, but I didn't think it was going to be me. I thought they were happy with me and wanted me to stay'. Christine is upset, angry, and sad when she talks to the coach.

COACH: 'So you think you were laid off because management isn't happy with you and the way you do your job?' The coach leans forward slightly and looks directly at Christine.

CHRISTINE: 'Yes. Even though they didn't say that in so many words, that's what I think. I have more seniority than many of the others'.

COACH: 'Then the layoff was really a shock for you. I know I hold my breath and feel tension in my body while I'm listening to you. How has this time since you were told you were being let go been for you?'

CHRISTINE: 'Yes, it was a shock, and it's been awful'.

Christine describes her turmoil, anxiety, and sense of failure to the coach. As she talks, she slowly beings to cry, and her voice starts to tremble. The coach listens, nods, and sometimes makes short comments to show Christine that she is there with her.

After a while, Christine wipes her tears, looks at the coach, and says: 'It feels really good to tell you how terrible I feel. I came here to find a new job, and instead I just sat here and cried like a baby in front of a complete stranger'.

COACH: 'It looks like that was what you needed right now. I know that I've been right here with you while you were talking—I was completely focused on your story. I held my breath several times and was very tense for a while. I noticed that I relaxed a bit when you began to cry, and it seems as if you're also more relaxed right now'.

CHRISTINE: 'Yes, I'm a little calmer, it's as if the air has gone out of the balloon. It's like it's a little easier to be me, although I still don't know what I'm going to do'.

COACH: 'It's good to hear that you feel a little calmer. I'd like to meet with you again and spend time talking about the future. I think it's important to take one thing at a time. We can start where you are and how you feel'.

CHRISTINE: 'Yes, it feels very different to be me now, I feel much calmer. I hope that by talking with you it will be easier for me to figure out what I'm going to do'.

In this conversation, 'what is' is the fact that Christine has lost her job. Naturally, she wants to find a new job and solve what she sees as her problem. The coach believes, however, that it is important to explore 'what is' and determine where Christine 'is' first, and that this can make finding a new job easier for her. The coach's questions and interested presence triggers many emotions and thoughts, and Christine shares these with the coach. It is completely natural that Christine was closed off to these feelings when the layoff was a fact. It was important for her to be able to deal with her everyday life with all its challenges and be able to think practically. When she had time and space to stop for a moment, it became possible for her to be in 'what is' and to acknowledge all the feelings and turmoil and her fear of the new and unknown. The experience of 'what is' changes into something new, a new 'what is'. When Christine's subjective experience of 'what is' changes, she gets a sense of being different than she was before she shared her feelings with the coach.

Supporting clients in therapy

There are many ways in which a therapist or coach can challenge and support clients. Many of the methods used in the coaching or therapy room that are illustrated in the preceding examples contain a combination of both. Fritz Perls was known for challenging his clients and helping them to remain in the impasse, while Laura Perls was interested in how the therapist could support the client, especially via body work and the breath. Her hypothesis was that anxiety was often caused by a lack of support, which led to shallow breathing, a lack of oxygen, and the client closing off her emotions and preparing for danger. (See Chapter 11 on experiments for more about challenge and support.)

There are situations where the therapist feels that a client does not have the resources and opportunities that are implicit in our theory of paradoxical change. This may be the case if the client is in a serious crisis; has experienced major and disruptive events such as death, accident, assault, or abuse; and is depressed or anxious. Clients might struggle when they are in the midst of a process where they have conflicting needs and have to make a choice. In these situations, they often need a lot of support and few challenges since they have enough to deal with in their everyday lives. They often lack the ability to be here and now, to endure suffering, to reflect on their own situation and be available for contact, and they tolerate poorly any attempts to hold them in discomfort and difficulty (Taylor, 2014). In fields with this type of client, the therapist can proceed carefully and work actively to support the client's ability to implement necessary changes rather than expect the client to do it herself. It is the therapist's ability to be aware of the client's responses and signals in the therapy room, together with knowledge of the client and her life history, that determines how and the degree to which the therapist supports and challenges the client. In the next chapter on creative adjustment, we discuss further how the therapist can meet and support clients who have been exposed to traumatic experiences of the type mentioned above.

Summary

Beisser's (1970/2006) theory of change is commonly referred to with the following quote: 'change occurs when one becomes what he is, not when he tries to become what he is not' (p. 77). This statement can be perceived as a cliché where the deeper meaning is lost. The challenge inherent in this statement, and indeed in Beisser's theory, is to look past the cliché and take the allegation seriously. One of the most challenging things we can do is to be what we are. It means putting aside all notions of how we should be or what we think others should be; it means seeing ourselves and others with openness and warmth, without prejudice. This process can be painful, frightening, and uncomfortable, but leads to spontaneous change that cannot be planned. You can occasionally hear someone say, 'You just have to accept it, that's how it is'. This is a misguided version of Beisser's change theory. It is not possible simply 'to be what one is'. As we have described in this chapter, it requires real knowledge of the situation.

In further examples in this book, Beisser's paradoxical theory of change is the foundation on which the therapist's interventions and experiments are built and influences her attitude in relation to how she meets her clients. This therapeutic attitude presupposes the therapist's genuine presence, in which she is continually aware of and attentive to what she perceives in the therapy room, both with the client, herself, and between them.

References

Beisser, A. R. (1970/2006). The paradoxical theory of change. In J. Fagan & E. L Shepherd (Eds.), *Gestalt therapy now: Theory, techniques, applications* (pp. 77–80). Gouldsboro, ME: The Gestalt Journal Press.

Braathen, E. (2011). Å akseptere det som er: om mindfulness og gestaltterapi [Accepting what is: On mindfulness and gestalt therapy]. *Norsk Gestalttidsskrift, 8*(2), 7–29.

Clarkson, P., & Mackewn, J. (1993). *Fritz Perls*. London: Sage Publications.

Hong, E. H., & Hong, H. V. (Eds.). (1998). The point of view. In E. H. Hong & H. V. Hong (Series Eds., Trans.), *Kierkegaard's writings* (Vol. 22). Princeton, NJ: Princeton University Press.

Krüger, Å. (2002/2008). Gestaltterapeutisk metode: Fenomenologi i teori og praksis [Gestalt therapeutic method: Phenomenology in theory and practice]. In S. Jørstad & Å. Krüger (Eds.), *Den flyvende hollender* [The flying Dutchman] (pp. 55–60). Oslo: NGI.

Perls, F. S. (1969). *Gestalt therapy verbatim*. Highland, NY: The Gestalt Journal Press.

Shapiro, S. L., & Carlson, L. E. (2009). *The art and science of mindfulness: Integrating mindfulness into psychology and the helping professions*. Washington: American Psychological Association.

Staemmler, F. M. (1994). On layers and phases. *The Gestalt Journal, 17*(1), 5–30.

Staemmler, F. M. (2009/2016). *Einige Gedanken zu dem Satz "Was ist, darf sein, und was sein darf, kann sich verändren"*. (Zweite, geringfügig überarbeitete Ausgabe) ["*Some thoughts on the sentence: 'That which is, can be, and that which can be, can change'*". (Second, slightly revised edition)]. Würtzburg: Author. [Monograph]. Retrieved from www.frank-staemmler.de/www.frank-staemmler.de/Publikationen_files/Was%20 ist,%20darf%20sein.pdf

Taylor, M. (2014). *Trauma therapy and clinical practice: Neuroscience, gestalt and the body*. Maidenhead: Open University Press.

van Baalen, D. (2013). Forskjellige paradigmer: om ulike tilnærminger i behandling [Different paradigms: On different approaches in treatment]. *Norsk Gestalttidsskrift, 10*(1), 68–79.

Wheeler, G. (1998). *Gestalt reconsidered* (2nd ed.). Cambridge, MA: CIGPress.

Zwiebel, R. (2009). Das Studium des Selbst: Psychoanalyse und Buddhismus im Dialog [The study of the self: Psychoanalysis and Buddhism in dialogue]. *Psyche, 63*(9–10), 999–1028.

Chapter 6

Creative adjustment

We all meet various challenges in life that we handle in different ways. These challenges can sometimes be big, such as losing someone we love, being exposed to abuse, experiencing illness, or being in an accident. Sometimes it can even be challenging to deal with good periods in life, when the sun shines, we have no financial problems, and we have everything we want or need. Regardless of whether the challenges are large or small, or we perceive them as good or bad, we find ways to deal with them. This does not mean that we are always happy or satisfied with how we adjust, and it does not always feel satisfying or creative. However, no matter how we deal with the challenges we encounter, even when we do nothing at all, we are adjusting to the situation. People who come to therapy are often in situations where they experience that the ways they adjust involve pain and suffering, and they therefore seek out other ways to relate to their environments.

In this chapter, we describe what is meant in gestalt theory by 'creative adjustment' and how the term is based on gestalt psychology and leads to several theoretical models that are useful in therapeutic practice. We begin with an example from a therapy session before we turn to the theory and explain the term.

LISA: 'I really regret my one-night stand with Kevin from work. It felt so right while it was happening, but seeing him again now at work is really awkward'.

The therapist nods and says: 'Can you tell me something about what happened?'

LISA: 'I was at the Christmas party with everyone from work. I had a great time. I felt good and was flattered that Kevin was interested in me. He's a good colleague and a really nice man. We danced together all evening and had a lot of fun. He walked me home, and I invited him up. One thing led to another, and we ended up in bed. The chemistry was good, and I was completely happy afterwards. But when I saw him again on Monday, it was awkward. I really just want to be his colleague'. Lisa looks down and is clearly sad.

DOI: 10.4324/9781003153856-8

> The therapist nods and repeats what Lisa says: 'I think I understand. You had a great time with Kevin, but Monday at work, it was awkward to see him again'.
> LISA: 'Yes, now that I've had sex with him, it'll be so complicated at work'.
> The therapist nods: 'Mmmm . . . and you maybe weren't thinking about that when you were having fun at the Christmas party?'
> LISA: 'Not at all, I was just having a good time. It was so nice not to think about anything and just have fun. I think I'm way too conscientious'. She sighs a little and looks at the therapist.
> The therapist nods and smiles a little: 'I can understand that you might regret what you've done. It's much easier to view a situation in hindsight than it is when we're in the middle of it'.
> Lisa nods.

The excerpt describes how Lisa adjusted to the situation at the Christmas party. The therapist is interested in exploring Lisa's experience so that she can become more aware of herself and her choices, and so that she herself, as a therapist, can gain an understanding of the sequence of events. It occurs to her that Lisa needs support to see the situation at the Christmas party with a new perspective, which hopefully can help her to recognise that her actions were something she chose in that situation. She did not about the consequences, she simply lived in the moment.

The theory of creative adjustment

The theory of creative adjustment is a basic tenant of gestalt therapy and is described in several chapters in the book *Gestalt Therapy: Excitement and Growth in the Human Personality* by Perls et al. (1951). The authors argue that human beings always adjust to their surroundings creatively, and that this adjustment can be described both as a situation and as a process in which adjustment is described from moment to moment. A therapist can either look at how the client adjusts to her surroundings over a period of time, how the adjustment—the process—takes place, or be interested in how the client has adjusted or can adjust to a concrete situation in the moment. In the processes of contact and experience (Chapters 18 and 19) we are concerned about the course of events: that which has been or may come. In the situation, we are concerned with the client: who she is, her needs, what she does, and who she becomes. The final model is the theory of self and is described in Chapter 7.

Our objective with this chapter is to discuss the very principle that underlies all therapeutic approaches, namely that everyone adjusts to her environment creatively. Perls et al. (1951) argued that 'the creative [is] coming to a new figure; it is to differentiate between "obsolete responses" and the unique new behavior called for' (1951, p. 375). We meet any situation again and again, because the figure-ground formation can only take place in the moment and is therefore continually happening anew. Perls et al. felt that 'a perceived figure is not bright and sharp unless one is interested in it and focuses on it and scans it' and that 'it is the organism-as-a-whole in contact with the environment that is aware, manipulates, feels. This integration is not otiose; it is creative adjustment' (p. 374).

In the example with Lisa, we see that she adjusts in one way together with Kevin at the Christmas party, in a different way with Kevin at work, and in a third way with the therapist in the therapy room. We will now hear more from Lisa as the conversation continues and see how she explores the different situations with Kevin.

THE THERAPIST answers: 'So now, when you look back on that night with Kevin, it's not really something you think you could have done differently?'

LISA: 'No, not really. It didn't occur to me at any rate, although I regret it today. It gets difficult when I think about what I'm going to do in terms of meeting him at work'.

THE THERAPIST answers: 'So now you regret that you invited him home, you didn't think about the consequences there and then, and when you now think about how it will be to meet him at work, it's difficult'.

Here, the therapist repeats what Lisa has told her, in order to make the two situations with Kevin clearer for Lisa.

LISA: 'Yes, that's it. I really don't know what I can do about it now'. Lisa looks sad.

THE THERAPIST answers: 'It doesn't sound easy, and now I hear you say that in a way, you accept what happened at the Christmas party. You're thinking that you likely wouldn't have done anything different there. That's an important realisation for you. I think that it gives you a better sense of yourself and your choice that night: you can accept that you invited Kevin home and had sex with him'.

When the therapist clarifies the situation at the Christmas party and shares what she thinks, it is easier for Lisa to acknowledge and accept her actions that night. Lisa did the best she could, given her awareness in the situation. During the session they talk about the fact that Lisa feels Kevin avoids her at work and that it might also be difficult for him to see her. After discussing it for a while, Lisa says: 'Hmm, Kevin and me at work . . . ' Lisa hesitates a bit; the therapist sits quietly, waiting for her to continue.

LISA: 'It's so embarrassing to see him and talk to him. I don't want anyone at work to find out what happened that night'.

THE THERAPIST answers: 'Is this something you can say to Kevin? Maybe he feels the same way?'

LISA: 'Yes, I probably can. I really wonder what he's thinking, if he regrets what happened, or maybe wants to have a relationship with me . . . ' Lisa's words hang in the air.

> THE THERAPIST says: 'I can understand that you wonder what he's thinking, and you can only find out by talking with him. I understand that you feel this can be a difficult subject to bring up. We can try out the conversation here first, as a way to prepare yourself for a real conversation with Kevin. Now that you're aware of the situation, you might regret not doing something about it'.
>
> The therapist and Lisa talk for a bit about what she can say to Kevin and how to say it, without Lisa trying anything out in the therapy room. By talking about it, it becomes clearer to Lisa what she would like to say and how she can say it. She also remembers that part of what she likes about being with Kevin is that it is possible to talk with him, and that he is quite sensitive.
>
> LISA: 'I think I can talk to Kevin at lunch tomorrow. We can probably find somewhere quiet, and he'll probably agree to talk when I ask him. It'll be good to finally talk to him and hear what he has to say. I've only been thinking about myself. It might well not be so easy for him either and he's pretty shy, so I don't think he'll take the initiative'.

The therapist is interested in helping Lisa see more ways she can adjust creatively in the situation with Kevin, and by talking back and forth about these possibilities Lisa becomes more aware of what she wants, and that Kevin is part of the situation. It is important that Lisa become aware that there are others involved, and that the relationships she has with colleagues at work affect her.

Lisa is neither aware that she affects Kevin nor how she was affected by him in the situation at the Christmas party. In the conversation with the therapist, however, she is more aware of herself, and by preparing the conversation she wants to have with Kevin at work she will adjust to the new situation more consciously than she did at the Christmas party.

Adjusting to life's situations is always a creative process even if we do not always feel creative. Much of what we do is repetitive and characterised by habits and routines; we often do not pay attention to our actions. This is helpful and appropriate in daily life and makes it possible for us to focus our attention and creativity on tasks we consider to be more important.

Creative adjustment and the law of prägnanz

We have previously described the laws of perception and therefore also the law of *prägnanz* (pp. 10–11). This was described after long experimentation with how people perceive the world around them and how phenomena are organised and structured in such a way that we understand them as meaningful wholes. Gestalt psychologists found that this process takes place in certain ways and according to specific laws, one of which was named the 'law of *prägnanz*'. This law says that we organise that which we perceive in the simplest, most natural form possible at any given moment. Later, this law was also applied to behaviour and actions, and can be expressed thus: we act in the simplest, most natural, and best way in the moment.

In the example above, the therapist wanted to help Lisa see that she chose her behaviour at the Christmas party, and that she had not been aware that she had other choices other than inviting Kevin home after they had had a good time together all evening. Afterwards, Lisa regretted her choice, but in the actual situation she made the best choice she was able to, based on her awareness and needs. The fact that she now thinks she could have acted differently that night does not change what she actually chose to do there and then. In retrospect, Lisa has more insight and knowledge about the situation at the Christmas party, but twenty-twenty hindsight does not change what happened. It is an experience she can learn from and remember in other, similar situations.

In the conversation with the therapist, Lisa takes responsibility for her choice and understands that it was the 'best form' she was capable of that night.

As already mentioned, we do not necessarily experience the way in which we adjust to our surroundings as creative; it is more often a result of our habits and routines. This is supported by the law of *prägnanz*. In other words, it is easier for us to act as we usually do. It is easiest and most natural to take the path we know rather than create a new path or form. In therapy, it is important that the therapist is aware of both sides of the law of *prägnanz* and creative adjustment. Clients always adjust creatively and in the best possible way to their surroundings, and at the same time, a change in this way of adjusting, when inflexible and inappropriate, can be demanding, as the example with Oliver illustrates.

Oliver has told the therapist about a traumatic childhood where both parents were unstable and drank for periods of time. He grew up with a younger sister whom he looked after and protected from their parents' uncontrolled outbursts of anger. He has sought out therapy because he is having problems in his relationships with his wife and children. In the sessions with the therapist, he has often been frustrated and upset over how he holds back when his wife complains and nags. It is as if he does not dare to respond to his wife.

Oliver describes an episode from the previous day, when Lydia asked him to make dinner. Oliver was sitting beside his eldest son helping him with his homework. Instead of saying no to Lydia and continuing to help his son, he got up and started to prepare dinner. While he cooks, he fumes inside; he would much rather be with his son than making dinner but does not dare say anything because Lydia spoke in such an authoritative manner.

The therapist and Oliver spend a lot of time exploring this episode together, among other things by Oliver imagining that he is back in the living room the previous day. He relives what happened with a focus on the feeling in his body when Lydia was talking to him. He is aware that he almost stops breathing, that he tenses his body as if to defend himself, and that he is scared and on guard.

OLIVER: 'It's clear to me that I hold back and that I don't want my son to know how frustrated and afraid I am'.

THE THERAPIST says: 'Do you think that he senses something?'

OLIVER: 'No, I don't think so, he's just mad at me because I have to stop helping him'.

THE THERAPIST says: 'I can feel that I'm holding my breath now. It sounds hard to want two things at the same time. You want to say no to Lydia and help your son, and at the same time you don't say no to Lydia because you're afraid your son will discover how frustrated you are'.

OLIVER: 'Yes, that's exactly how it is. When you say it out loud, I stop breathing too, it's really uncomfortable. It's as if I'm back home with my parents when they were fighting. I held my breath then, too, and did as they said so they would leave my little sister alone'.

THE THERAPIST says: 'So you recognise the unpleasant feeling in your body and that you stop breathing from when you were a child at home with your parents? I can understand that, based on everything you've told me about your upbringing. So it's as if you adjust to the situation today with Lydia in the same way you did at home when you were a child?'

OLIVER: 'Yes, it's obvious now that we've talked about how I felt at home yesterday'.

THE THERAPIST says: 'As far as I've understood what you've told me, you felt that the best and safest way to survive with your parents was by holding back and doing as they said, almost becoming invisible. Is that correct?'

OLIVER: 'Yes, absolutely. I tried to fade into the woodwork. When they didn't notice me, they left me alone'.

THE THERAPIST says: 'So when you were a child, you really adjusted in the best way you could in a very unstable and unsafe environment. You actually got good at being invisible and avoided a lot of trouble that way'.

OLIVER: 'Yes, that's absolutely true. I'm very good at adjusting to changing conditions. I notice my surroundings, see what's needed, and manage to do a lot without being noticed'.

Here, Oliver is aware of how the way he adjusted to his surroundings as a child helped him to avoid problems with his parents when they were drunk or unruly. He is also mindful that by adjusting in this way, he has developed characteristics or qualities in terms of being flexible and aware of his surroundings.

> The session continues, and Oliver returns to the problems he has with his wife. It becomes clear to him that he adjusts to his wife in the same way he did with his parents. This is something that has worked for a long time, but that he is no longer happy with. It is as if he is not able to act differently.

Oliver's previous experiences and creative adjustment today results in his feeling stuck and frustrated. The therapist wants Oliver to be aware of his bodily sensations and needs in the situation with Lydia. It is our needs, as noted elsewhere in this book, that govern most of our actions (Chapter 4). It is therefore important for Oliver to be aware of the needs he has and to understand, with the help of the therapist, how his need for change is in conflict with his need for stability and security. Oliver's original creative adjustment to his parents was both appropriate and the best he could do. These experiences are with him in adulthood, and the way he adjusts to new situations is built on his previous life experiences. It is understandable that Oliver's survival strategy from childhood permeates his life and actions in adulthood, and that finding new ways to adjust can be very demanding and create anxiety. At the same time, it is necessary now, because he is in a new situation with other people with completely different needs and requirements.

We stop our example here. In later chapters, we demonstrate how the therapist works with clients throughout change processes (Chapter 20).

Self-regulation

Fritz Perls' claim that all living beings are by nature self-regulating builds on several theories (Clarkson & Mackewn, 1993). Among these are Lewin's idea of organic self-regulation (p. 17). People have basic needs that they spontaneously attempt to satisfy. If they are not disturbed in this process, they will immediately search for a way to meet these needs, without having any sort of plan. If, however, people are interrupted in the process of satisfying their needs, they will do whatever is necessary to meet their own needs in their environments and with the available resources. If there are conflicting needs, the dominant or most important need will be met first.

People are social beings, however, and there may be situations in which it is necessary to postpone the satisfaction of one's own important needs for the sake of the needs of other. Fritz Perls emphasised that an important aspect of self-regulation is taking into account the needs of others, because together they create the relational field they are a part of (Clarkson & Mackewn, 1993). Perls' understanding of self-regulation is a backdrop for the theory of creative adjustment and is, in principle, simply another way to formulate the same theory. Self-regulation makes it possible for us to be more aware of a person's needs and how they are met, and creative adjustment is the focus of the contact with—and form of—adjustment to the environment. In the example with Oliver, we see how the therapist is interested in how Oliver's needs are met, his self-regulation, and how he creatively adjusts as best he can in the situation.

Is all adjustment creative and 'the best we can do'?

Often, we can marvel over whether all adjustment is actually creative and the best we can do in the situation. When we look at our own actions and the world around us, this can be difficult to accept. At the same time, we can see that the fact that we adjust creatively does not necessarily mean that our adjustments are always the most optimal in a given situation. Adjustments that were perhaps appropriate when we were growing up can cause pain and suffering today, and sometimes be directly harmful to us or our surroundings. For example, it was good and even necessary that we could be vocal about our frustration and anger as children; it was the way we could ensure that we were seen and heard. As adults, however, this behaviour is inappropriate, and we react negatively to people who behave as if they were children.

As we have emphasised previously in this chapter, learning new forms of adjustment requires considerable effort and attention, something the following example with Ingrid shows.

Ingrid is in the therapist's office. Her head is bowed, and she is crying quietly. She tells the therapist how horrible things are. She lost patience with her daughter; she yelled and hit her and is struggling with a bad conscience. She recounts that it was like a blackout; she did not know what she was doing until after the fact.

INGRID: 'As soon as I hit her, it was like I woke up from a trance. I didn't realise what I was doing until I heard Charlotte scream. That's when I stopped and began to comfort her. It was almost like I wasn't the one who was so angry; I was a different person. I don't know what to do'.

Here, we hear Ingrid's despair over having lost control and hit her daughter. Despite the fact that she knows she should not hit her child, she was not able to stop herself. Can we then say that in this case, she did the best she was capable of? The therapist thinks so, even though she realises this is not an excuse to hit a child. She is interested in what it was in the situation that caused Ingrid to lose control and to act contrary to her own convictions. We see here that the therapist distinguishes between ethical norms and rules in society that dictate that violence against children is unacceptable, and Ingrid's creative adjustment with Charlotte. The therapist explores this further with Ingrid.

In the course of the session, Ingrid tells the therapist about how exhausted she was at the time. Charlotte had been ill and had cried for long periods that night. Ingrid had felt helpless and alone because her husband was out of town. All the emotions had overpowered her, she had been scared and angry and had completely lost control. She cries as she tells her story, and the therapist supports her by saying that she understands how difficult this situation was for her.

To express emotions that have been held back, as Ingrid does here, is important in therapy. The next step on the road to learn other ways in which to act, is for the client to realise and acknowledge what she has done and acquire an understanding of and insight into how she acts when she is scared and tired—and that she did the best she was able to in this situation. Ingrid will need time in therapy to be more aware of who she is when she is with Charlotte and to become familiar with her fear, loneliness, and helplessness. It is only when she experiences that she can feel her fear without needing to find a way to avoid that fear that she will be able to more easily withstand Charlotte's crying and emotional outbursts.

The question we initially asked in this paragraph, whether all adjustment is creative and the best we are capable of, has only partially been answered with this example. It is as if Ingrid's creative adjustment with Charlotte is interlaced with all of her earlier experiences—her relationship to her husband, to her child's illness, and many other factors she is not aware of. This is true for others as well. They are influenced by their upbringings and the environments in which they live and adjust in the way that is simplest and easiest for them, and thus as best they can in the situation. It is important that we are aware that the 'simplest' and 'easiest' is an important part of the law of *prägnanz*, and that the 'best form' in the situation is independent of ethics, right and wrong, and what is best for the client's surroundings.

Unfinished business

One of Fritz Perls' famous phrases is what he called 'unfinished business', which we call 'unfinished situations' or 'unfinished gestalts'. These are concepts that gestalt therapists often use when clients bring up the same events again and again in therapy.

The term 'unfinished situation' alludes to a phenomenon Goldstein (1939) called 'self-actualisation' (p. 13). He viewed all needs as specific cases of a fundamental tendency towards fulfilment or completion. This was a continuation of the way in which gestalt psychologists viewed perception with its basis on the principle of completion: unfinished or incomplete situations require completion and will continue to emerge until completion occurs (see Chapter 1). Gestalt psychologists explained that this is due to the fact that people have a need to organise sensory input meaningfully, and that the same principle applies to human behaviour. Until this organisation is completed, we will continue to be reminded of the incomplete situation.

'Unfinished situations' or 'unfinished gestalts' are also a result of the Zeigarnik effect, which states that unfinished or interrupted tasks are remembered better and more often than are completed actions (see pp. 18–19). In real life, we can see that there is a big difference between the tasks we try to solve that we do not complete and events that originate outside ourselves that are experienced as meaningless and incomplete. The need to shut down and be done with the unpleasant and painful sensations, thoughts, and feelings that can arise from unfinished situations is, however, the same. Regardless of whether we have a task to be finished at work or we experienced something difficult in our childhood, the need to be 'finished' is the same, and we adjust creatively to both situations as best we can. When we finish a task at work, it fades into the background and we begin a new task. We cannot, however, finish painful or traumatic experiences from the past in the same way. These can continue to plague us to a greater or lesser extent throughout our lives.

Perls and the Zeigarnik effect

Laura and Fritz Perls argued in their theory that health can be characterised by repeated experiences that reach completion, while illness is a state of a constant lack of completion. They took the notion of a gestalt as a perceptual pattern and organised whole, and developed it to mean a psychological, emotional, and cognitive experience within an oral–digestive model:

> If people are not able to organize a childhood experience fully into their lives—to chew and assimilate it—they will forever be plagued by it. It will be a 'disturbance' in their field—the so-called 'unfinished business' of the Zeigarnik effect. At the simplest level, we can say that the Perlses created a therapy to complete unfinished experience—to make them whole inside of us—so we can move on with life.
>
> (Zinker, 1994, p. 49)

There and then, here and now

In gestalt therapy, we believe that recognising the situation as it was in the past and as it is experienced now can help reduce the experience of discomfort and suffering in the moment. This is described in the theory of paradoxical change (Chapter 5).

Common to all topics that deal with unfinished situations is the extent to which clients can acknowledge what has been inflicted on them and become aware of what they themselves can do in such situations. Many clients suffer unnecessarily because they struggle to acknowledge that they have adjusted to difficult situations earlier in their lives 'as best they could', and that it is natural that these situations continue to return in an attempt to be completed. They often think that 'I should be done mourning my husband by now' or 'I shouldn't need to think about my unhappy childhood anymore'. As therapists it is important that we are aware that a client's need to be finished with earlier painful experiences is natural, and that it is only in recognition in the moment that she can experience that the pain diminishes and something new can emerge. We see from experience that when a client explores and gains an increased awareness and understanding in 'unfinished situations' over time, these events recede to the background and eventually create less suffering in the client's life.

In the session with Oliver, we see how he creatively adjusts to difficult situations today and how each adjustment carries with it all previous experiences from childhood. In gestalt therapy we say that childhood shows up here and now. When it does, the therapist chooses whether to explore and work on the childhood experiences or concentrate on today's challenges. With Oliver, the therapist does a little of both. She brings childhood experiences from there and then to here and now by allowing Oliver to relive emotions and share thoughts and feelings from past experience. The correlation between how he adjusted creatively in his childhood and how he adjusts to his life today becomes clearer to both of them. In the first example with Lisa, we show how the therapist works here and now with the future on the basis of Lisa's insight into how she behaved with Kevin at the Christmas party.

It is important that the therapist sees the connection between the past and the future, how earlier traumatic experiences and crises are activated by new crises, and that events today can function as triggers for painful experiences from the past (Joyce & Sills, 2014). The therapist is interested in making sure that the new crisis or traumatic experience does not retraumatise the client; in other words, that it does not becomes an automatic reaction where the client is without contact with reality here and now.

Creative adjustment and traumatic events

There are situations where the process in the therapy room repeats itself, and the therapist and the client do not make progress. In other words, they stagnate. In these situations, it is not enough to increase the client's awareness. This usually happens in work with clients who have experienced severe traumatic events, as in the examples in the previous chapter. In these cases, the therapist becomes aware that the response she is getting from the client is not what she expects. The therapist may be more cautious and supportive as she experiences that the client is vulnerable and aware of her explorations and proposals for experiments.

Gestalt therapist Miriam Taylor (2014) writes in her book that it is important that gestalt therapists have knowledge of and are conscious of the challenges that arise when working with traumatised clients in therapy. According to Taylor, trauma is defined as being events that are 'life-threatening, exceeding the victim's normal resources. . . . There is usually an overwhelming sense of shock and an inability to escape in the face of unforeseen events' (pp. 2–3). The term 'creative adjustment' can also be described as the ways in which we adjust to survive crises and traumatic situations, even though this adjustment may have had a high price. Taylor emphasises that there is a big difference in how clients handle traumatic events and whether these events are repetitive or one-time events. For example, war experiences or repeated, repressed sexual assaults are more serious and more difficult to treat than a rape or an accident. In cases of minor trauma, the therapist can often work with the client as she otherwise would in cases of unfinished situations that need to be concluded. This is described earlier in this chapter (see the example of Oliver). Taylor stresses, however, that a single trauma can also trigger previous, unprocessed traumatic events, and that the treatment of a single trauma must be seen in a coherent context with the client's earlier life.

Many severely traumatised clients have experienced unimaginable degrees of shame and struggle to acknowledge and appreciate that their adjustments were the best they could do in the situation. It can be extremely challenging for these clients to see new and other ways in which to adjust creatively (Taylor, 2014). Taylor argues that the therapist must spend time creating safety and stability between herself and the client and that the field between them is fragile and vulnerable. The field provides little space in which to challenge and keep the client's experiential focus firmly in that which is uncomfortable in the situation. She says that the client needs time to acknowledge that the adjustment to the unbearable situations was the best the client was able to do, and that it can be challenging for the client to recognise herself and the way she adjusted creatively. However, this recognition is an important prerequisite for the client to be able move forward in life and learn how to adjust to new situations. In a field that includes a traumatised client, it is important that the therapist provides guidance, is supportive, educational, and uses her understanding and knowledge of how traumatic events affect the client as well as the therapist. Being able to cope with hearing the client recount a painful experience, seeing her tears, shame, and bodily discomfort, while putting aside one's own experiences and keeping a certain distance, is a demanding situation in which the therapist's phenomenological attitude is put to the test (see Chapter 3 on phenomenology). In such situations, it is important that the therapist seek guidance, both so that she herself is not overwhelmed by the client's feelings, anxiety, and depression, and to maintain a professional approach, thereby ensuring good treatment for the client (Joyce & Sills, 2014).

Today considerable attention is paid to how we can treat clients who have had traumatic experiences, who are in crisis, or who have been diagnosed with post-traumatic stress disorder. We have chosen not to write specifically about the various theories and treatment of trauma and crisis in this book, but rather to focus on the gestalt theory of creative adjustment and how gestalt therapists work in clinical practice with clients who experience these challenges. However, we recommend therapists who have traumatised clients in therapy to seek additional knowledge about this subject and read the books we refer to in this section.

Creative adjustment in the therapy room

Creative adjustment is closely related to how the field we are a part of is organised at any given time. How we organise our experiences is described in gestalt psychology in terms of figure-ground, as explained in Chapter 1. We organise everything we sense and perceive in a field in such a way that something becomes a figure against a background.

In much of what we do in everyday life, in our creative adjustments, there is no clear distinction between figure and background. Our lives are too complex for this to be possible. What matters is what we do in the context of all the possibilities that exist at the moment. How we adjust to the situation and what we do can give an indication of what we are interested in and the figure that emerges for us in the situation (Brownell, 2010).

When we speak the words we use are important, but how we speak is equally important. For example, we convey two different meanings if we say we are going to cut the grass tomorrow while we wink and smile as opposed to saying the same thing seriously while maintaining eye contact and nodding. We form our understanding based on the entirety of what is said, the way it is said, and the body language of the speaker. It is this whole that gives context and background to the figure in the foreground and is essential to how we act and adjust creatively (Brownell, 2010).

In therapy, therefore, the therapist is aware of how the client speaks, how she moves, and the content of what she says. It is through these aspects that it is possible not only to form an understanding of the client's needs, but also of what is not expressed—which is the background. The therapist is also aware of sensations in her body, her thoughts, and feelings. It is in this way she becomes conscious of what she sees as a figure, what she is interested in, and what she and the client need in the situation (Brownell, 2010). What happens between the therapist and the client in the session and how they adjust to each other is also an expression of

The therapist meets Thea in the waiting room. Thea phoned to make an appointment a week ago and mentioned that she has problems in her relationship with her parents. The therapist greets Thea by shaking her hand and introducing herself. Thea shakes the therapist's hand, but quickly pulls her hand back while saying her name softly as she glances sideways at the therapist. The therapist becomes aware that she holds her breath for a moment as she leads Thea to her office.

the figure that emerges between them (Skottun, 2005), as the following example with Thea shows.

In this sequence, the therapist becomes aware of many figures. The first figure she notices is how Thea takes her hand, the second is that Thea barely looks at her, and the third is that she speaks softly. The therapist can interpret this behaviour as holding back and that Thea may be shy or afraid to come to therapy. The way Thea behaves in the first moments of their meeting, how she adjusts, captures the therapist's interest. This interest is supported by the fact that she herself stops breathing and chooses to lead the client to her office instead of letting the client go first, as she often does. She is aware that she is careful and nurturing with Thea. Here we see an example of how what captures the therapist's attention in the first encounter with Thea becomes the figure for her and is the starting point for how she walks to the therapy room with the Thea. We see how the therapist creatively adjusts to this first moment with her client.

In the conversation in the therapy room, the therapist can continue to be interested in the first figure, or this figure can go to the background as she and Thea talk. The therapist may be more interested in Thea's relationship with her mother, because that is what Thea is interested in and is the reason she has come to therapy. The therapist explores how Thea experiences her mother and their relationship in several ways. In a later session, the therapist can choose to bring up her own experience with Thea from their first meeting to see if there is anything Thea recognises in other situations and whether it relates to growing up with her mother. The connection between the figure 'how Thea is with the therapist' and the figure 'how Thea was with her mother' can be explored as one figure, and possibly give Thea new insight into her relationship with her mother, how she adjusted to her, and her creative adjustment to her environment in general. The therapist may also be interested in what the client fails to address in the sessions—the underlying issues. If Thea continues to talk only about her mother, the therapist might become curious about the relationship she has with her father. Maybe Thea fails to talk about this because the relationship with her father is painful and difficult, or because the relationship is good, and Thea is not conscious of how important her father has been to her as she grew up. When the therapist begins to be curious about Thea's relationship to her father, this becomes the figure, and the other subject they spoke of goes to the background.

Many examples in this book show how the therapist chooses between several possible figures in conversation with the client. In some cases, this choice is deliberate and clear, while other times the therapist chooses the background of sensations and an awareness what is happening in the situation between herself and the client. In these cases, she might become aware of the figure or figures later, on reflection. The relationship between the therapist's awareness and attention in the therapy room influences her choice of figure and what she chooses to explore at any given time. It also influences how the two creatively adjust to the situation in the therapy room (see Chapter 7 on the theory of self and Chapter 18 on contact processes).

Much of the therapist's task is to clarify and increase the client's attention to what she sees as important in her life, the figures that emerge between them, and issues that are outside the client's awareness. Because we can only be aware of one figure at a time, there will always be something outside of our awareness, making new discoveries possible. Clients' view of the world around them is often limited by the figures to which they have grown accustomed. By exploring new possibilities, seeing new figures, or making existing figures clearer, the client can understand situations in a new way (Brownell, 2010).

Summary

In this chapter, we have explained that the term 'creative adjustment' implies that all of our adjustments to new situations are innovative and are always done in the way that is the easiest and best as possible under the prevailing circumstances. The therapist and client adjust to each other on the basis of where their interests lie at any given time—that is, on the basis of the figure there and then. The therapist can choose to support the work being done with the client on the theoretical model of figure-ground or on the model of creative adjustment. She may want to use a combination of both, which we will show in examples later in this book.

In the next chapter, we will describe the theory of self and how Goodman and Perls formulated the relationship between this theory and the concept of creative adjustment.

References

Brownell, P. (2010). *Gestalt therapy: A guide to contemporary practice*. New York: Springer Publishing Company.

Clarkson, P., & Mackewn, J. (1993). *Fritz Perls*. London: Sage Publications.

Goldstein, K. (1939). *The organism: A Holistic approach to biology derived from pathological data in man*. New York: American Book Company.

Joyce, P., & Sills, C. (2014). *Skills in gestalt counselling & psychotherapy* (3rd ed.). London: Sage.

Perls, F. S., Hefferline, R. F., & Goodman, P. (1951). *Gestalt therapy: Excitement and growth in the human personality*. London: Souvenir Press.

Skottun, G. (2005). Figur/grunn: og dannelse av gestalter nok en gang [Figure/ground: And the manifestation of gestalts once again]. *Norsk Gestalttidsskrift, 1*(2), 37–42.

Taylor, M. (2014). *Trauma therapy and clinical practice: Neuroscience, gestalt and the body*. Maidenhead: Open University Press.

Zinker, J. (1994). *In search of good form*. San Francisco: Gestalt Institute of Cleveland.

Chapter 7

The theory of self in gestalt therapy

Sharon is hostess for a large sixtieth birthday celebration with family, friends, and colleagues. As is customary, many of the guests hold speeches during the course of the dinner. They speak about Sharon in different contexts, depending on how they knew her. Because this is a celebratory occasion, most of the anecdotes in the speeches are pleasant episodes and highlight positive aspects of Sharon's personality. However, Sharon notices that her reactions to the speeches vary, depending on the extent to which she recognises herself in the different ways she is portrayed. Some guests who have known her since she was a child describe her as they remember her from years ago, while others describe situations from later periods of her life. As various parts of her life are highlighted throughout the evening, she realises that the guests have very different ideas of who she is today. While Sharon can recognise herself and how she was in the anecdotes the guests tell, it occurs to her that she is a completely different person today at the age of sixty.

This example illustrates a deep, existential question in relation to who an individual thinks she is, and is directly related to the gestalt concept of self. Attempts to answer the question of who we are can be found in philosophy, religion, and psychology. Philosophy and religion tell us, for example, that humans have a soul or that there is a God or a divinity within or around us.

Freud founded psychology's concept of self based on his theories of the structure and dynamic of the personality, which included the *id, ego*, and *superego*. Those who came later developed a different, and to some degree contradictory, view of our basic drives, and put a greater emphasis on the ego. Some of Freud's successors are referred to as ego psychologists and were also interested in sociocultural factors. Heinz Kohut (1913–1981) developed his theory of the self in the 1970s. A principle of his original understanding of the self is that each individual possesses a core that can be analysed and explained. With a point of departure in Freud's way of thinking, Kohut developed a central concept that he called the

DOI: 10.4324/9781003153856-9

'core self': humans have a constant core of characteristics that can be explained and categorised (Teigen, 2004/2015). Later theorists discussed and criticised the idea that people have a core self.

How does the concept of gestalt therapy fit into this? At the time they developed their own self theory, Perls and Goodman were perhaps more than ever committed to developing a theory that stood in contrast to psychoanalytic thinking. It was important for them to emphasise the fundamental distinction between psychoanalytic and gestalt therapeutic theory (Perls et al., 1951). Their self theory was therefore pioneering and is challenging for all who study and practice gestalt.

In this chapter, we describe our understanding of the concept of self in the theory and method of gestalt therapy with examples from clinical practice.

The theory of self

Perls and Goodman were influenced by trends in philosophy, psychology, and religion when they developed their theory of self. As a result, their original theory spread in many directions. Especially Goodman was influenced by two varying philosophies: American pragmatism and neothomism (Skottun, 2008). He derived the idea of the self as an emerging or growing function of a total experience from American pragmatism. His dualistic idea of the self as being split between mind and matter, where the soul was seen as the creative power of matter, came from neothomism. We rely mainly on theories taken from American pragmatism, which were further developed by Isadore From, one of Perls' students.

As mentioned earlier, the founders of gestalt therapy wanted to distance themselves from the psychoanalytic theory of a core self. They argued that self is not something people have inside themselves, but rather something that is created when people meet and interact. The term 'self' in gestalt theory is therefore closely linked to the gestalt principle of the organism's self-regulation (p. 13). This principle describes how people regulate themselves in relation to their needs in the environments in which they find themselves, for instance when they allow themselves to speak with their fellow passengers on the tram when they have a need to socialise, or when they take out their cell phones and check their messages because of a need to distance themselves from those around them. Therefore, in contrast to some theorists, we do not describe self as a noun, but rather as something that is acted, created, or expressed (Staemmler, 2016; Wollants, 2012). In gestalt theory, self is described as a function of a situation in order to clarify that it is not something people are. A function can be explained as potential or an opportunity that exists in the situation in an individual who is present, and that is manifested in how the individual acts and thinks (Perls et al., 1951).

Aspects of self: id, ego, and personality

Although Perls and Goodman rejected Freud's theories of self, they took their point of departure in the terms 'id', 'ego', and 'superego' from psychoanalysis. They renamed the terms 'id', 'ego', and 'personality', and gave them a new meaning. This choice has been the cause of much confusion and disagreement within the gestalt milieu as to how the concepts should be interpreted. For Perls and Goodman, self was related to the creative adjustment that happens in the situation. It described their view of how the various aspects or functions of self are active in the various phases of the contact process (Perls et al., 1951). In Chapter 19, we describe the process of contact; here, we elaborate what is meant by the terms id, ego, and personality, and how they manifest themselves in a situation.

Three functions of self: impulse, personality, and I-function

From developed Goodman and Perls' theory of self further. His goal was to develop a model that therapists could use in clinical practice (Müller, 1984). As with Perls and Goodman, From used the terms id, ego, and personality for the functions of self. These are closely linked to the psychoanalytic concept of a tripartite self. We think that this is confusing and distracting for the understanding of the theory of self in gestalt therapy, and rely instead on Hanne Hostrup's descriptions, which we believe are better suited to a gestalt-oriented terminology. We therefore refer to them as the *impulse function*, the *personality function*, and the *I-function* (Hostrup, 2010, pp. 122–124).

From described the three functions as follows: what the individual wants to do or what the individual's needs or spontaneous impulses are (impulse function), who the person is or becomes (personality function), and what the person chooses to do or not do (I-function) in a situation (Müller, 1984). In the example of Sharon and her confusion about who she really is, her memories of how she behaved with various people throughout her life were an expression of the personality function. It gave her a sense of being different than she was at the time of her sixtieth birthday, but at the same time she was able to recognise the descriptions of how she had been at other times and in other situations. Her emotional reactions during the speeches are an expression of the impulse function; her reflections and the speech she gave after hearing the other speeches are an expression of the I-function. We will now describe each function in more detail in order to provide a deeper understanding of these complex concepts.

The impulse function is the comprehensive, bodily awareness of how a situation is implicitly charged with sensations: that we perceive and recognise our surroundings with all of our senses. At the same time, we often notice our bodily sensations and impulses without being fully aware of what goes on in and around us (see Chapter 8 on awareness). By becoming more aware and conscious of this bodily process, we also become more aware of our impulses and the underlying needs—the id function of the situation (Wollants, 2012).

As we become more familiar with our impulses and needs, we can regulate whether to act on them and allow them to be expressed. This is useful for therapists when working with people who have too much or too little impulse control, and for all of us who sometimes struggle with this regulation. With practice, we can learn to 'choose our feelings'. By this, we mean that when are aware of our emotions and impulses, we can regulate what we choose to express in different situations. Allowing emotions and impulses to be expressed is not always appropriate, and the ability to regulate helps us to avoid unnecessary conflict and create better relationships and cooperation, both in close relationships and in the workplace.

The personality function is me the way I perceive myself: how I am, how changes affect my experience of coping with the given situation now, and how it will continue to affect my understanding of myself and the situation. The personality is also a set of characteristics. Characteristics are expressions of biological (innate) aspects of who I am. These include gender and appearance, roles I am assigned or take (such as marital status, being a parent, sibling, etc.), and the roles and functions that develop during my lifetime (such as being patient, irritable, scrupulous, wise, uncertain, and so on). The personality is me as I prefer to define and describe myself, to present myself to the world around me, and to let myself be seen. The personality affects my interaction with the environment and what I experience, what I become aware of, or what I risk. It allows me to make sense of the world based on what I have experienced and believe in up to now, and the ideas and explanations I give myself based on the experiences I have (Wollants, 2012).

The personality function does not correspond directly to the core self in psychoanalytic thinking, but it is the function it most closely resembles.

This theory illustrates that we can act in different ways, be different personalities, or play different roles. In practice, this means for example that we have the opportunity to be 'a quiet person' in one situation and be 'the outgoing person' or 'the person who takes a lot of space' in another situation. When we know ourselves and all our possible personalities, we can choose the 'me' or the aspect of 'me' that is best suited to the situation (Polster, 1995). There are examples of this later in the chapter.

The I-function, or ego function, is the 'I' that explores my implicit knowledge of my situation. This function looks for solutions and how I can change or rearrange the situation. 'I' includes the me who acts, chooses, and orients myself; who gives direction, thinks, plans, and chooses what I do and do not want; and who evaluates my choices (Wollants, 2012). The I-function relies on the impulse and personality functions to provide direction so that I can act (Hostrup, 2010). The I-function is expressed in situations where we use the personal pronoun 'I' in such statements as 'I want this; I'd like to do it this way' or 'I love you'. The I-function is also evident when we *perform an action* (act) such as go to work, read a book, or talk to a colleague.

Creating and being shaped by the situation— together

Implicit knowledge of ourselves is something that can be developed by being attentive to and conscious of how we think and act. It is closely linked with awareness of impulses and needs, and therefore the impulse function. Increased awareness of who we are in the situation, the personality function, is necessary in many situations in order to choose and act. The ability to choose who we want to be and which needs and impulses we act on or express leads to what we choose to do. Simultaneously, how we choose to act influences who we are in the situation. It is therefore not always clear whether the personality function, who we are, and the I-function, the action we take, come first or last. Both functions are often implicit in our actions.

To illustrate what we mean by creating and being formed by the situation while bringing all of our previous experience into the situation, we will give an example from a family that consists of a mother, Caroline; a father, Frank; and their two-year-old son Ross.

> The whole family is asleep. Suddenly, Ross, who is in the room next to his parents' room, starts crying. Caroline jumps out of bed and runs to Ross's room to see what is wrong. She adjusts his blanket and strokes his head. Ross continues to cry, so she picks him up and rocks him in her arms. He settles down in Caroline's arms, and after a while Caroline lays him back down and sits down next to the bed. Eventually, Ross falls back asleep, and Caroline returns to her own bed. Frank woke up when he heard Ross's cries, but stayed in bed.

If we apply the theory of self to this situation, we see that when Ross begins to cry, he expresses his needs and impulses: this is the impulse function. He cries based on his experience that this behaviour will summon someone who will comfort him. This is the personality function—in this situation, he is a crying child. The fact that he cries is his action: his I-function. Caroline acts (I-function) on her impulse when she hears Ross cry, and she becomes mother-of-the-crying-child (personality function). She attempts to calm Ross down in various ways, based on her earlier experiences of his nighttime crying. It is likely the way Ross cries that causes her to choose to pick him up. Maybe Caroline thinks that he has had a bad dream or is cold. Because Ross cannot yet explain his needs in words, Caroline has to act based on her past experiences with him (personality function). In this situation, Frank remains in bed (I-function) because he and Caroline have an agreement that it is her turn to get up if Ross wakes up (personality function). He notices an impulse to get up (impulse function) when he hears Ross cry, but at the same time there is another impulse to stay in bed, based on the agreement he has with Caroline (personality function).

This is an example of how family members adapt to each other in a specific situation and thus 'co-create' the situation (Slagsvold, 2016). In this situation, it could have happened that Caroline did not manage to calm Ross down, and that he continued to cry. In that case, Caroline would likely have tried many different things, like giving him milk or changing his diaper. Maybe Frank would have become irritated that Ross's crying prevented him from sleeping, and might even have yelled at Ross and Caroline. How Caroline and Frank together manage to cope with Ross's crying depends largely on the degree to which they are able to be patient when they are not able to meet Ross's needs. Caroline and Frank's handling of this situation is also influenced by how their parents acted when they were infants and cried at night. Are they able to be two parents who try together to meet Ross's needs, or do they become a couple where Caroline is a desperate, helpless mother and Frank is an irritated, tired husband? It is also possible that Frank might choose to get up and comfort Ross and ask Caroline to go back to bed, because he thinks that the situation needs something other than what Caroline is doing. He might be calmer and more patient than Caroline, who could feel like an exhausted and helpless mother.

Frank and Caroline might seek out a therapist because they feel that they need help and support in order to be parents together. This can also make it easier for them to be spouses. They might get help to see how the impulses and irritation they feel together with a crying Ross can be linked to experiences they bring with them from their own lives. Becoming aware of previous experiences might make it easier for them to hold back impulses such as anger, irritation, and impatience. Later, we will show how this can be done in practice.

Self and creative adjustment

In the above examples, there are many possible scenarios for how the parents separately and individually can adapt creatively to Ross and his crying, and how Ross relates to his parents' efforts to provide care and comfort. In Chapter 6, we describe how people always regulate and adjust to each other creatively and as best they can in the situation in which they find themselves. The terms 'self' and 'creative adjustment' are described by Perls and Goodman (Perls et al., 1951) as a theory in which any creative adjustment begins with the impulses and needs people have in the situation (impulse function), as we see in Ross and his parents. People choose and act (I-function) depending on who they feel they have been or are in the situation (personality function), as we can see in the example above. In the same chapters on creative adjustment, Perls and Goodman describe a model for the course of the process that in this book is described as two models: the process of experience (Chapter 19) and the process of change (Chapter 20).

Conflicting needs in the situation

There are situations in which we struggle to choose because we have conflicting needs or face major challenges. In these cases, it may be useful to sort our needs and be aware of how we are stuck in our perceptions of who we are, or who the people around us are. We illustrate this in an example with Katrine and Peter.

Katrine and Peter are in their early thirties and live together in a small apartment. Both work quite a bit and are active in their spare time. After living together for a year, Katrine wants to have children. She is aware that she has a limited window of time in which to get pregnant and give birth. Peter feels this is not a good time to have children; they have considerable debt and his career is at a crucial point. They decide to wait a bit, because—in addition to the other reasons—Katrine is unsure if she will be a good mother.

Here, Katrine and Peter choose together to wait to have children because they feel or are unsure about how children will fit into their life. At the same time, they become aware that there is a limited time in which they can choose to have children. In this example, the desire to have children is the impulse function, which creates a new situation for and between Katrine and Peter. Since this desire has come up, it is necessary that both of them explore what they want. They do this (I-function) by taking a look at who they think they are in the situation (personality function). Peter's focus is their debt and his career, and Katrine wonders whether she will be a good mother. Their action (I-function) is to delay having children. We can then say that Katrine and Peter do not yet need to have children. However, the situation will be different two years later, when Katrine is approaching forty and the choice of whether to have a child together needs to be made before time runs out. If they choose to have children, the situation will need them to be less concerned about careers and finances and to feel that they can be good parents. In this example, we see how Katrine and Peter create the situation together when Katrine brings up her desire to have children, and how the topic of children affects and shapes them both.

The theory of self in clinical practice

The theories of self and creative adjustment are useful in practice both as a therapist and coach, as well as in daily life. In Chapter 8, we describe how to increase awareness of the ways in which we contact our environment, and that the realisation this can lead to is the cornerstone of the gestalt-therapeutic method. Increasing attention to how people regulate, co-create, and adapt to their surroundings is therefore both a goal and a method for therapy and coaching. In practice, this means that the therapist works to increase her own and the client's attention to impulses, bodily sensations (impulse function), which roles or functions therapist and client experience together (personality function), and what they choose (I-function). In this way, the relationship between therapist and client is instrumental in making the client more aware of herself in her interaction with the therapist. The therapist can also focus on relationships the client brings into therapy and explore and raise awareness of these in relation to self functions (impulses, sensations, feelings, who she is, and what she chooses to do in the situation).

The therapist will therefore be concerned with who she feels she is in the meeting with the client and who she thinks the client becomes in their meeting. By that, we mean the type of roles or functions they have in the therapy room and the needs and impulses that manifest themselves. The therapist can choose to be and act in many different ways with her client, depending on what she thinks the client needs.

From the first moment, the therapist is interested in the client's nonverbal body language, tone of voice, pace, and emotions, but is also aware of her own bodily sensations and emotions, where everything is an expression of the impulse function. She is also interested in what the client says and how it is said. In this way, the therapist receives information about the id of the situation (impulse function) that catches her attention, what they do together (I-function), and who she feels they are together (personality function). She will also hear the client's story of what brings her to therapy. The therapist can choose to work with the theme client brings in or with the relationship between herself and the client. What the therapist chooses to work with depends on what the client wants and what the therapist thinks the client needs and will benefit from. This is illustrated in the following example.

Tina has come to coaching for the first time. At one point in their first session, the coach notices that Tina does not look at her when she speaks; she stares into space or looks at the floor. The coach also notices that she has a hard time understanding what Tina is talking about. In a low and gentle voice, she says to her: 'You know what, I notice that you look out into space or at the floor when you talk, and I'm having a hard time understanding what you're saying. I'd really like to understand you'.

Tina sits up in her chair and looks straight at the coach, her eyes wide. 'I didn't realise that. I look away to concentrate on what I want to tell you. I've never been aware that I don't look at the person I'm talking to, but I've often heard that others don't understand what I say'. Her voice becomes livelier as she says this to the coach, and the expression on her face changes.

The coach notices that she feels happy. She smiles at Tina, and says: 'I feel happy when you tell me that. It's nice that you heard what I said, and that you didn't experience it as criticism. When you look at me now, I really feel you see me'.

In this example, the coach noticed that Tina's impulse (impulse function) was to look away when she spoke (I-function). The coach thought (impulse and I-functions) that Tina was not aware of how it affected the relationship between them. In this situation, the coach was someone who did not understand, and Tina was someone who looked away when she spoke (personality function). When the coach chooses to point out (I-function) that Tina does not look at her when she speaks and that she wants to understand her (impulse function), Tina becomes aware of the fact that she looks away when she speaks. She spontaneously changes how she sits and looks at the coach as she speaks (impulse and I-functions). She becomes someone who sees and talks to the coach, and the coach becomes someone who smiles and understands. The relationship between them has changed and they have both gained a new understanding of the other and themselves.

Choosing who I am in the therapy room

In transitions in life, such as moving house, starting a new family, starting a new job, retirement, or illness and death, it is natural that feelings of insecurity about one's own identity and how we experience who we are can arise. It is important to take these feelings seriously; the premise of the theory of self is that we become who we are in our meetings with others (Slagsvold, 2016). Not knowing who we are is therefore an understandable and normal response when we lose the people we have around us. We illustrate this through the example of Anette and Simone.

Anette and Simone are both twenty-four years old and have been living together for three years. Lately, Simone has been dismissive and angry, and one day she announces that she has met someone else and wants to end their relationship. Anette is devastated and does not understand how Simone can behave this way. Anette consults a therapist to help her sort through her feelings and figure out what to do. The therapist helps Anette discover that she is very angry and that she feels she has been treated unfairly.

In one of their sessions, the therapist asks Anette to notice where in her body she feels anger. Anette notices that she tightens her whole body and holds her breath. She begins to move her hands and feet. The therapist asks Annette to exaggerate her movements, which she does. Anette kicks her feet on the floor and claps her hands on the armrests. The therapist then asks Anette to stand up so she can express what she feels in her body to an even greater degree. The therapist stands as she asks Annette to stand and begins to move along with Anette, mirroring (making the same movements as) Anette. Anette tells the therapist that she is very angry. The therapist asks Anette to repeat what she just said, exaggerating with her voice.

THERAPIST: 'You're SO angry with Simone!'
ANETTE SCREAMS: 'Yes, I am SO incredibly angry with her!'

In this sequence, the therapist supports Anette to express her anger physically and with her voice. The actions of kicking, walking, and screaming are triggered by Anette's spontaneous impulses, which the therapist chooses to support. In this way, Anette feels and finds an outlet for the trapped emotions. Anette becomes aware that she is angry: this is the personality function. The therapist becomes someone who supports Anette in the situation—this is also the personality function. They continue the session.

THERAPIST: 'Can you imagine that Simone is here in the room right now? Can you see where she is?'
ANETTE: 'Yes, she's just inside the door'.

Anette appears to sink into herself and begins to cry quietly. Her whole body changes. She goes from walking upright to stopping and slumping over.

THERAPIST: 'What would you say to Simone if she were here?'
ANETTE cries as she says: 'Why are you leaving? I feel so betrayed and so alone'.
    The therapist then asks Anette to play the part of Simone, in order to become aware of what she unconsciously assumes about her. As Simone, Anette says in a sad voice: 'I'm so sorry, I didn't want to hurt you and haven't been able to find a way to tell you how I was feeling'.

When Anette pretends that she is Simone, she becomes aware of how sad she feels as Simone. She understands that it might not have been easy for Simone to end the relationship. She feels less rejected and has a better understanding of why Simone had been so angry and dismissive recently. Furthermore, in the therapy room, Anette is able to experience that while she is still angry and upset, she feels calmer and more sorrowful. It becomes apparent to her is that she is afraid of a future without Simone because she has relied so much on her. She continues to work on this in later therapy sessions.

In this sequence, the therapist thought that Anette's notion of who she was in relation to Simone could be expanded to something more than feeling angry and rejected, which Anette experiences when she plays the role of Simone and acquires insight into Simone's situation (personality function). Anette discovers a new understanding of how it is to be Simone by noticing Simone's sadness in her body (impulse function). By gaining greater awareness of feelings, bodily reactions, and her own fear of being alone, it is easier for Anette to acknowledge and own these reactions, and she is able to change her views of both Simone and herself in the situation they are in. In the therapy situation, the therapist works with the relationship between Annette and Simone on the basis of her own impulses and what she notices she wants to do with Anette. The therapist becomes a therapist who listens, suggests experiments, reinforces and supports, while Anette becomes a client who explores and tries things out together with the therapist.

In Chapter 11 on experiments and Chapter 14 on projection, we show how role-playing and chair work can be useful techniques for expanding clients' attention. In the example of Anette, we show how these techniques can also be used when the therapist thinks it might be appropriate to extend the client's perception of who she is in different situations. The client can become aware that there are many potential roles to play, and that she can be herself in many different ways, such as Anette experienced through role playing. Experiences like these can give Anette insight into how she can choose who she will be, depending on the situation. Perhaps she will be the angry, spurned Anette; the grieving and understanding Anette who sees her own part in the relationship; or someone else entirely.

When the I-function is lacking

Many people seek help when they are in the midst of difficult choices and do not know what to do. They can feel paralysed and frustrated and be interested in looking for solutions. This is related to what we call the I-function, and is referred to in the theory of self as a *lack of ego function* (Perls et al., 1951; Müller, 1984). In the gestalt method it is important for the therapist to explore either the impulse or personality functions rather than to look for solutions. In practice, this means that when faced with a client who describes a situation in which she needs to make a choice (personality function), the therapist works to raise the client's awareness of bodily sensations, such as breathing, tension, motion or lack of motion (impulse function), and the client's (sometimes conflicting) roles and needs in the situation. This exploration can take place between the client and therapist and in the relationship the client brings to therapy, which creates her inner conflict. This is the case with Luke in the following example.

Luke has done very well in his job in Oslo. He has climbed the corporate ladder and has been offered a management position in Stavanger. He contacts a gestalt coach because he does not know whether to accept the position. In the first session, the coach notices that Luke's body is tense, that his breathing is shallow, and that his face lacks expression. Luke says that he is flattered to be offered this new position but is afraid he will not be able to live up to expectations and is not sure about moving from Oslo, where he has friends and two adolescent children. He asks what the coach advises him to do. The coach is aware that her stomach is tense and that she is barely breathing. She says to Luke: 'I notice that my stomach muscles are tense and that I'm barely breathing. When I look at you, it seems that you're also very tense. I think this is an important and difficult choice, and I'd like to explore it with you'.

Here, the coach shares what she feels in her own body and what she observes when she looks at Luke. Her purpose is to increase his attention on his own bodily sensations, and thus work with his impulse function. Moreover, she tells him what she thinks about the choice he has to make, and that she would like to explore it with him (I-function). She wants to be someone who supports so Luke can feel supported (personality function). They work with the relationship that exists between them (I-function).

LUKE responds: 'It's good to hear that you'll help me find a solution'.

He feels supported and is still searching for a solution. The ability to choose is still lacking (I-function). They talk for a while about how Luke feels about the job he has today, his relationship with this friends and children, and what he knows about the new job he has been offered. It becomes apparent to both Luke and the coach that this he has already talked a lot about this with others.

At the end of the session, the coach says: 'When I listen to you, it seems that you've already explored many aspects of the choice you have to make, and still don't know what you want to do'. By pointing out that Luke does not know what he wants, the coach emphasises what is apparent in the situation without trying to find a solution.
LUKE answers: 'Yes, I know at least that I don't know what to choose. That's even clearer to me now'. His body seems to sink into his chair as he breathes more deeply. 'I feel a little less tense, it's as if it helped to say it out loud, that I don't know . . . '

Here, Luke has new, spontaneous insight into himself and the situation he is in (impulse and I-functions). This spontaneous insight leads to a paradoxical change in the way he looks at his choice; he is not focused on a solution and can reflect on his situation. There is no longer a lack of I-function; he becomes a person who reflects and explores his choices (personality function).

In the fourth session, the coach proposes an experiment in which Luke first imagines that he is in Oslo, then in Stavanger. The coach says: 'Now, Luke, by thinking and imagining, we've explored what you know about living and working in Oslo and what you know mentally about moving to Stavanger. Now I want you to imagine that this space in the room is Oslo', she indicates one corner of the room, 'and that here, you are in Stavanger. I want you to begin by standing in the corner that symbolises Oslo'.

Here, the coach thinks that Luke has an opportunity to explore who he is (personality function) both physically and emotionally in the different cities (impulse function).

> While in 'Oslo', Luke says: 'As I stand here, I don't notice much in my body. Maybe I'm a little tired or feel a little heavy'. He moves over to the area that represents Stavanger, straightens up slightly, looks at the coach, and says: 'How weird, here I feel lighter, I feel curious and want to move'.

Here, Luke becomes aware that he has different sensations depending where he is in the room. The impulse function gradually makes itself known, and the coach continues the experiment.

> The coach asks Luke to stand midway between the two places, repeats to him what he said at the different locations, and describes the change she saw in his body in order to reinforce and clarify his experience. She asks him what he thinks about the experiment, if it gave him information. Luke says he became more aware that he would really like to move to Stavanger—to something new, a contrast to the familiar and mundane. He had not been aware of how heavy he often felt at work.

Here, his desires and needs make themselves known (impulse function), built on the sensations he experienced in the different areas in the room.

> Luke often feels that he should do more for his children. They are, however, seventeen and nineteen years old and rarely have time to spend with him. Maybe they would even think it would be fun to see him in a new city, to be with him on an oil platform, and get to know each other in a new way.

Here, Luke reflects on who he is when he is with his children (personality function), which also affects his decision.

> After talking a bit more about the experiment and the choice Luke has to make, they finish their conversation. They meet a few weeks later, at which point Luke has accepted the offer and started negotiations with his employer.

We have shown examples of how the coach has experimented with and explored different situations between herself and Luke, and between Luke's job options, in order to increase his attention to his bodily sensations. When he became more aware of his bodily sensations, he also became more aware of his impulses and underlying needs (impulse function) and who he wanted to be (personality function). This enabled him to make a choice (I-function) about his workplace.

In a later session, Luke tells the coach how his fear and his uncertainty as to whether he is the right person for the position constantly pops up. He begins to wonder if being in his old job, where he knew who he was (personality function), would be better after all. Together they first explore in different ways Luke is in the old job, where he feels safe. He then talks about some meetings he has attended in his new job. When he compared his experiences in his old and new jobs, he sees that while he perhaps felt safer in the old job, he is more engaged and eager for something new. Gradually, he becomes aware that he was afraid when he thought about what it would be like to be in the new job. Luke has a few more coaching sessions before moving to Stavanger.

In the last part of the example, the coach explored Luke's notions about the new job and the various ways he could be in the new job (personality function). Luke then compared this with his experiences from his old job. He is not paralysed by his uncertainty (a lack of I-function); rather, it helps him to stick to his choice when he becomes aware that he has the potential to be more and something different in the new job.

Working with the personality function

When we as therapists or coaches talk about needs we or our clients have, we should be aware that what we call 'needs' might actually be impulses coming to the surface, possibly impulses that are being held back. When we use the phrase 'Who do I become together with you?' we mean for example what we do together and how are we together. In some situations, we might become a teacher and the client a student, or mother and daughter. If the situation in the therapy room is stuck, and for example we always become a responsive caregiver and the client always becomes helpless, we may ask ourselves what the situation needs now.

The following example is taken from a supervision group for six high school teachers, led by a gestalt therapist with post-graduate training in supervision.

Katy has told the others how tired she is and how difficult she's finding the senior class. They are preparing for final exams. As Katy speaks, the supervisor sees that she seems sad and serious. When she mentions this, Katy responds that it matches how she feels. She feels that final exams are a big deal and is unsure if everyone will pass. The students are also uncertain, and the uncertainty affects the atmosphere in class. The supervisor says that she understands, and asks if Katy is willing to try an experiment. She asks her to imagine that the five participants in the group are her class and to talk to them about the exam, as she has done in her own class.

After the experiment, everyone in the group says that they feel serious after hearing the information Katy gave them about the exams. The supervisor then proposes that Katy repeat the information she gave the others about the exam, but this time experiment with smiling to the group, looking up, and speaking with a lighter voice. Katy does as the supervisor suggests and smiles at the others. They smile back, and the atmosphere in the room becomes lighter. Katy also notices that she was much lighter and happier this time and was surprised by the reaction from the others. She feels she is a different kind of teacher, as opposed to when she started the experiment.

The supervisor has a hypothesis that Katy's seriousness affects the students. She suggested the experiment because she wanted Katy to notice that there are several ways to be a teacher (personality function). In the experiment, we see the impulse function in the seriousness that Katy and the others in the group felt while Katy spoke (I-function). When Katy changes the way she is by smiling (I- and personality functions), it affects her colleagues in the group. The impulse is to smile, which they do (impulse and I-functions). This affects Katy and she smiles back (momentary I-function), and the other group members become happy together with a happy colleague (personality function).

It is of course not always this easy to change the mood of a class or between people. Research shows, however, that when we change our facial expression, it affects our environment (Staemmler, 2007). On pp. 174–175 we write about mirror neurons and resonance, which explain in part how humans are affected by facial expressions and tone of voice.

An example of a different approach involves Violet, a participant in a therapy group.

Violet is part of a gestalt therapy group with five members, which has met twice. As the session progresses, the therapist notices that Violet has not said anything thus far and asks how she is. Violet smiles and says that she is fine, and that she has looked forward to coming to the session. The therapist is surprised, because Violet is huddled on her chair and a muscle near her eye is twitching.

Here, the therapist observes a lack of correlation between what Violet says and her smile (I- and personality functions) on the one hand, and how she sits and the twitching muscle in her face on the other (impulse function).

> The therapist says she is confused by what Violet says, and that her words and smile do not match the way she is sitting. She also mentions the twitching muscle near her eye. Violet shakes her head slightly and continues to smile while her eyes fill with tears. The therapist tells her that it is okay to smile and have tears at the same time when she is in the group.

Here, the therapist emphasises the situation they are in together—a therapy group (personality function, who they are together)—and that it okay to cry there (I-function). She hopes doing so will make it easier for Violet to follow her impulses and her need to cry (impulse function).

> Violet now bursts into tears and says that her mother is seriously ill. She tried to push her feelings away, but they became intrusive here, together with the group and the therapist. The therapist and group members support her by telling her that she can go ahead and cry if that is what she needs. Violet continues to cry, but after a while she sits up, breathes, looks at the others, and says that she feels calmer. In the discussion afterwards, it becomes clear that the members of the group are also calmer, and that they had initially been uncertain when there was no correlation between what Violet said and how she behaved.

Her impulses and need to cry become clearer for Violet when the therapist tells her that the therapy group is a place where she can cry. The therapist and group members are supportive towards her, and she welcomes and accepts their support (personality function). When Violet stops crying, the relationship between her, the therapist, and the participants changes. They feel calmer together; they know who they are as a therapy group, with a leader (personality function) and where they have few impulses and needs at that moment beyond being calm (impulse and personality functions). In this example, Violet needed to show her emotions together with the therapist and other group members, and not hold back. She had the support to do what she needed in the situation.

When impulse control is lacking

Many clients seek therapy because they struggle with impulse control at home or at work. The therapist will often work to increase the client's attention to what it is in the situation (impulse function). This enables the client to lose control and helps her notice signals in her body that can warn her in advance. Sometimes this involves training the client to observe and use her vision and hearing as she learns to recognise the bodily reactions that occur as a result of external stimuli (see Chapter 9 on contact functions). Therapists also frequently work with clients in such a way that they can learn to calm themselves down by being aware of how they breathe, feeling their feet on the floor, or feeling the surface they sit on, in order to hold their impulses back. Here is an example of a way to sort impulses.

Harriet has come to therapy because she is quick to anger with her children and colleagues at work. She wants to be calmer and have more self-control. She tells the therapist about many episodes in which she loses her temper and lashes out. She speaks quickly, in a loud voice, and with large arm movements, which the therapist points out along the way. Harriet says that she feels stressed, is always pressed for time, and feels that she is losing control over her life. The therapist notices that she almost stops breathing, her body is tense, and she feels sad. She chooses to share what she notices about her body, and then asks Harriet about what she is aware of in her own body. At first, Harriet starts to say that she does not notice anything, but then she stops herself and says that she is breathing high up in her chest, and that she feels very tense. This is the start of a long process in which the therapist explores Harriet's bodily unrest and tension. She works to raise Harriet's awareness of what is going on in her body (impulse function) and how she talks without being aware of reactions in her surroundings. Eventually, it becomes evident to Harriet that she does everything very quickly, whether at work or at home. This means that she often has to wait for someone else (I- and personality functions). Waiting makes her impatient and irritated, which her surroundings react to. When Harriet becomes aware of how quick she can be and how this affects her and surroundings, she is sad and relieved at the same time.

By exploring her impulses together with the therapist, Harriet becomes more aware of what she was doing and how she was doing it (I-function), and that she can choose how to act and who she will be (personality and I-functions).

Summary

In their self theory, Fritz Perls and Goodman wanted to make a distinction between gestalt therapy and psychoanalysis. They succeeded to a great extent by distancing themselves from the theory that humans have a core self. Instead, they developed a theory that humans are created and become who they are together with others, and that what is perceived as self is constantly changing. However, their theories, as described in their book (Perls et al., 1951) are contradictory, unfinished, and not well enough thought through, which has caused difficulties for their successors. In this chapter, we have chosen to present parts of their theory of self as it has been further developed by their descendants.

We have described how self can be expressed in gestalt therapy as a verb or a function and not a noun, and that together we create the situation we are in and are shaped by what we do in the moment. Self is divided into three functions: the impulse function is expressed in a situation as sensations and impulses, which result in thinking, considering, and acting. This is called the 'I-function', and who we are together, which 'me' I am when I am together with you, is called the 'personality function'.

There is still a major challenge in the theory as it is presented today: the concept of function. This is understood as a verb that expresses what you and I do together in a situation, and can never be understood as your or my personal function. It is important to take into account that the concept of self includes the idea that we are created and shaped by the environment as we create and form that same environment, and that we are in a constant process of change that we influence and by which we are influenced (Slagsvold, 2016).

References

Hostrup, H. (2010). *Gestalt therapy: An introduction to the basic concepts of gestalt therapy* (D. H. Silver, Trans.). Copenhagen: Hans Reitzlers Forlag.

Müller, B. (1984). Isadore from: His contribution to the theory of the self, ego, id and personality function. *The Gestalt Journal, 14*(1), 6.

Perls, F. S., Hefferline, R. F., & Goodman, P. (1951). *Gestalt therapy: Excitement and growth in the human personality*. London: Souvenir Press.

Polster, E. (1995). *A population of selves*. San Francisco: Jossey-Bass.

Skottun, G. (2008). Arven etter Paul Goodman og teorien om selv nok en gang [Paul Goodman's legacy and the theory of self once again]. *Norsk Gestalttidsskrift, 5*(2), 22–32.

Slagsvold, M. (2016). *Jeg blir til i møte med deg* [I become me together with you]. Oslo: Cappelen Damm.

Staemmler, F. M. (2007). On Macaque monkeys, players, and clairvoyants: Some new ideas for a gestalt therapeutic concept of empathy. *Studies in Gestalt Therapy, 1*(2), 43–63.

Staemmler, F. M. (2016). Self as situated process. In J.-M. Robine (Ed.), *Self: A polyphony of contemporary gestalt therapy* (pp. 103–121). France: L'Exprimerie.

Teigen, K. H. (2004/2015). *En psykologihistorie* [A history of psychology]. Bergen: Fagbokforlaget.

Wollants, G. (2012). *Gestalt therapy: Therapy of the situation*. London: Sage.

Chapter 8

Awareness

> My first encounter with gestalt therapy and the concept of awareness was an important awakening. Until then, I had thought that I was a good listener, that I met others with openness, and that I had good self-understanding. Now I realised how limited my attention actually was when I was together with others, and how, for example, my thoughts tended to wander when my feelings became too strong. The importance of practicing awareness in teaching and in my own therapy has been crucial to how I meet others today, both in terms of my awareness of myself and of my development as a therapist. Sharpened senses and increased awareness in a situation not only help me to see and hear others, but also gives me a heightened awareness of who and how I want to be in a given situation.
>
> (Skottun, 2012, p. 7, our translation)

We tend to push our bodily sensations into the background; we are consumed by everything we need to do and remember in the course of a day in our hectic lives. We forget to be truly present with all our senses, to see, hear, and know what we experience in the moment, and to be aware of the choices we make, as we make them. Everyday habits often make us spectators rather than participants in our own lives.

We shall now take a closer look at what is perhaps the most basic concept of gestalt therapeutic theory and practice: being aware, sometimes formulated as having awareness of something, or more precisely, being aware of something in the situation. The concept undoubtedly has a direct connection with phenomenologists' and gestalt psychologists' call to return to the senses (Clarkson & Mackewn, 1993), which also has support in Zen Buddhist thinking (Kolmannskog, 2018).

To be aware

To be aware is a vague bodily sensation of some aspect that is sensed in the situation, something that cannot yet be expressed in words. The possibility of discovery and recognition lies in the body's sensory apparatus. To be aware

DOI: 10.4324/9781003153856-10

can thus be defined as that sensory feeling in the situation before what is sensed and perceived becomes a conscious thought. Joyce and Sills (2014) argue that 'in Gestalt, awareness is not about thinking, reflecting or self-monitoring' (p. 30).

It is as if the body's sharpened senses understand something that both transcends and precedes words. In this way, the body is the messenger of unexplained experiences; a precautionary sense that Wollants (2012) describes as 'bodying forth' (p. 51). We become aware of our bodies—the body reveals us to ourselves, before we have time to describe our experiences in words. The body senses; our experiences are manifested in the body and are expressed in, for example, raised shoulders, a clenched jaw, or a stomachache, which becomes the body's own language. This body language affects us and is influenced by us in every situation we find ourselves. The body is inevitably present in the here and now. This link between the body and our thoughts, between bodily sensations and our conscious reflections, can often be heard in everyday conversation, in phrases such as 'body language' or when we say someone 'thinks through his body' (Wollants, 2012, p. 75). These phrases reflect that our thoughts are not just in our heads but originate from an awareness that begins in the body—likely more so than we are aware. Laura Perls (1992) emphasised that awareness implies a collaboration of all sensory and motoric functions. She also worked extensively with body awareness, such us breathing, posture, coordination, and continuity and fluidity in movement. This is supported by Joyce and Sills (2014), who say: 'At its best, awareness is a non-verbal sensing or knowing what is happening here and now' (p. 30).

From awareness to consciousness: the awareness–consciousness continuum

Let us look at a simple example of the process from awareness to consciousness.

Simon is on a morning walk in the forest with his dog early in the spring. As he walks, he is aware of the forest smells, he hears birds singing, and sees the trees and foliage around him. He is aware of his body as he moves, his mind wanders, and he registers a feeling of calmness and presence without paying attention to any particular aspect of his surroundings or himself. Suddenly, his attention is caught by the first flower he has seen this year, next to the trail, and he stops to look at it. He starts to look around; his gaze is sharpened. Now he is only looking for more flowers on the forest floor—everything else is forgotten. As he walks slowly along looking for flowers, his dog comes running and starts to bark; it is impatient to continue the walk. Simon's attention now turns to his dog, and he becomes aware that he has stopped to look for flowers and forgotten both the dog and where he is. He pets the dog as his eyes move from the dog to the flower and the forest around him. It is as if he suddenly has a sense of himself in the woods with his dog, the flower, the birdsong, and smells, and he feels lighter and more comfortable in his body. At this moment, he becomes aware that he enjoys being right where he is, while acknowledging that it is time to move on.

In this example, Simon has noticed the flower without having chosen to do so—that is, without awareness. The flower suddenly becomes figure; it captures his interest, and his sensations and awareness now have direction. He has become aware of the flower, and follows this interest by looking for more flowers as the rest of his surroundings becomes background. When his dog comes running, he becomes aware of the situation he is in and that he has a choice: he can choose to have his attention directed to the flower or to continue on his walk.

Here we show how awareness and consciousness are a 'multi-sensory, whole-body phenomenon' (Wollants, 2012, p. 77). One is a function of the other, and neither exists without the other. Bloom (2019) explains that awareness is 'our initial awakening to what is . . . the fringe around the focus of our consciousness'. When we contact something or someone in our surroundings, consciousness 'emerges seamlessly from and never loses awareness. They are inseparable' (p. 33). As Simon senses the forest around him and himself in it, what he senses begins to take shape when he sees the flower; the flower organises itself as foreground as the rest of his surroundings and bodily sensations become background (see p. 11). Awareness, the body's sensory presence in the situation, is shaped and becomes a dawning attention to the flower. It continues to develop into a consciousness and understanding of the fact that he sees the flower, and that he has a choice. Consciousness is 'an important, inextricable constituent of contacting within the awareness–consciousness continuum' (Bloom, 2019, p. 39). This process is not linear, where one aspect follows another, but rather a coherent whole, where one aspect interacts with the other in a figure-ground duality as it takes on form and meaning in the situation. The example of Simon also applies to therapy. From an initial awareness of the situation, something new emerges for client and therapist. They gain a new understanding and a new meaning takes form. The process for this gestalting can thus be described as a continuous circular process that goes from an unclear, sensory awareness to a beginning awareness that gradually finds direction, before becoming a conscious acknowledgement.

This process of awareness can of course also begin with a conscious decision to pay attention to how we breathe. By paying attention to the breath, we become aware of where in the body we feel our breathing, and whether it stops or flows freely. In this way, we can have a

'moment to moment' experience of breathing and an awareness of how we breathe in the moment. When you consciously focus your awareness, you are

> 'paying attention' and it is this directed awareness that is the central therapeutic activity of the Gestalt counsellor.
>
> (Joyce & Sills, 2014, pp. 30–31)

The steps of this process can also be found in awareness exercises and meditation, among other things.

In brain research, there is a great deal of focus on consciousness—what it is, where it is located, and the connection between memory and how changes in the brain create changes in our consciousness. The words 'awareness', 'attention', and 'consciousness' can be found in abundance in the English-language research literature when consciousness processes are described (Nunn, 1996; Posner, 2009). Attention and consciousness are different from awareness in that the first two phenomena have direction and intent, and are about something in particular, whereas awareness is understood to be an activity in the brain where we are conscious of the fact that we are aware of something.

History of the term 'awareness'

The concept of awareness has etymological roots to the Old English *gewær* (watchful, vigilant), which comes from the proto-Germanic *gad-waraz*, which is related to the modern *gewahr* (Bloom, 2019). The English term 'awareness' was, however, only brought into use in this context after Perls came to the United States. Therefore, when he wrote the book *Gestalt Therapy* (1951), it was natural to give the term an English-language equivalent. He chose 'to be aware', or 'awareness'. Laura Perls (1992) points out that the ancient Greek word *aisthesthai* means to be aware. It is used as an active verb and implies the collaboration of all sensory and motoric functions.

Our intention when writing the first Norwegian edition of this book was to translate the concepts of 'awareness' and 'to be aware' into Norwegian. When doing so, we realised that awareness in English is an overarching concept that covers awareness, attention, and consciousness. We found Bloom's critique of the use of 'awareness' useful (see later in this chapter). He points out that gestalt literature is published today in many languages other than English:

> It is nonsense to consider translations as merely secondary or best efforts at grabbing hold of what the founders discovered/invented, which could only be accurately articulated in English—as if 'authentic' Gestalt therapy belongs in English. . . . Awareness or consciousness? While this distinction has more significance in English than in other languages, a discussion in terms of these English words offers a perspective on how we ordinarily understand fundamental Gestalt concepts. We are always 'translating' experience.
>
> (2019, pp. 21–22)

The Norwegian translation we decided on, the verb *å være var* and the noun *varhet*, have their origin in the Norron word *varr* and the Old English word *gewær*. *Varr* can be translated as to be aware of something. An even earlier version, to see with *varre* eyes, emphasises the aspect of sensual awareness implicit in the concept. When translating the Norwegian word *varhet* to English, we decided to keep this limited understanding of awareness and add attention and consciousness to the awareness continuum formulated by Laura and Fritz Perls.

Words and concepts with different or overlapping meanings

We have already explained that to be aware or have an awareness of something is fundamental to gestalt theory. We call what happens next a beginning attention, in which we pay attention to something in the situation when it captures our interest. However, paying attention to something is not the same as being aware or awareness (Posner, 2009), precisely because it is the starting point of the process. In the example of Simon, we see how his attention becomes focused on the flower and his interest in it is aroused. It is the first flower he has seen this season, and he wants to see if he can find more. He begins to look without thinking about what he is doing. Perls used the example of a floodlight and a dark theatre stage, where the floodlight is a metaphor for attention. It is possible to either randomly sweep the light over the stage and see what catches our attention, or to purposefully illuminate the actors so that we can see the play on the stage (van Baalen, 2002/2008). Both the example of Simon and the metaphor of the floodlight show how attention and the formation of a figure against a background are mutually dependent. There is no figure without attention, and no attention without a figure.

The concepts of 'becoming aware of something' and 'consciousness' are closely related to the recognition of sensation. They are derived from phenomenology and in particular Merleau-Ponty (2005) (see Chapter 3). This understanding of the concept of consciousness must not be confused with Freud's theory of the unconscious. Simon becomes aware of the flower, and it affects him so much that he stops. He then consciously recognises the whole situation in the forest, which includes sounds, smells, flowers, his dog, his own body, and the fact that he has a choice. In this context, consciousness is used to denote the cognitive acknowledgement he has of himself and his choice in the situation.

Fritz Perls' reckoning with Freud: back to the senses

In the history of gestalt therapy, we find traces of a discussion related to the awareness–consciousness continuum. It is especially in connection with the use of concepts such as consciousness that Fritz Perls' criticism and refutation of the Freudian idea of the subconscious are expressed. He and his wife Laura were interested in making clear the necessity of phenomenological sensation and awareness for discovery and insight, influenced by Zen Buddhist thinking of being here and now (Perls, 1947/1969; Clarkson & Mackewn, 1993) (see Chapter 3).

Fritz Perls himself was educated as a psychoanalyst and was thus also well acquainted with Freud's concept of the unconscious. This is where his criticism is sharpest. Fritz Perls wanted to highlight a phenomenological and sensory understanding, which both Laura and Fritz knew from the work of the gestalt psychologists. For both, awareness is the whole of our ability to be in touch with everything of which we are conscious, both in ourselves and in our surroundings: that which is spontaneous and immediate, before planning and action occur (Perls et al., 1951).

This distinction between gestalt therapy and psychoanalysis also seems evident in the initial choices of the name of the therapy form. While Fritz Perls was still in Germany, he chose to call this therapy form 'focus therapy', a name that suggests the importance of paying attention here and now rather than delving into childhood experiences. Later he used the term 'concentration therapy', which may also indicate a demarcation from Freud's theories and which suggests the here-and-now perspective in the therapy form. This emphasis on the importance of awareness can also be found in the introduction to Perls et al. When they wrote the first fundamental book about this therapy form in the United States, they devoted several pages to free association in the here-and-now situation, a description that encouraged the reader to pay attention to the senses here and now (see Chapter 3).

Later, Fritz Perls and his colleague Paul Goodman changed the name to gestalt therapy and then concluded that they:

> had to shift the concern of psychiatry from the fetish of the unknown, from the adoration of the 'unconscious', to the problems and *phenomenology of awareness*: what factors operate in awareness, and how faculties that can operate successfully only in the state of awareness lose this [property]?
>
> (Perls et al., 1951, p. xxv, our emphasis)

There is no doubt that this distancing from an analytic point of view was successful. The challenge, however, was that the emphasis on 'being aware', the sensory here and now, may give the impression that this form of therapy is only concerned with our cognitive assumptions, and that our understanding thus becomes incomplete. It is precisely this that has also been pointed out in the years since, and thus been challenged (Wollants, 2012; Bloom, 2012, 2019).

Newer generations have developed the therapy form in several ways, and naturally re-examined and reformulated the original tenets. Some of this criticism is aimed at Fritz Perls' generation's understanding of the concept of awareness. Bloom (2012, 2019), among others, has pointed out that Perls' unilateral emphasis on the importance of the senses and of awareness as the only valid point of view has historically been detrimental to gestalt therapy. Bloom's claim is that the therapy form ended up being so critical of the Freudian concept of the unconscious that the concept of consciousness in gestalt therapy came to be seen as an unbalanced theory where everything is awareness, without consciousness. The continuum was interrupted.

Bloom (2012) points out that consciousness—'knowing', understanding—is toned down and is in fact largely absent in Perls' interpretation. This missing link or gap in our theory puts gestalt therapy far too much at risk of becoming a form of therapy that only focuses on awareness, the non-verbal, and the sensual. Awareness is more than a sudden 'eureka!' experience; it also includes knowledge and insight. Bloom (2019) states that awareness is too broad a concept to describe the experience of being human. He disagrees with gestalt therapy's expansive understanding of awareness as being everywhere. He is critical to the awareness continuum and suggests that it should instead be called the 'awareness–consciousness continuum'.

In this discussion, it is important to realise that Fritz and Laura Perls had different points of view in practicing the awareness continuum. Fritz practiced, according to Laura (1992), 'just a free association or a free dissociation, hopping from one thing to another. Now I'm aware of this. Now I'm aware of that' (p. 13). From Laura's point of view, the awareness continuum is 'the freely ongoing gestalt formation where what is of greatest concern and interest to the organism, the relationship, the group or the society becomes Gestalt, comes into the foreground where it can be fully experienced and coped with' (p. 138). Bloom (2019) points out that Laura Perls is not clear whether there is a conscious reflection about experience during the awareness continuum.

Many theorists argue that awareness is both the method and outcome of gestalt therapy (Perls et al., 1951; Yontef, 1993). van Baalen disagrees and makes this clear in his article 'Awareness is not enough' (van Baalen, 2002/2008, p. 70). With this statement, he points out that gestalt therapy is more than simply a description of our sensations here and now. This point of view is supported by Bloom's arguments in his two articles (2012, 2019) about meaning-making and the use of mind and thoughts in this process. Herrestad (2014) argues that this process also includes conscious choices. He points out the importance of the therapist taking the time to reflect on the client's increased awareness in the therapy session, so that the client can take responsibility for her actions and act on the basis of conscious choices. Later in this chapter you will see examples of how the therapist and client work with this awareness process.

Being aware and attentive in the therapy room

Increasing awareness of the body's sensations, attention, and awareness of oneself and one's choices is fundamental in gestalt therapy (Perls et al., 1951; Yontef, 1993; Joyce & Sills, 2014). In this awareness and attention lies the possibility for the client to make new discoveries and gain new insight, which is fundamental to what we have previously described in Chapter 5 as paradoxical change, and to make conscious choices, as we show in the following example of Karen in the therapy room.

Karen has been going to therapy for a few months. She has told the therapist about the challenges she has at home. She is tired, and tired of the fact that her husband is so withdrawn.

KAREN: 'He totally withdraws, and I have to do everything! I'm so tired of being the one who always has to take care of things'. Her voice is loud and irritated.

As the therapist nods and listens, she notices that Karen is leaning forward on the chair, as if she is tilting. She also becomes aware that she herself is barely breathing—as if her involvement in Karen's story takes her breath away. This immediate awareness causes the therapist to choose to interrupt Karen in the middle of her story, in order to point out what has become obvious to her.

THERAPIST: 'Karen! Do you notice how you're sitting?'
   Karen stops speaking. She becomes quiet and looks at the therapist; it is as if time stands still for a moment.
KAREN: 'Oh! I'm sitting on the edge of the chair and balancing!'
THERAPIST: 'How are you balancing?'
KAREN: 'I hold my position—and I need to relax . . . ' She slides back into the chair, exhales as her back comes into contact with the back of her chair, and say spontaneously: 'Ohhh, I need to rest. I need to let go . . . '

At this point, the therapist becomes aware that she was holding her breath and that Karen was sitting on the edge of her chair as she spoke. The content of the client's story goes to the background and her bodily sensations become foreground. The body makes itself heard—it expresses itself in the situation. The body is the carrier of information, and it is this information the therapist brings to Karen's attention. When Karen becomes aware of how she sits and spontaneously associates it with 'holding her position', she realises what she needs at that moment, namely rest. This spontaneous realisation is a paradoxical change in Karen's understanding of herself and her relationship to her husband (Chapter 5). She has not previously been aware of how tired she is and that she needs rest. Here we see how awareness and attention are prerequisites for spontaneous realisation and change, and how realisation and insight occur in the moment, in what we call the here and now between therapist and client.

Mindfulness, meditation, and gestalt therapy

The gestalt therapist's most important task is thus to help increase the client's awareness of what she thinks and feels, what she senses in her body, and how she is in contact with her surroundings. In recent years, other forms of therapy have also emphasised the importance of sensory awareness in the therapy room. 'Mindfulness' is a relevant concept in this respect (Braathen, 2011; Endsjø, 2010). Here, emphasis is also placed on supporting the client to take an observant perspective in the here and now and to acknowledge what she notices without prejudice. It is interesting to note that in mindfulness, the stages in the process are not described as being in a prescribed order.

Recent brain research clearly shows how useful meditation is in therapy. Meditation also helps to increase clients' ability to be in the moment, to withstand stress and discomfort, to accept what is, and to feel more empathy and a greater sense of belonging. As Joyce and Sills (2014) point out, there are several similarities between this form of attention and the gestalt therapeutic 'awareness'. The difference is, however, clear: in gestalt therapy, increasing awareness is directly related to the figure-ground process in the field. Mindfulness emphasises the ongoing process in which one figure flows over to the other without a particular preference. Emphasis is placed on supporting the client to notice and glean information from what is experienced, while in mindfulness the intention is to flow with that which is sensed.

When awareness becomes conscious thought

The body's language is more diverse and complex than spoken language. 'Speaking is but a refinement of the body feeling' (Merleau-Ponty in Wollants, 2012).

When awareness and sensation are given verbal expression, we can acknowledge them. At that point, we can know and put into words that which previously was only perceived vaguely. In the example of Karen, we see how she becomes aware of her body when the therapist asks her about it and how she gains a new understanding of herself when she describes how she sits. This interplay between body and thought is also highlighted in modern research on how the brain integrates and shapes sensory impressions into meaningful entities (Staemmler, 2012).

The therapist's task is not only to help the client to be aware and attentive in the situation but also to support her verbal descriptions of her experience and discoveries. In other words, the therapist supports the client's process from vague, sensory experience to expressed verbal insight. The body senses the whole situation. We illustrate this in the following example, where Peter is in just such a process in therapy.

This is Peter's fourth therapy session. He feels that the last two sessions were more confusing than clarifying, and as he approaches the therapist's office, he thinks this will likely be his last session. He feels he is not getting anywhere. The therapist is fine, but they spend a lot of time talking about the same problems.

And so begins this session. Peter immediately starts talking about problems at work in the same way he has done previously. There are many problems to deal with, but at the same time he is a little tired of the whole thing. As Peter explains, the therapist senses a vague feeling of unrest in the vicinity of her diaphragm, and it occurs to her that she is tired of hearing the same story again. Her impulse is to interrupt Peter, but as she is on the verge of stopping him, she becomes aware that the inner turmoil is intensifying, and chooses to hold back.

Peter, on the other hand, feels a vague irritation about not being interrupted. Still, he continues to talk, noting that the irritation becomes confusion. Peter stops talking. And as it gets quiet, the therapist is also confused. The therapist's turmoil intensifies, but at the same time she recognises a possibility that something new is happening. She chooses to let silence prevail.

Peter sighs heavily and looks sad.

THERAPIST: 'I hear you sighed . . . ?'
PETER: ' . . . I'm tired of being alone with everything . . . '
THERAPIST: 'Are you alone with everything now, do you think?' The therapist sits a bit further toward the edge of her chair, as if she wants to approach Peter.
PETER: ' . . . Yes!' (His confusion increases.)
    The therapist is aware that her own turmoil is still there and that she feels sad. At the same time, an image pops into her head. She chooses to describe this image to Peter.

THERAPIST: ' . . . I get a picture of a man in an open boat on a stormy sea . . . a life preserver is thrown out to him . . . '

As she says the words 'life preserver', Peter's eyes open wider. He looks directly at her and his eyes are filled with tears.

The therapist feels focused as well as a strong will and desire to be present with Peter.

THERAPIST: 'I see your tears . . . and I feel tears in my own eyes . . . I feel sadness and sorrow . . . '

PETER: 'Yes, I feel sad, and I want to cry even more . . . I suddenly understand that it's like the open sea at work, too. I'm lonely, alone. And there's no life preserver'.

THERAPIST: 'Is the life preserver here now, do you think? I know I want to be a life preserver for you'.

PETER: 'Yes! It's as if it's possible to grab onto what you said, as if you threw me a life preserver . . . maybe I've been waiting for you to say something or interrupt me so I don't have to be so alone. It's like I felt alone here, just like the way I feel at work. And I think I lack a life preserver at work. It's like nobody ever asks me about myself or shows any interest in me'.

THERAPIST: 'Yes, I also thought you were waiting for me to interrupt, but I was confused and didn't know what to say until I pictured you in the boat. It was as if I didn't know what you needed from me'.

PETER: 'That's absolutely true, I was waiting for you to say something . . . Maybe I'm waiting for my colleagues to say something too, for someone there to throw me a life preserver'.

In this example, both Peter and the therapist become aware of their bodily sensations, unease, and irritations as they become clearer, and these cause confusion in both of them. The therapist observes something in Peter that she also notices in herself and which seems to be unarticulated in the field. She therefore chooses to introduce a metaphor, and the two of them explore this via the idea of a life preserver. Through this metaphor, Peter has an 'aha' experience which he is able to describe in words. He becomes aware that he has been given a 'life preserver' by the therapist, and that this is what he lacks at work. Peter gains new insight when the therapist tells him that she suspected he was waiting for her to interrupt his story. It is as if the therapist's words immediately make sense to him, and he gains a spontaneous insight into how what he does with the therapist is the same thing he does at work.

Practicing awareness and attention

Gestalt therapy places particular emphasis on developing the capacity for awareness and attention. The possibility of movement, new discoveries, and development lies precisely in paying attention to the information we receive from our senses. By gestalting our experiences, we increase this sensory awareness. In other words, the emphasis is on the process of experiencing, as we described in the example of Peter. Increasing awareness is thus both about what the client says and how she says it. The ability to be aware can be learned, and for the gestalt therapist, practicing paying attention to the senses is vital. There are many ways in which to practice, such as meditation, mindfulness training, yoga, breathing techniques, or the Alexander Technique and Feldenkrais method (Skottun, 2012). These methods can help us to become more aware of and attentive to our breathing, movement, bodily sensations, and how thoughts and emotions can affect each other. In some cases, the methods can be used in groups, while others are practiced in individual teaching and in the therapy room. What you choose will depend on whether you want to focus on silence and practice an introverted mindfulness method or a more active and participatory approach, where movement and interaction is desirable. There is much useful information on these methods available online.

Athletes, actors, and musicians also practice awareness of bodily sensation and to be conscious of the connection between thoughts, emotions, and movement in order to perform better (Fagerheim, 2016). Such awareness training is of course useful for all of us, not only in order to perform better, but also to become more aware of the choices we make and how we live with the opportunities and limitations that life gives us.

Awareness zones

In their book *Gestalt Therapy*, Perls et al. (1951) included descriptions of exercises we can do on our own to increase our awareness and become more conscious of our behaviour. Fritz Perls was, as mentioned earlier, very concerned that people should live a more conscious life and be aware of their own bodies and the surrounding environment. The exercises describe how we can consciously focus attention on bodily sensations, surroundings, and thoughts in order to increase awareness of these phenomena. In *Gestalt Therapy Verbatim* (1969), Perls describes the body's sensory presence from three perspectives, or so-called zones: the outer zone, the inner zone, and the middle zone. In practicing awareness, he recommends allowing sensory attention to flow from moment to moment through the three zones. In this flow there is a process from a growing awareness to conscious knowing in all three zones. Here we describe the awareness zones and the process that can be experienced.

The outer zone

Contact through the senses with that which is experienced in the world around us here and now: what we see, hear, smell, taste, and touch.

> Example: Right now, I become aware that I see the computer screen, hear the sound of the keyboard, feel my fingertips make contact with the plastic

keys, smell the trapped air in the room around me, and hear cars on the road outside.

The inner zone

Contact through the senses with that which is experienced in the body's muscles and breath.

> Example: Right now, I become aware that I feel tension in my fingertips, tightness in my shoulders, my stomach is bloated, my breath is shallow, and when I move my head, I notice that my neck relaxes.

These two awareness zones, outer and inner, describe how something is experienced in the body here and now. Because the description is purely phenomenological, it is reliable in the sense that it describes empirical facts of what is experienced in the moment. Regardless of what others may think about what I am experiencing, it is a pure description and thus not open for debate. The moment I put words to the experience, I have a conscious knowledge of the sensed experience. This leads us to the third zone, which is very different from the phenomenological description of the outer and inner zones.

The middle zone

The middle zone includes all the thought activity that goes on and leads away from a sensory experience of what is happening here and now. It involves all kinds of explanations, interpretations, assumptions, and memories of the past, thoughts of the future, fantasies, and dreams.

To be aware of inner zone activity is different from being conscious of the content of the activity, the thoughts, feelings, etc. Here there is also a process from a beginning experience of something going on in the head (mind) to knowing that there is thinking. When we know that we are thinking, we are more or less conscious of the activity and can explore the content.

> Example: Right now, I become aware that I wonder how long it will take to write this book. I have an idea of when we will finish the book, and I wonder how it will be received. I think about what to wear for dinner, and how much time to devote to writing today.

The middle zone also includes our interpretations of bodily sensation and the way we describe sensations as emotions. In such situations we use the word 'feel' synonymously with 'think'. Emotions belong to the inner zone only when coupled with bodily sensation.

> Example: 'Right now I feel tired' is an interpretation of 'Right now my body is heavy'.

'I'm tired of reading' is an interpretation of 'My body is uneasy; it is difficult to sit still, and I am unable to concentrate on what I read'.

The three zones in practice

Awareness is always a whole; all zones are mutually dependent and interconnected (Joyce & Sills, 2014). Splitting awareness into zones can be understood as a metaphor or a map the therapist uses to keep track of which zones are being explored at any given time. The therapist notices for example how the client moves, sits, or uses her eyes. She is also aware of what she herself feels, how she breathes, her impulses, and what she thinks and feels. The information the therapist becomes aware of by paying attention to the zones helps her to make conscious choices in the field with the client (Skottun, 2012).

The therapist can increase the client's awareness of the zones with awareness questions. For example, she might point out what she becomes aware of, and ask: 'I see you take in a big breath; what happens to you when you do that? What do you notice when you move your chair? I see you sitting in the chair with your feet on the floor; what do you notice in your body? How is it for you when you do this? How is it for you when I say this?' In addition to pointing out what the therapist becomes aware of, what is obvious in the situation, and asking awareness questions, she can use experiments and exercises to increase the client's awareness of herself in the situation. Many exercises and experiments designed to raise awareness can also be done in groups. In Chapter 10, we show examples of such exercises and experiments, how they can be performed, and the situations in which they are suitable.

From the middle zone to the outer zone and back to the middle zone

Thea has recently been hired as a professional supervisor at a health institution. She was very happy when she got this job—she had wanted it for a long time, and getting it was like a dream come true. However, not everything has been as expected. She is tasked with leading a professional group with four participants, whom she experiences as silent and introverted. Nothing seems to work, and she seeks coaching to explore the problem.

THEA: 'I'm so frustrated! They just sit there in their offices, and when there are meetings they just read from their documents and report separately on what they've done!'

Thea speaks in a loud and annoyed voice. The coach has a feeling that Thea is talking to herself more than to the coach, who is after all in the room with her.

The coach tries to get Thea's attention. She interrupts her and says: 'Can you see me? I notice you're looking up in the air as you speak'.

Thea, slightly irritated: 'Sure, I can see you!' She then continues to talk.

The coach interrupts again: 'When I hear you tell me about your work, I notice I barely breathe and feel alone. It's like you're not talking to me, it's almost like you're talking to yourself more than to me'. As she says this, Thea looks right at her. It is as if she sees the coach for the first time.

COACH: 'Now you're looking at me, and I feel myself breathing more easily. What's happening to you?'

THEA: 'I realise you're here and we're both here in this room. In one way this is obvious, in another, it's not. I disappeared inside myself in all my frustration. I think I barely took a breath while I talked'.

COACH: 'Is this something you also notice in the group you lead?'

THEA: 'Yes, it is; with the group, I also become introverted, I'm mostly interested in thinking. That's probably what the others do as well. So if I get them to turn their attention outwards, as you did to me just now, I might be able to enjoy being together with them'.

Together with the therapist, Thea discovers that all of her attention goes to thoughts of how things are at work, to the middle zone. She was not aware of the therapist (outer zone) nor was she aware of her voice, or what she feels in her body (inner zone). When she sees the therapist (outer zone), she becomes aware that they are both in the room and that she had not really seen the therapist up to this point. With the help of the therapist's questions, she realises that the way the group is may have to do with the participants being in the middle zone much of the time, just as she herself was with the therapist. Through reflection with the therapist (middle zone) she sees that the possibility of development in the group may lie in the members learning to focus more attention on each other, on the outer zone. With the help and support of seeing and listening to each other, as she did together with the therapist, she can have a new experience and change can happen. In this process, Thea became aware that she has choices in how she contacts the group members, which is part of the awareness and consciousness process we have described previously.

From the middle zone to the inner zone

Ingrid is at her second therapy session. She has told the therapist about the challenges she faces as a single mother for two young children combined with a demanding job. The therapist becomes aware that she holds her breath and frowns as she listens to Ingrid. She looks at Ingrid and notices that she also wrinkles her forehead and sits stiffly in her chair as she speaks very quickly. She wants to increase Ingrid's attention of her body expression and thinks it must be done with caution.

The therapist slowly strokes the wrinkles on her own forehead, breathing and looking at Ingrid as she says: 'I realise that I wrinkle my forehead, and I'm stroking it now. How is it for you when I do that?'

Almost automatically, Ingrid's hand moves to her own forehead, and she says: 'I'm trying to iron out my wrinkles. I didn't realize I was wrinkling my forehead until I felt it with my hand'. She begins to explain why she did it.

The therapist is still stroking her forehead with her right hand; she puts her left hand on her chest, and says: 'I stroke my forehead and put my hand on my chest to see how I'm breathing. What's going on with your forehead and breathing?' Ingrid stops talking and puts her hand on her chest. It is as if she senses something in her own body. She continues to stroke her forehead slowly with the other hand.

Ingrid: 'It's so strange, I didn't realise how little I breathe and how tense I am in my body. When I hold my hand on my chest, it's as if there's more room for my breath, and as I stroke my forehead it's as if my forehead and entire face release the tension I felt'.

Ingrid and the therapist smile at each other as they sit together. Both have one hand on their foreheads and the other on their chests. Both breathe more freely, and it is as if silence and calmness descend on the room.

The therapist becomes aware that Ingrid is in the middle zone when she speaks, and that she herself is wrinkling her forehead and holding her breath (inner zone). She would like to increase Ingrid's attention to her inner zone and creates an experiment in which she strokes her forehead and then puts her hand on her chest. Her impulse is to do this to Ingrid, but instead she chooses to do it to herself, as she imagines it can be frightening or startling for Ingrid if she gets so close. The therapist has an idea that when Ingrid sees her stroke her forehead and put her hand on her chest (outer zone), she can become aware of her own forehead and chest (inner zone). In addition, she asks awareness questions both so that she as a therapist can gain information and to increase Ingrid's attention to her inner zone. The attention between them moves between the zones, where they think, look at, and interact with the body, which results in them both remaining quiet as the relationship between them changes.

Exploring activity in the middle zone

Sean has been to coaching a few times. He has told the coach about his worries at work and at home, and how he struggles to fall asleep at night.

Through these sessions, he has become aware of how he constantly thinks. The coach asks if he has a picture or metaphor for all his thoughts.

SEAN: 'It's like I have a hive in my head where the bees buzz around and around all the time. I can almost see my thoughts moving around, almost completely without purpose and meaning. I get a headache when I see how busy the thought bees are. It's no wonder I can't get to sleep when this is going on'.

The coach asks Sean to draw the hive, which he does with great zeal. As he draws bees flying in and out of the hive, he realises that he is not thinking, but is only interested in drawing. When the coach asks him to stop and look at the drawing, Sean says with a big smile: 'It really is a good picture of how I felt, but right now it's very quiet in my head. It's as if the thoughts just disappeared as I drew. I feel lighter in my body and my headache is gone'.

Sean has become more aware of how much he thinks, and is in the middle zone through the first conversations with the coach. This allows him to create a metaphor for his thoughts and to illustrate the metaphor. In the process of drawing, Sean turns his attention from his thoughts to the drawing, and without being aware of it, his thought process changes. He has moved from the middle zone, where he constantly thought about everything that was difficult and all his worries, through the outer zone by drawing the bees, and to the inner zone, where the body feels lighter and the headache is gone. Through this process he also becomes aware that he has choices. He can choose to remain in an awareness of how he thinks or he can instead let his mind and thoughts continue to whirl around like bees. He can then assume the role of observer towards himself and reflect on the thought process.

Summary

Both phenomenology and Zen Buddhism are fundamental to gestalt therapy's understanding of the concept of awareness (Braathen, 2011). Being present with our senses here and now, practicing awareness, and becoming more conscious of the present moment can be found in both theories. In this chapter, we have described what we mean by awareness and the process from awareness to acknowledged consciousness, both theoretically and in clinical practice. Elsewhere in this book you will find many examples in which the therapist works to increase the client's awareness and attention, either by awareness questions, phenomenological descriptions, or various exercises and experiments. This increasing of awareness in the client is fundamental regardless of theoretical model. Becoming self-aware causes a change in how the client views herself and her problems, which in turn leads her to become aware that she has more choices in the situation she brings to therapy (Staemmler, 2012).

Examples of awareness questions related to the zones

The following awareness questions can be used to raise awareness of the inner zone:

- Do you sense how you breathe now?
- Can you sense whether you are breathing high in your chest or far down in your stomach?
- Can you breathe more slowly and sense how your breath changes, or breathe faster?
- Do you feel what is going on in your body now?
- Are there any places you feel tension, pain, or discomfort?
- Are there any parts of your body that you are more aware of than others?
- How are you sitting on the chair? Do you feel the seat under you? The backrest?
- Do you feel the floor under your feet?
- Can you move your hands, arms, and legs or get up and walk? What do you become aware of when you make these movements?

The questions can be combined with the therapist's observations:

- I see wrinkles in your forehead. Do you sense that?
- I see you move your legs. Are you aware of that?
- When you talk, it looks like you're holding your breath.
- I see you're leaning forward. Describe what you see. Are you aware of that?
- I hear you say that you're sad (angry, sorry). Where in the body do you feel it?

Questions for raising outer zone awareness:

- Can you describe what you see in the room?
- Can you see me? What do you notice when you look at me?
- Do you see me smiling/looking serious?
- Do you hear what I'm saying?
- Are you aware of the surroundings at work/home?
- What does your husband look like? (your children, your friends)

Questions can be combined with what the therapist is aware of:

- I notice you look down at the floor as you speak. Do you see anything there? Can you look at me instead?
- I know I'm smiling when I talk to you, do you see that? I hold my hand on my stomach, do you see?

- I notice you kept talking after I said . . . I wonder if you heard what I said? Can you repeat that?

Questions for raising middle zone awareness:

- Are you thinking now?
- Are you aware of whether you are thinking or feeling now?
- Are you trying to find solutions by thinking?
- Is it easy for you to think and look for solutions?

Questions combined with what the therapist is aware of:

- I see you look up in the air when you talk. Are you thinking?
- I hear you're talking really fast. Are there many thoughts in your head at once?
- Now I can't follow what you're saying, it sounds like you associate very quickly. Do you realise how your thoughts changes?
- I hear you're talking a lot, and it seems like your mind is jumping from one thing to the other. Is that right?
- Now you're talking very softly/loudly, and I wonder if you're thinking about something sad/difficult.
- Now you're speak loudly and quickly. Do you feel attacked by what I say? It's as if you're defending yourself. What do you think about what I just said?
- Now you're very quiet. Are you thinking?

References

Bloom, D. (2012). Sensing animals/knowing persons: A challenge to some basic ideas in gestalt therapy. In T. Levine (Ed.), *Gestalt therapy: Advances in theory and practice*. New York: Routledge.

Bloom, D. (2019). From sentience to sapience: The awareness-consciousness continuum and the lifeworld. *Gestalt Review*, 23(1), 18–43.

Braathen, E. (2011). Å akseptere det som er: Om mindfulness og gestaltterapi [Accepting what is: On mindfulness and gestalt therapy]. *Norsk Gestalttidsskrift*, 7(2), 7–29.

Clarkson, P., & Mackewn, J. (1993). *Fritz Perls*. London: Sage Publications.

Endsjø, C. (2010). Øyeblikkets magi: Awareness og mindfulness i parterapi [The magic of the moment: Awareness and mindfulness in couples' therapy]. *Norsk Gestalttidsskrift*, 7(2), 5–21.

Fagerheim, B. (2016). Jeg må ivareta det relasjonelle perspektiv i prestasjonsutviklingen. [I have to consider the relational perspective in performance development]. *Norsk Gestalttidsskrift*, 13(1), 80–87.

Herrestad, H. (2014). Awareness og fortolkning [Awareness and interpretation]. *Norsk Gestalttidsskrift*, 10(1), 77–84.

Joyce, P., & Sills, C. (2014). *Skills in gestalt counselling & psychotherapy* (3rd ed.). London: Sage.

Kolmannskog, V. (2018). *The empty chair*. London: Routledge.

Merleau-Ponty, M. (2005). *The phenomenology of perception* (C. Smith, Trans.). London: Taylor & Francis e-Library. (Original work published 1945)

Nunn, C. (1996). *Awareness: What it is, what it does*. London: Routledge.

Perls, F. S. (1947/1969). *Ego, hunger and aggression*. New York: Vintage Books.

Perls, F. S., Hefferline, R. F., & Goodman, P. (1951). *Gestalt therapy: Excitement and growth in the human personality*. London: Souvenir Press.

Perls, L. (1992). *Living at the boundary*. Gouldsboro, ME: The Gestalt Journal Press.

Posner, M. I. (2009). Attention, awareness and mindfulness in psychotherapy. *Studies in Gestalt Therapy*, *3*(2), 13–36.

Skottun, G. (2012). Awareness, teori og praksis [Awareness, theory and practice]. *Norsk Gestalttidsskrift*, *1*(9), 7–25.

Staemmler, F. M. (2012). *Empathy in psychotherapy: How therapists and clients understand each other* (E. J. Hamilton & D. Winter, Trans.). New York: Springer.

van Baalen, D. (2002/2008). Awareness er ikke nok [Awareness is not enough]. In S. Jørstad & Å. Krüger (Eds.), *Den flyvende hollender* [The flying Dutchman] (pp. 70–77). Oslo: NGI.

Wollants, G. (2012). *Gestalt therapy: Therapy of the situation*. London: Sage.

Yontef, G. M. (1993). *Awareness, dialogue & process*. New York: The Gestalt Journal Press.

Chapter 9

Contact

We live and move constantly in and out of different environments, such as family, friends, the city in which we live, work, our school, or new and unfamiliar surroundings. These various settings influence and affect us in different ways, just as we influence and affect our environment. We experience this type of influence in our encounters with others, where a meaningful conversation, a hug, or a smile affects us. We smile back, feel our muscles relax, and experience joy in the moment. We are affected differently by loud, angry voices, angry facial expressions, and words that contain accusations or criticism. These can cause us to hold our breath, take a step back, or go on the attack. We are influenced because we have or initiate contact with each other. In this chapter, we describe what we mean by contact and contact functions in gestalt therapy, how they are expressed in everyday life, and how models can be used in therapeutic practice.

Contact in gestalt therapy

The term 'contact' originates from the Latin word *contingere*, which means 'affect emotionally, move/touch'. One of Perls and Goodman's many definitions of contact relies on this definition: 'Contact is touch touching something' (Perls et al., 1951, p. 373). This definition is recognisable from daily life; we talk about what kind of contact we have with each other, the quality of the contact, how we feel touched by others, and the kind of connection that exists between us. Laura Perls (1992) stressed that: 'contact is nothing one *has*, or *is*, or *stays in* or *out* of. . . . We *make* contact by acknowledging and tackling the *other* and experiencing ourselves in doing so. It is a continuous shuttling or oscillating between *me* and the *other*' (p. 144). The French gestalt theoretician Serge Ginger (1995/2004) described gestalt therapy as the art of contact and claimed that people can learn to become more aware of when they are affected and how they are connected with each other via gestalt therapy.

In gestalt therapy, contact is referred to as 'the simplest and first reality' (Perls et al., 1951, p. 227). According Staemmler (2011), this sentence establishes the

DOI: 10.4324/9781003153856-11

basis for gestalt therapy's intersubjective approach. This means that 'we are always in contact with our surroundings through our senses and have been since we were in the womb. We see, hear, smell, taste, feel touch to the skin, and know movement—we are touched' (Slagsvold, 2016, p. 167, our translation). Human beings are created and shaped by and in our surroundings and cannot live in total isolation over time. Nature, social relations, culture, and politics are important factors that we are a part of. From the beginning, the founders of gestalt therapy were more interested in seeing human beings as part of a field and in a wider context than simply studying the individual in isolation (Kolmannskog, 2018). This is illustrated in the example below in the situation between Beth and Pierre.

Beth is in the kitchen making dinner while her partner Pierre is in the living room, checking his cell phone. Beth is becoming increasingly irritated; she and Pierre had an agreement that they would make dinner together. Pierre is so absorbed in a message that he has completely forgotten the agreement he had with Beth. They are each in their own worlds: Beth in the kitchen, in the midst of dinner preparations and with expectations, and Pierre in the living room, with his cell phone and message.

There are several possibilities for how this situation can develop.

Option 1: Beth decides to go to the living room to Pierre, to see what he is doing. When she sees him sitting with his phone with a worried expression, she strokes his back and says in a friendly voice: 'It looks like you got some bad news.' Pierre looks up, smiles, and says: 'Yeah, I got some news that surprised me, and completely forgot about you and making dinner. I'll be there as soon as I finish answering the message'.

Option 2: Beth shouts from the kitchen with an irritated tone of voice: 'Get in here right away! Have you completely forgotten our agreement?' Pierre does not respond—he is still busy with his phone. Beth storms into the living room, grabs the phone out of Pierre's hand, and shouts: 'I'm so tired of you and that damn phone! It's absolutely impossible to talk to you' and starts to cry. Pierre gets up without a word, takes his phone back, and slams the door as he leaves the room.

We have shown two possible ways in which the situation with Beth and Pierre could go. Both versions say something about the contact between them, how they 'touch' each other. In the first example, Beth goes into the living room to see what is keeping Pierre. She is clearly affected when she sees Pierre's facial expression and is able to put herself into his situation; she sees and hears him. Pierre sees Beth's worried facial expression, hears that she speaks to him in a friendly tone of voice, and senses that she touches his back. This causes him to smile and respond in a pleasant manner. In the second example, their contact is completely different; they neither see nor hear each other. Beth yells from the kitchen while Pierre's attention is entirely geared towards his phone. We recognise that each of these ways of reacting has its basis in the relationship between them, how they were 'connected' to each other, before Beth began making dinner. We also see that the relationship between them changes depending on how they perceive the contact between them.

Contact as an interpersonal phenomenon

These examples show that contact is an interpersonal phenomenon characterised by how individuals see, hear, and understand each other, and the expectations each brings into the situation. It is apparent that Beth and Pierre have differing levels of attention to each other and to the contact between them (see Chapter 8 on awareness). Beth's attention is focused outwards, towards Pierre and dinner, while Pierre's attention is focused inwards, towards the thoughts and feelings he has as he reads the message on his phone. This is a recognisable example of how we sometimes shut out our surroundings and turn our attention inward. In these situations, we have more contact with ourselves than with our environment. The examples also show two ways in which Beth and Pierre regulate the contact between them: in the first example they come nearer to each other, and in the second they create distance between themselves.

Contact with oneself

The expression 'to have contact with oneself' is used in everyday speech to mean being aware of what we feel or know about a situation. If you say: 'Now I have contact with sadness inside me, it is easy to think that you have contact with your feelings. However, this is an indirect way of describing what you perceive, and it is not obvious to the environment what you have contact with. If you instead say: 'Now I feel a lump in my throat and tears are flowing', you give a more precise and phenomenological way of describing the same experience. In addition, it may well be easier for those around you to understand. In gestalt therapy we therefore prefer to say 'to have contact with oneself' as a phenomenological description of what this contact actually means, for example 'I feel a lump in my throat and tears are flowing'.

The term 'contact' in gestalt therapy

The term 'contact' is described in several ways in gestalt theory. For Perls and Goodman (Perls et al., 1951), contact is an encounter between one person and another, or the meeting of a person and her surroundings, in which a form of exchange exists between the two. Contact is the point at which a person meets someone who is different from herself. Perls and Goodman argued that by being aware, we can control our behaviour towards that which is new and possible to assimilate (digest), and avoid that which cannot be digested. They viewed contact as dynamic and creative. They were concerned that we should not act automatically and without attention, but rather stay in touch with ourselves and the world by seeing every situation as new and unique, in which contact is creative adaptation (see also Chapter 6 on creative adjustment).

Polster and Polster (1974) define contact differently, and give an example from the first moments of life:

> In the womb we had it made. All we had to do was swim in the benevolent environment. The catch was that growth beyond a certain limit put an end to the tenancy; we had to get out and, willy nilly, learn to make our own way in a less solicitous world. Since our umbilicaletomy, each of us has become separate beings, seeking union with that which is other than ourselves.
>
> (p. 98)

They go on to say that from this point on, we seek closeness and solidarity on the basis of this experience of separateness. They call this the paradox that we constantly strive to resolve. They argue therefore that 'the function which synthesizes the need for union and for separation is contact' (p. 99). This means that we always have the opportunity to meet our surroundings again and again through contact, through meeting and then ending contact, or through a new meeting with a new ending. People exist between two conflicting needs that are fundamental to contact: the need for distance and for closeness.

The Danish gestalt therapist Hanne Hostrup (2010) describes contact thus:

> Contact consists of three factors: initiation, being with, and withdrawal. Contact requires difference and motion and can be described as a meeting between at least *two separate individuals that includes an exchange* of feelings, words, thoughts, gaze, actions etc. An exchange that produces a *particular meaning*, which each of the parties is able to perceive, interpret (gestalt formation) and respond to.
>
> (p. 134)

Contact in the therapy room

The term 'contact' is often used in gestalt therapy as a description of how the therapist and client meet and interact in the therapy room (Clarkson & Mackewn, 1993). They are always in contact, but the contact can be experienced differently from their individual standpoints and over the course of a therapy session. The therapist will be interested in the nature of the contact she has with the client and will spend a good deal of time examining and increasing the client's awareness. The relationship between them is formed and developed as a result of their being aware and paying attention to the nature of the contact between them. This is illustrated in the following example.

> Marie is new to therapy—this is her first session. She took the initiative by calling the therapist and booking an appointment. She begins to speak as she enters the therapy room, before the therapist has had time to say anything other than her name. Marie sits down on one of the chairs in the room as she speaks, without noticing the therapist or the surroundings. The therapist sits down in a chair opposite Marie and listens to what she says. She is aware that Marie looks straight ahead as she speaks.
>
> After a while the therapist interrupts, 'Hi, Marie. I am glad that you want to tell me all this, and I understand that you need to tell me. But I want you to know something about the person you're talking to, so you can be sure that I'm someone you can confide in. I don't know how accustomed you are to telling strangers about yourself, or if you've been in therapy before'.

Here, the therapist interrupts Marie in the middle of her story because she thinks that Marie is not aware of her and that this affects the contact between them. The therapist is aware that she is not emotionally or physically touched when she hears Marie speak, and thinks that this is a sign that Marie is more absorbed in herself than in contact with the therapist, without being aware of the distance it creates between them. The therapist wants to get closer to Marie and thinks that one way to do so is to join the conversation by saying something about her thoughts, and to ask Marie about her experience with gestalt therapy. This is also a way to bring the relationship between Marie and the therapist into the therapy room here and now.

> MARIE looks briefly at the therapist, and says: 'No, I've never been in therapy before, and I thought that I should tell you about myself and what was difficult, and that your job as a therapist is to listen to me'.
> THE THERAPIST nods and smiles slightly: 'Yes, I also think that I should listen to you, and that you should tell me about you. At the same time, I think you might find that there's a difference between talking to a

person you know well and one who is completely new to you, as I am. It may be that you find it easier to talk about yourself to a stranger, and that you already feel confident enough in me to tell me what's important to you'.

MARIE: 'I guess I haven't thought so much about it . . . I'm the kind of person who just talks away . . . '

And in this way, Marie continues to talk about herself and her problems.

Marie has an idea about how she should be as a client in therapy, which influences the contact between herself and the therapist. The therapist thinks that Marie has a need to be seen and heard during her first therapy session, and that she is not aware of the psychological distance that is created when she simply starts talking without seeing or hearing the therapist. The therapist chooses not to interrupt her a second time, because she believes that it is good for Marie to be able to tell the therapist her story in the way she had planned to.

The session is almost over; the therapist decides to stop Marie, and says: 'Marie, the session is coming to an end, and I think it's important that we book a time for another session. I've enjoyed listening to you, and I think it would be good if you were to spend some more time with me, exploring what you've been talking about. What do you think about that?'

MARIE looks a little surprised, and says: 'Oh, the session is over already, I feel like I've just started getting into what I want to tell you. Yes, I would like to come again, it's been nice to talk to you. I feel like you've been listening to me, even though you haven't said anything'. She looks across at the therapist and smiles slightly. The therapist smiles back and suggests a time for a new session the following week.

At the end of the hour, the contact between Marie and the therapist has changed. They smile at each other, and it seems as if they have come closer to each other compared to when they started. The therapist's choice to listen meant that Marie's initial need was met—namely to tell her story. She felt she had been heard when therapist did not interrupt her. The therapist in turn noticed that Marie looked at her when she did not talk about herself, and that she was able to direct her attention both inward, towards herself, and outward, towards the therapist. The therapist thinks that it is possible to develop the contact between them, something she imagines also can be useful for Marie in her relationships with her environment and the issues she talked about during this first session.

Contact functions

The function of the senses is to develop contact. The term 'contact functions' emphasises this close relationship between the senses and contact (Polster & Polster, 1974). These senses include sight, hearing, taste, smell, physical sensation, touch, motion, and the use of the voice. By training our awareness and attention to how the contact functions are used, we also train our attention to how we are in contact with ourselves and others. How contact is in a given situation is thus related to both what and how we perceive (see Chapter 8 on awareness).

Sensations and interpretations

In gestalt therapy we distinguish between sensation and the meaning or interpretation we create on the basis of our perceptions. What is sensed and how sensation is organised is explored in gestalt psychology as perception and processes of perception (see Chapter 1). Contact functions as described in gestalt theory are based on the theories of the importance of the senses in gestalt psychology, and how we create meaning based on perception. It is important to see that all perception seeks to form meaningful wholes, as formulated by the gestalt psychologists. On the basis of the laws of perception, gestalt psychologists found that the meaning we assign our perceptions does not always match reality, and that two people who see the same tree do not describe that tree in the same way. The fact that we perceive—and organise what we sense—differently, provides innumerable challenges and opportunities for misunderstanding. This is why the gestalt therapist is focused on raising the client's awareness of how she uses her contact functions: how she sees, hears, perceives, and moves, and the meaning she gives to that with which she is in contact.

Wanting to *understand* the other thus involves both sensing and giving meaning to, in the form of interpretation of what is perceived. In the meeting with the other is the possibility of what might be called 'good contact', where conversation flows freely and is unhindered. In this type of meeting we meet the other with good intentions: we intend to listen to what is being said in order to respond, as the first example with Beth and Pierre illustrates. However, despite our good intentions, we can experience that what is said or heard is misunderstood and misinterpreted. This is often called 'bad contact'. One person in the conversation may have expressed herself unclearly, or perhaps the other did not listened carefully enough to what was said. Body language can be confusing, and thus be interpreted differently than intended. In addition, there are also situations in which we do not have good intentions, or are angry, irritated, and in no way willing to see or hear what the other person says, as the second example with Beth and Pierre illustrates. Such situations create fertile ground for further quarrelling and misunderstanding between people, and often require great effort from both to be able to listen to and see the other in a new way.

Misunderstanding and misinterpretation are often the background for what in daily speech is called communication problems, which is related to how people use their contact functions and how they interpret the resulting information. Clients often come to therapy or coaching because they are struggling with communication or contact in their intimate relationships. It is therefore important to acquire knowledge and understanding of what creates good communication, and how it can go wrong.

Working with contact functions in couples' therapy

We return to the beginning of the chapter, where Beth yelled at Pierre and he left the 'scene of the crime' in anger. For the sake of discussion, we imagine that they have continued to argue, and decide to seek out a gestalt therapist.

At one point during the session, the therapist asks the couple to talk together while she listens. It becomes clear to the therapist that neither of them hears what the other says. They look at each other only now and then and sit partially turned away from each other. The therapist tells them what she observes, and asks them, as an experiment, to sit farther apart and turn even more away from each other. They do this and initially continue to talk, but their conversation stops after a short while.

BETH turns more towards Pierre, and says: 'You aren't listening to what I say'. Pierre also turns, and responds: 'That's right, and you're not listening to me, either'.

The therapist asks them to talk about how it feels not to be heard. They continue to experiment by sitting closer to each other while they talk. With support and guidance, they manage to tell each other that they feel lonely and alone, and how scared they both are that the other does not love them anymore. Slowly, they manage to look at each other and take in the significance of what the other says.

In this example, the therapist notices how Pierre and Beth talk to each other, the words they use, the distance between them, and how they position themselves physically. The therapist helps them to try out different ways to talk to each other and to experiment with sitting with varying distance between them. The purpose of this testing and experimentation is to increase their awareness and attention, and to help them experience something new about themselves and each other. The foundation for development in the relationship between Pierre and Beth lies in attention to the phenomenon of 'how we communicate with each other'. This allows them to see each other anew.

This is a constructed example; the process rarely goes so quickly. However, this example does demonstrate that it can be useful to raise awareness of the contact functions in couples therapy: how and whether the clients look at each other, talk and sit, and how seeing the other anew can be easier when they sit in a 'new room' with a 'new person'. (See Chapter 11 to see how experiments are used and attention can be developed.)

Working with contacts functions in therapy

Johanna has come to therapy because she is frightened and has anxiety attacks. She sits with the therapist and talks about how incredibly frightened she can be, especially when she is alone. As she speaks, the therapist notices that Johanna does not look at her. Her breathing appears to be shallow, and the therapist wonders if her muscles are tense.

THERAPIST: 'It looks like you're scared now. Can you feel how you breathe, and notice that you're not looking at me?'

JOHANNA: Glances at the therapist for a few seconds, and almost stops breathing. She says: 'Yes, I'm scared now. I don't know what you think about me, I feel so ashamed . . . '

THERAPIST: 'That sounds like it must be very hard for you. I have tears in my eyes and am holding my own breath as well. Perhaps you can see it if you look at me just for a moment?'

JOHANNA: Looks quickly at the therapist again. 'Yes, but I don't know if I believe you completely, you probably just feel sorry for me'.

THERAPIST: 'I don't feel sorry for you. I'm sitting here with a lot of good feelings for you, have tears in my eyes, and am smiling at you, all at the same time'.

JOHANNA: Looks up at the therapist for a bit longer. She breathes a little more deeply, looks down, then up again. 'Yes, I can see now that you have tears in your eyes and are smiling. It was hard to believe, but I do believe it now'. Johanna smiles hesitantly, breathes, and settles back on her chair.

It helps Johanna to see the therapist and hear what she says; this helps her to move beyond the fear she feels. The therapist also shares what she herself senses, so that Johanna receives information about this (through her sense of hearing) and feels that it is easier to look at her. Here, the therapist deliberately contacts Johanna's contact functions of hearing and sight. It is important that the therapist is sincere about what happens to her so that Johanna can have a new experience of seeing and hearing, and thus can let old experiences and fantasies move to the background. In the therapist's approach we see that a total support that increases the client's attention beyond using her senses, and at the same time appeals to her thoughts and understanding of their situation, gives the client an increased awareness of herself.

The regulation of the contact between therapist and client is important both as part of the therapy process and for the relation between client and therapist (Joyce & Sills, 2014). Knowledge of how this regulation can happen, based on the therapist's understanding of the situation and the use of contact functions, is therefore fundamental. In later chapters on contact, contact forms, and contact processes, we describe how the therapist consciously uses her knowledge of various aspects of contact in her meeting with the client in order to create confidence and increase the client's awareness of what is. Confidence in the therapy room is a prerequisite for the client and the therapist to explore and develop a good relationship, and simultaneously creates confidence in the interaction between therapist and client while the relationship develops.

The contact boundary—a concept in gestalt therapy

In gestalt literature, the term 'contact boundary' is used to describe the distinction between what is 'me' and what is 'you' (Perls et al., 1951). Polster (1974) describes the concept in this way: 'The contact boundary is the point at which one experiences the "me" in relation to that which is not "me" and through this contact both are more clearly experienced' (pp. 102–103). Laura Perls (1992) found the experience and the concept of the *boundary function* most useful when working with patients. She stated:

> The boundary where I and the other meet is the locus of the ego functions of identification and alienation, the sphere of excitation, interest, concern, and curiosity, or of fear and hostility. . . . A small child, before becoming socialized, lives on the boundary: looks at everything, touches everything, gets into everything. He discovers the world, expands his awareness and means of coping in his own pace.
>
> (pp. 149–141)

Latner (1973) has emphasised that this boundary is flexible and is an event created in the moment. He uses the point at which beach and sea meet as a metaphor to describe how we meet our surroundings. In this image, the shoreline is constantly changing, but at the same time consists of both water and

(Continued)

land. The challenge with this image is that it is mainly the water that moves and adapts to the shore it meets. In our view, the same opportunity for movement and flexibility exists for both parties in situations between people. The second challenge is that contact is defined as a boundary phenomenon rather than as a function of the field. A boundary phenomenon can give associations to either-or formulations, such as 'disturbances in the contact process' or 'bad or good contact' (Jørstad, 2002/2008, our translation). Wheeler (1998) argues that we need definitions that refer to the quality of the contact, and notes that the discovery that 'I am me and you are you' needs to be integrated as a phenomenon in itself. Also Staemmler is critical to the use of boundaries in gestalt therapy (1996) and argues viewed against the background of the recent pandemic experiences, that there is no clear boundary between people (2021)

In our opinion, the contact boundary between us is a metaphorical term that refers to my experience of the contact that exists between me and my surroundings. This metaphorical boundary often manifests as various bodily sensations of discomfort when we feel experience that the other comes too near, either physically of psychologically, or there is too much distance between us. Supported by Laura Perls' point of view, we think that the experience of a contact boundary is thus closely related to what were called contact functions in the previous section in this chapter.

Summary

In this chapter, we defined and illustrated the term 'contact' in gestalt therapy and discussed how people's experience of being in contact with each other is closely related to their awareness and attentiveness to each other. Contact functions and contact boundaries were described and the importance of how the senses are used to experience contact with the environment was emphasised.

Contact, contact functions, and attention are key concepts for the therapist in her meeting with the client. The therapist is aware of what happens with the client and herself, how the contact between them is, and how it evolves. The therapist notices how the client contacts her, uses her contact functions, and the extent to which the client sees, hears, and is aware of her surroundings. The therapist regulates the physical and psychological distance between herself and the client, depending on what she thinks is useful in the given situation.

The term 'contact' is fundamental in all gestalt theory and has therefore occurred in several places in this text. The direct relationship between the terms 'contact' and 'contact functions', described in this section, appear later—in Part 3 (contact forms) and Chapter 19 (contact processes).

References

Clarkson, P., & Mackewn, J. (1993). *Fritz Perls*. London: Sage Publications.

Ginger, S. (1995/2004). *Gestalt therapy: The art of contact*. Paris: Marabout-EPG.

Hostrup, H. (2010). *Gestalt therapy: An introduction to the basic concepts of gestalt therapy* (D. H. Silver, Trans.). Copenhagen: Hans Reitzlers Forlag. (Original work published 1999)

Jørstad, S. (2002/2008). Oversikt over kontaktformer [Overview of contact forms]. In S. Jørstad & Å. Krüger (Eds.), *Den flyvende hollender* [The flying Dutchman] (pp. 128–139). Oslo: NGI.

Joyce, P., & Sills, C. (2014). *Skills in gestalt counselling & psychotherapy* (3rd ed.). London: Sage.

Kolmannskog, V. (2018). *The empty chair*. London: Routledge.

Latner, J. (1973). *The gestalt therapy book*. New York: Julian.

Perls, F. S., Hefferline, R. F., & Goodman, P. (1951). *Gestalt therapy: Excitement and growth in the human personality*. London: Souvenir Press.

Perls, L. (1992). *Living at the boundary*. Gouldsboro, ME: The Gestalt Journal Press.

Polster, E., & Polster, M. (1974). *Gestalt therapy integrated*. New York: Vintage Books.

Slagsvold, M. (2016). *Jeg blir til i møte med deg* [I become me together with you]. Oslo: Cappelen, Damm.

Staemmler, F. M. (1996). Grenze? – Welche Grenze? – Zur Problematik eines zentralen gestalttherapeutischen Begriffs [Boundary? – Which boundary? – On the pitfalls of a central term in gestalt therapy]. *Integrative Therapie, 22*(1), 36–55.

Staemmler, F. M. (2011). Kontakt som første virkelighet: Gestaltterapi som en intersubjektiv tilnærming [Contact as a first reality: Gestalt therapy as an intersubjective approach]. *Norsk Gestalttidsskrift, 8*(1), 7–20.

Staemmler, F. M. (2021). Det finnes ingen innside/utside – Om sammenviklingen av det kroppslig selv og det biososiale miljø som grunnlag for tilhørighet og medfølelse [There is no inside/outside – On the entanglement of bodily self and biosocial environment as a basis for connectedness and compassion. *Norsk Gestalttidsskrift, 18*(1), 10–19.

Wheeler, G. (1998). *Gestalt reconsidered: A new approach to contact and resistance* (2nd ed.). Cambridge, MA: GICPress.

Chapter 10

Polarities

> Alice is quiet and shy. When together with others she usually stays in the background and lets others talk and keep the conversation going. Paul, however, is outgoing. He is able to start up a conversation easily, and often does so when together with others. These are two different ways of being; both Alice and Paul have the potential to be more than just one of them. In some situations, Alice can also be outgoing, especially when together with her best friend. In those instances, she finds it easy to talk—she says a lot and takes a lot of space. Paul can be shy and hold back when he is asked to give a speech in large gatherings.

The story of Alice and Paul is an example of how people can be more than one thing, depending on the field in which they find themselves and the needs they have at a given moment. In this ability to be more than one thing lies the potential for development and discovery. When Paul becomes familiar with and recognises that he is extroverted and Alice sees that she is quiet and shy, the opportunity arises to discover the other polarities, where Paul can be shy and Alice talkative. Polster and Polster (1974) define polarities in this way: 'Whenever an individual recognizes one aspect of himself, the presence of its antithesis, or polar quality, is implicit' (p. 61).

In this chapter, we show how Fritz Perls used ideas from Lewin's field theory, Friedlaender's theory of the organism, as well as holistic and Buddhist ideas, and elaborate the concept of polarities in light of needs, fear and desire, detecting contrasting and developing flexible polarities, 'topdog–underdog', and discuss polarities as an existential theme.

Polarities and needs in the field

Opposites are interdependent: light cannot exist without darkness nor darkness without light; they predetermine each other and are interconnected polarities (Clarkson & Mackewn, 1993). Polarities therefore occur in pairs, described as opposing complementary forces, subject to each other. Friedlaender's philosophic

DOI: 10.4324/9781003153856-12

theory of creativity and polarities (Frambach, 2003) has its point of departure in his idea that all phenomena must be different from and oppose something else in order to be recognised and appreciated. This difference—or 'differentiation', as he called it—creates 'the world of figures' and has to do with how phenomena form. The most basic principle of creation, which structures the unique differences in a given phenomenon, arises in polarities. All reality can be explained in polar relationships, such as plus and minus, in and out, big and small, high and low, near and far, etc. (see Chapter 3).

When opposites are illustrated as two polar extremes of a line with a zero point of pre-differentiation in the middle, they are seen to be essential aspects of each other, as shown by Fritz Perls' example (1947/1969, p. 19).

	Zero point	
Beginning	Middle	End
Past	Present	Future
Convexity	Flatness	Concavity

Contrasts or polarities are needed in order to form clear, strong figures of interest against an indifferent background. This way of thinking of polarities is a holistic conception of difference. In gestalt therapy we are interested in both the qualities that separate and the qualities that bring together the polar aspects of the field. We explore the differences and the interdependences within the organism/environment field.

As human beings we organise our needs in *polar opposites*, where we constantly explore which needs are important to meet, which need is in the foreground and which can go to the background (Clarkson & Mackewn, 1993). A need or desire creates immediate fear and resistance. These are polar needs in the field where the need for the new is in conflict with the need to maintain the status quo.

In addition to field theory and figure-ground formation, the gestalting process—which describes how we regulate our needs—is also important for the understanding of what is meant by polarities in gestalt therapy. With reference to biology, Perls felt that humans always seek to maintain a balance, an equilibrium, in what we experience. When the organism is fatigued, it will put a great deal of effort into seeking wakefulness. Perls called this organismic quest for balance the principle of homeostasis. It is this quest to meet the basic need for physical and mental balance that is the core, the driving force, for all life. Perls believed that there will always be opposing forces that affect this need for balance, whether the interference is external or comes from within the person himself. Hunger, excitement, and emotions will continually bring us out of balance. There is an ongoing process between the forces within us that wants to contact and integrate that which is new and resistance to experiencing that which is new (Perls, 1947/1969; see also Part 1, Chapter 3).

The therapist can work with these conflicting forces or needs by alternately creating a safe or challenging environment for the client. In gestalt therapy we are interested in both the forces that unite us and those that divide us, and in the qualities that bring the polar aspects of the field together. We explore the differences and interdependence of polar opposites with the client in the therapeutic situation.

The desire–fear model

The tension that is created between multiple and conflicting needs means that we must make choices that can often be challenging. The choice that is the most natural and easiest for us is what is known and safe (see the law of *prägnanz*, pp. 10–11). Life has taught us to adjust creatively and to create security and predictability (see Chapter 6 on creative adjustment). The model in Figure 10.1 shows the relationship between the desire and the need for something new, and its opposite: fear of what the new can entail. On one hand we see the desire and the need to perform a specific action, and on the other we see the counterforce that is experienced as resistance or fear of what the action might trigger.

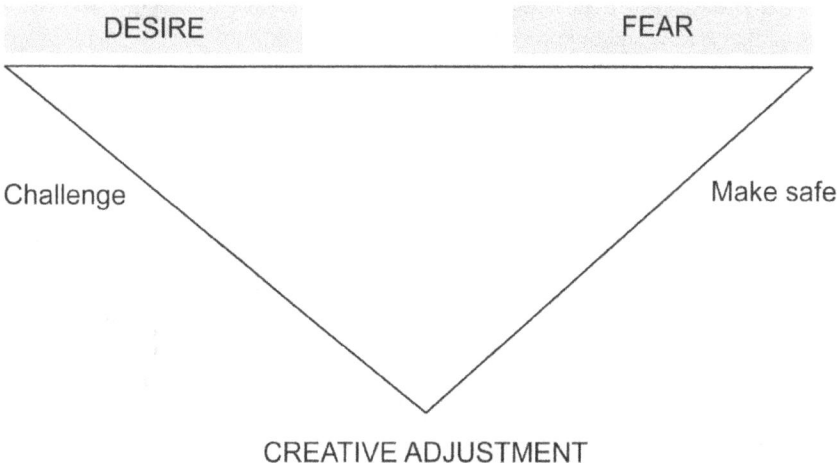

Figure 10.1 The model for desire – fear.

In order to dare to choose something new, the need for 'new' must be more appealing than 'the usual'. In therapy, it is often important to explore and raise awareness of one or both sides of the model so that the client can make a more conscious choice. This is illustrated in the following example.

Therese is a gentle woman who takes time making decisions, even when it comes to going into therapy and choosing a therapist. At the first session, she tells the therapist about how much time she spends making choices and how burdensome she feels it is to have to make choices at all. She sits on the edge of her chair and speaks softly. In conversation with the therapist, Therese becomes aware that she can choose, but that it takes time when she is afraid. Fear is often predominant, and it can be difficult to sense desire. She has avoided many challenges due to fear and has instead chosen that which felt safe.

She tells the therapist that her partner wants children, but she does not know if she dares. She is afraid to give birth and of the responsibility involved in caring for a small child. She has had a painful and difficult childhood herself and does not know if she will be a good mother. Therese decided to go into therapy when one of her friends told her she was pregnant. She felt a twinge of envy and wanted to take the feeling seriously. It occurred to her that although she was afraid and uncertain, she perhaps also had a desire to have children.

Here, Therese tells the therapist that it was the twinge she felt when her friend told her she was pregnant that triggered her choice to go into therapy. She has a feeling that is new and unknown to her, and wants to explore whether she perhaps wants, and is not only afraid, to have children. She becomes more aware of her need to go into therapy, which leads her to her book an appointment with a therapist.

The therapist focuses on the situation in which Therese felt a twinge of envy, and asks her to tell more about the physical sensation. Therese says that it was like a stab in the chest. She felt actual pain and indicates where the pain was located with her hand. The therapist asks her to keep her hand on the area where she felt pain as she notices the pain and describes what she senses as she talks about her friend and the fact that she is pregnant.

THERESE: 'When I hold my hand here, it's like the twinge is more like a vague pain. At the same time, it's like my skin softens under my hand'.
THERAPIST: 'So you feel a vague pain and that your skin softens?'

THERESE NODS AND SAYS: 'Yes, it's like the pain is a kind of longing in my chest, maybe I actually want to have children . . . ' She moves her hand against her skin.

THERAPIST: 'Just take a moment to feel what it's like to move your hand'.

After a bit, Therese says she feels calm; it's as if she feels the desire to have children without the accustomed feelings of insecurity and fear.

The therapist chooses to explore the unknown pole by asking Therese to be aware of the twinge she felt by placing her hand on her chest. This allows Therese to bring the experience she had with her friend to the situation here and now, together with the therapist. She experiences that the twinge changes, and the yearning for and the desire to have children becomes more prominent.

After exploring one pole (the desire to have children represented by the twinge in her chest), the therapist and Therese explore fear, which is the other pole. Because Therese is already well acquainted with this fear, it may be that the therapist and Therese can experiment with letting the desire to have children face the fear, and thereby clarify her choice.

Polarities and conflicting needs

The following is an example from a coaching session in which the client experiences conflicting needs.

Bonnie is on sick leave for the first time in her life. She is conscientious and likes her job. She has three children and a new partner, and she says that she is torn between having to satisfy many different needs at home and at work and doing things she herself enjoys. She sleeps poorly and is very tired. Her colleagues want her back at work, something she herself would like. At the same time, she feels exhausted and that she really wants to give in to her need to be at home.

The coach follows up what Bonnie said about her needs and asks if they can explore the theme; Bonnie says yes.

THE COACH extends her arm out to the side and says: 'On the one hand, you feel like being at home'. She then stretches her other arm out to the other side and says: 'On the other hand, you feel you should return to work'.

BONNIE looks at her, stretches out her arms, and says: 'It's as if I'm a scale that's trying to balance, but I don't feel like I'm balanced right now'.

> She lowers her right arm and lifts the left up. She says: 'I'm really out of balance in my life!' She continues: 'My feeling of duty is way up here, it dominates me, and my desire and need for rest and to just be is missing. Or maybe it's the opposite right now; now my fatigue and the desire to rest is up, and it's my sense of duty that's down'.
> She shifts position: her left arm goes up and her right arm goes down. 'Maybe I should do what my doctor says and stay on sick leave'.

Bonnie's choice of metaphor for her imbalance and the excitement she felt between her conflicting needs helped her to become aware of how she struggles. It is not easy for Bonnie to stay on sick leave, but at the same time it is as if this work with polarities allows her body and entire being to become aware of how tired she is. Through her 'scale' movements she has a bodily experience and an insight into the imbalance she experiences, and into what she needs to create more balance in her life.

Here, we see the poles to need to rest/be on sick leave, and the need to work/go to work set up on each side. It is the tension between these polarities that is explored in therapy and coaching, as the example above and Figure 10.2 illustrate.

In therapy and coaching, we are interested in the client being able to identify with both poles, even if she prefers one over the other. A lot of energy is tied up when we do not recognise that both sides are parts of us (Clarkson & Mackewn, 1993).

Discovering opposite polarities

There are an infinite number of possible polarities in us at all times. Polarities can be explored, and can be described as different sides of ourselves, such as: 'I can be kind and easy going, but also angry and rough. I can feel hurt, and I can hurt others'. It is also true that a single side of a personality can have several possible polarities, depending on the individual and the field she is a part of. For some, the opposite of being angry is to be kind, while for others it is to be patient. In the example above, Bonnie acknowledges that she can be a person who is on sick leave and a person who can go to work, even though she prefers one over the other.

It is not uncommon to become acquainted with only one aspect of who we are, and thus be locked into a one-sided perception of ourselves. The assumption is that we ignore the opportunity to discover and acknowledge the range of diversity in ourselves. It is as if we have a tendency to freeze (Polster & Polster, 1974, p. 61) or be locked in a socialised conception of ourselves: 'I am someone who

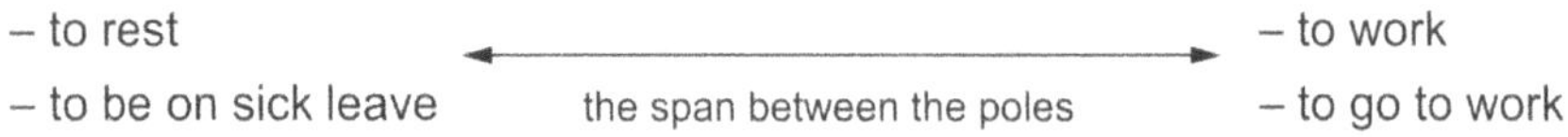

– to rest		– to work
– to be on sick leave	the span between the poles	– to go to work

Figure 10.2 Two poles and the span between them.

is never taken by surprise' or 'I could never hurt my child'. It is as if this frozen form defines us and perhaps even become an obstacle to discovery and insight. In gestalt therapy, emphasis is placed on developing better balance in life by facilitating processes where the client can explore unknown aspects of herself or ways of being. The work done in the therapy room makes it possible to discover new sides of oneself and expand one's repertoire, which in turn allows the individual to react spontaneously to situations as they occur, and to make good choices based on an attention to the here and now (Dyrkorn & Dyrkorn, 2010). The following is an example of gestalt supervision, where Grete explores new aspects of herself.

Grete becomes familiar with her voice in gestalt supervision

Grete is a newly qualified elementary school teacher. Being a new teacher is demanding and is the reason she chooses to be part of a regular supervision group. She enjoys her pupils, but sometimes struggles with discipline.

Her gestalt supervisor notices that Grete speaks softly; she often finds it difficult to hear what she says. When Grete talks about the challenges she faces in the class, her supervisor wonders if discipline in the class is in some way connected to Grete's soft voice.

SUPERVISOR: 'I notice that you speak softly, Grete, and that I have to concentrate to hear what you say'.
GRETE: 'Yes, others have made the same comment. Typical me. I don't know ... '

The supervisor knows that Grete's voice has an opposite pole, and invites her to participate in an experiment. Grete is familiar with this way of exploring and is eager to try.

SUPERVISOR: 'How would you describe the soft voice, do you think?'
GRETE: 'It's quiet and also a little introverted'. She stands up and shows the introvert, with bowed head and neck. The supervisor encourages her to experiment with exaggerating this introspective position.
GRETE: 'The soft voice feels like protection, like I don't have to be so specific'.

The supervisor encourages her to take a few steps forward to create some distance from the 'soft voice'. Grete walks a few metres away and stands there.

SUPERVISOR: 'Can you still sense "the person with the low voice" standing there?'

GRETE: 'Yes! This is weird. I see her standing quietly with her head bowed, she's kind of introverted. But when I stand here now, I'm more outgoing and louder!'

The supervisor supports this discovery and encourages Grete to experiment with 'loud'.

After they have marvelled together over this discovery and Grete has tried out the two positions again, the supervisor encourages her to stand in an intermediate position, between 'soft' and 'loud'.

SUPERVISOR: 'Is it true for you that you're both soft and loud?' The supervisor asks Grete to take her time so that she can make this discovery her own.

GRETE (after having first searched for the right words): 'I have a soft voice, and I can be loud. And maybe I can practice being loud together with some of the boys in the class', she concludes with a smile.

Here we see how the supervisor first points out Grete's soft voice and then proposes an experiment to make her aware of what her body expresses when she speaks. When Grete moves a few steps away from where she stood as 'soft voice', she becomes aware that the soft voice has an opposite pole, 'to be loud'. Upon further experimentation with the unknown pole, she experiences how she can speak in a loud and powerful voice. When she stands in an intermediate position, she becomes aware that she can speak with both soft and loud voices. Grete understands that this discovery is important in her work as a teacher, where there is a need to be loud. This is the background for her need for supervision.

The theory of polarities emphasises that inherent in any pole is its opposite. To explore polarities is to become familiar with a range of opportunities in oneself and in meetings with others. When we become acquainted with opposite poles, their differences are made clearer to us. This clarification of each of the poles facilitates the integration and recognition of the possibility of a situation where both exist. Polster and Polster (1974) point out that this integration of poles is also seen in the dialectic theory of how thesis and antithesis are integrated into synthesis.

Polarities and the dialectical process

The theory of polarities has deep roots in gestalt-therapeutic theory and practice. Perls saw living as a continuous process between being close to and retreating from others. Latner (1986) describes this close relationship between life and polarities as the very basis of the organism's adaptation to its environment (see Chapter 5 on creative adjustment).

Polster and Polster (1974) point out that this inseparable connection between two poles—that one pole does not exist without the other—describes a dialectical process. When two poles are markedly different, the stage is set for a process whereby the opposite could evolve into something completely new and result in new insight: 'The relationship of the opposites is that the existence of one necessarily requires the existence of the other.... The interaction between polarities functions as a dialectical process' (Latner, 1986, p. 29). Any thesis always involves an antithesis and allows for a synthesis. Thus, the theory of polarities links gestalt therapeutic theory to our existential roots and dialectical thinking.

Developing flexible polarities

In polarity work we seek to develop flexibility. Zinker (1977) uses the expression 'stretching the self-concept' (p. 202), or more precisely, stretching our notion of ourselves, as the example with Grete illustrates. By being in contact with her 'soft-voice' self, Grete is able to amplify it and to clarify what it actually means to her to be quiet and introspective. In this way, the opposite pole—being loud—has the opportunity to emerge. When something is amplified and clarified there is also a possibility that its opposite might appear. Grete recognises that she is quiet and introverted. When she gives this experience increased attention, she finds the space to see that she can also be powerful and talk loudly.

An experience of shame can come to the surface in polarity work. There may be aspects of life that are not easy to recognise and accept—sides of our personalities that are buried and forgotten because they are not consistent with how something 'should' be. For example, it can be challenging to realise that the polarity of being generous is being stingy. When we were children, we might have experienced that shame was associated with being stingy. This may seem trivial to some, but for others it can be important to acknowledge that this 'stinginess' that is associated with shame is part of being oneself. It is important that we experience support and recognition for the unacceptable aspects of ourselves as we explore them in therapy. When the feeling of shame can be shared, the feeling may change, and it can become easier to see a side of ourselves we previously might have avoided. As we acknowledge and realise that we contain both polarities, it creates greater insight into who we are and opens up the possibility to be ourselves. This creates greater flexibility in the way we meet others.

Joyce and Sills (2014) point out that to acknowledge and realise an opposite pole does not always mean the client puts this experience into practice. Recognising aspects of ourselves, such as 'I'm homicidal' or 'I'm jealous' does not mean that we put this knowledge into practice, but rather that we recognise and realise that this capacity exists within us. It is therefore important that the therapist or coach clarifies this in therapy or coaching.

Discovering oneself in the other

Not acknowledging sides or polarities in ourselves can easily cause internal conflicts between the sides we do not like. These inner conflicts can also evolve into conflict in relationships (Zinker, 1977), as the example of Grete shows. Most of us can probably recognise that it is easier to see sides that we like and dislike in others than it is to recognise them in ourselves (see projections in Chapter 13). It is often more immediate and perhaps even more convenient to accuse others than to face our own bad sides or even recognise our own strengths. Clients who come to therapy because of difficult relationships with their partners or associates often benefit greatly from exploring what annoys them in others. This can enable them to discover that their irritation has to do with aspects of themselves they neither know nor like.

Zinker (1977) reminds us of the fine line between condemning others and rejecting and condemning ourselves. The challenge is to turn our focus inward and become familiar with the projection. In this way, we can experience that both sides reside within ourselves, also when together with others. We can also look for those aspects or features we miss in ourselves in other people. This often manifests itself when we fall in love, as the following example illustrates.

Hannah is shy and reticent and has had low self-esteem as long as she can remember. She has lived alone for quite some time and thinks that this is because she is shy and is not comfortable with taking initiative, such as taking the first step in getting to know men.

One day she enters the therapy room breathless, smiling from ear to ear. She met a man! Patrick! He is just amazing. *He* takes the initiative. He waits on her hand and foot and makes her feel good. She tells the therapist excitedly that it feels as if something has fallen into place in her, something she previously lacked. 'He fills out the picture I have of myself. It's as if he makes me a whole person'. Hannah is over the moon.

The therapist rejoices with Hannah. They talk about what it means to her that Patrick 'fills out her picture of herself'. It is as if Hannah feels that 'Patrick is perfect' and 'I'm not perfect'. When this thought occurs to the therapist, she proposes to explore these statements in chair work (see Chapter 10 on experiments).

The therapist and Hannah set out two additional chairs, one representing Patrick and one for Hannah. Hannah moves between the chairs, speaking alternately as herself and as Patrick.

HANNAH: 'Patrick, you're perfect!'

PATRICK: 'I'm not sure what you mean when you say that I'm perfect'.

HANNAH: 'What I like best is that you take the initiative. I would never dare to ask you out, as you did with me'.

PATRICK: 'Yes, I can be outgoing in situations where I know people . . .'

Hannah stops and is silent. The therapist suggests that she go out of the experiment and return to her original chair. Hannah looks at the therapist, still quiet.

THERAPIST: 'You became quiet. What do you notice?'

HANNAH, still wondering: 'I notice strength and a strong energy when I play Patrick'.

THERAPIST: 'Your strength?'

HANNAH: 'Yes, it's my strength'. She stands up with outstretched arms and hands and says: 'Yes, it's my power!'

THERAPIST: 'Yes, your power! Can you repeat that as you remember the feeling you had when you initially were yourself?'

HANNAH: 'I am strength . . . and I'm also still shy and cautious. I'm powerful, and I'm shy. Both fit me right now!'

Hannah becomes aware that she feels strength when she plays Patrick, and she acknowledges that this strength is in herself. She can thus gradually integrate both the new, 'I can be strength', and what was known, 'I can be shy and cautious'. This recognition opens the possibility for contact with the fact that she can be both, an experience of integration that provides new opportunities for insight.

Various theories of polarities in gestalt therapy

The theories of polarities we have described have some fundamental differences, which we briefly elaborate here. Opposites are seen as complementary and interdependent in dialectic thinking. There is a thesis and an antithesis, which will hopefully lead to a synthesis. One does not exist without the other, as we described previously and as is illustrated in the examples of Grete and Bonnie.

In Lewin's field theory this interdependence is seen differently. Tension is created in the field when there are contradictory needs. Needs in the field organise themselves in figure-background processes, as we described earlier. We can see the organisation of the figure against the background of a field as two polarities, where our needs attract our interest and come into the foreground while the needs of others enter into the background (Perls, 1969).

(Continued)

Which of these theoretical models a therapist chooses in a therapy situation will depend on the situation the client brings in. This will in turn affect how the therapist works with the client, and how she intervenes and experiments. In therapeutic practice the therapist uses these models interchangeably, often without even realising she is doing so. In many cases the therapist can begin by exploring the client's different needs in order to discover that two of the needs are particularly contradictory, as we see in the example of Bonnie.

The therapist often chooses polarity work when clients bring in aspects of themselves that they do not like or when there are sides of themselves with which they are not familiar, and there is a need to integrate and learn to live with and acknowledge oneself as one is. In the example of Grete, we see how the therapist senses a polarity in Grete that may be helpful for her to become familiar with in her work as a teacher. In the field with her students, Grete needs to speak loudly to create discipline, and we see how this need becomes figure for her through an 'aha' experience in the example.

When clients are in situations where they are faced with choices, where tensions between conflicting needs are prominent, the therapist works less with polarities per se and more on raising awareness of the conflicting needs in the field. By enhancing one or more of the needs, the client's choices may become clearer to her. Thus, one figure becomes more pronounced than others.

We show how the polarities 'topdog–underdog' are complementary and formed by the needs of the client in the field.

Topdog–underdog

Perls (1969) has formulated a classic and easily recognisable description of how polarities can present themselves, which he called 'topdog–underdog'. The term is a metaphor for a conflict that can be either between sides in ourselves or between two or more people.

The expression is taken from the description of how dogs check the power relationship between them when they meet: who is at the top of the hierarchy, and who is below. This distribution of power becomes clear when the dog that subjects itself to the authority of the other lies down flat on the ground as the other stands over it, snapping and growling. If we transfer this metaphor to human beings, we see that the power struggle has to do with how we attempt to stay in control and determine whose wishes will prevail. The 'topdog' is the stronger, the one who shows authority and knows best. The 'underdog' is the one who can be managed and decided over by the other, and who allows herself to become a victim. Perls (1969) points out that it is not obvious that the topdog is always the one with the most power, even though it might appear so. Although the topdog gives strict orders, the underdog can choose to become passive and helpless. As Perls points out, the underdog strategy can be equally effective: 'The underdog usually is very canny and controls the topdog with other means like *mañana* or "You're right," or "I try my best," or "I tried so hard," or "I forgot," things like that' (p. 106).

An example of a 'topdog–underdog''relationship is often seen among parents and children, in which the mother, the topdog, asks her son to clean his room, and the son responds as the underdog: 'Sure, right after I . . . ' A little later she asks again, and now she is annoyed. The son apologises and says he just needs to do something first. Often it ends with the mother becoming angry and starting to clean herself, or that the son cleans, but is cross. Whatever the result, it is uncomfortable for the mother, and the son has shown his strength in the power struggle.

Topdog–underdog in therapy

Both therapists and coaches meet the topdog–underdog phenomenon in the therapeutic field. Often it manifests itself as an internal conflict between one who is very critical, knows best, and gives advice, and another who is apologetic, gives up, and is helpless. In therapy the client can speak very critically about herself and everything she ought to but does not manage to do, and how hopeless she is. At the same time, she excuses herself and explains how difficult things are for her. We show an example of this from a therapy session with Hannah that takes place after Patrick has ended their relationship.

Inner dialogue between 'topdog' and 'underdog'

Hannah is distraught and angry that Patrick broke up with her. She criticises herself because she could not hang on to him. She feels that it was her fault that he left and that she will not be able to find a new boyfriend. The therapist explores Hannah's inner power struggle in chair work, where one chair is called 'the critic' and the other 'helpless'.

CRITIC: 'You'll never be able to get a new boyfriend, you're just pathetic and helpless'. Hannah moves to the other chair.
HELPLESS: 'Don't be so critical, it makes me sad, and there's no way I can do anything when you're so strict'.
CRITIC: 'You sound like a victim, as if you can't manage anything. You have to pull yourself together and start to look around right away'.

> The dialogue continues in this way, going back and forth between criticism and defensiveness. The therapist asks Hannah to get up and stand with her, and to look at the two chairs and reflect on what she 'sees and hears' as well as on the 'relationship' between the chairs. Hannah says that it does not feel good to look at them; they are so entrenched in their opinions and the conversation is not going anywhere. She adds that she recognises this in herself—she feels that she has stagnated and would rather feel movement in her life.
>
> With her point of departure in Hannah's own words, the therapist asks her to try the chairs as two versions of herself, one that has 'stagnated' and one that is 'on the move'. Hannah explores the two new positions and experiences that she is capable of both stagnating and being in motion, and that this is more meaningful for her than being critical and helpless.

In the initial chair work, Hannah becomes aware that she stagnates. The 'top-dog' critic and the helpless 'underdog' form each other in a relationship that lacks movement. As Hannah becomes aware of stagnation, she discovers the need for movement. This leads to spontaneous insight and *paradoxical change*.

The therapist wonders if the desire for movement might be an important need, and explores this with Hannah in the second round of chair work. In the second dialogue, Hannah experiences that she is capable both of being in motion and of being someone who has stagnated. Here, we see two polarities that have tension between them, a tension Hannah can explore in subsequent therapy sessions.

The internal polarisation between topdog and underdog can also be expressed between the client and her surroundings in different forms of power struggle. We can imagine that this might have been the situation between Hannah and Patrick when he ended their relationship. If the therapist thinks that this is the case, the chair work between the client and the person with whom the client is in conflict can be a way to make the client aware of the underlying conflict she has. Instead of having an internal conversation with herself, Hannah might for example have a conversation with 'Patrick' in an empty chair. In this way, she can recognise aspects of herself in the conflict with Patrick. This can in many situations be equivalent to working with projections, as described in Chapter 13.

Polarities and existential themes in therapy

Life's major questions make themselves known in polarity work. Conflict is inherent in life themes: life and death, meaning and meaninglessness, loneliness and a sense of belonging, responsibility and denial of responsibility, and the wish to be perfect and not being good enough are themes clients often bring into therapy. These issues can at times can be perceived as urgent and existential (see Chapter 2; Masquelier, 2002). Clients can come to therapy because they are in an existential crisis, or they can become aware of an existential crisis during therapy (Ingersoll, 2005).

When clients bring in existential themes or crises, therapists often look for possible polarities. In a situation where a client has just lost her husband, the therapist will first explore and be present in the grief and loss, then go to what it is like for the client to be alive. If a client is not sure that she wants to live, the therapist will explore the client's relationship to death and what she has to live for. There are also many clients who come to therapy because they feel that they are inadequate and are afraid to make mistakes. In those cases, the therapist often sees that a fear of not being perfect can be found below the surface. Here we discuss the contradiction between perfection and doing the best we can. Meaning and meaninglessness are also two polarities that appear in different forms in therapy, as the following therapy session with Hannah shows.

Hannah has come to a new session. She talks about how miserable and sad she feels after her relationship with Patrick ends. She is no longer angry with him, but no longer sees a reason to live; it is as if everything is grey and drab. The therapist takes hold of what Hannah says, and asks her to tell more about what grey and drab mean to her. Hannah does so, and after a while, the therapist asks her to describe the opposite of grey and drab. Hannah hesitates, but eventually responds that there are lots of colours, a lot of movement, and joy. As she speaks, she smiles slightly, and there is a bit more movement in her body. The therapist asks her to describe a situation in which she has experienced colour, movement, and joy. Hannah immediately responds that that was how it was when she was with Patrick and describes several situations where she felt happy and colourful. When she says, she smiles. The colour returns to her face, and she moves in her chair. After a short while she stops smiling and again becomes sad and serious. She is back in the second polarity.

The therapist asks Hannah to stand and repeat the following sentence while moving between two points on the floor: I can be depressed and sad, and I can be colourful, in motion, and happy. Eventually, Hannah ends up standing in the middle between the two points. She says: 'I'm depressed and sad, and I'm colourful, in motion, and happy, and that's me right now. She smiles a little as she looks at the therapist and says that it's true, she is both, and now she feels the future holds meaning and hope.

Here, the therapist explored Hannah's experience of meaninglessness. As she explored the polarity of being depressed and sad, the opposite polarity appeared spontaneously: colours, movement, and joy. When Hannah acknowledges that both poles are known to her, and that she contains both poles, she is experiencing meaning and hope—the opposite of meaninglessness. We recognise that Hannah's desire to live increases when she says that she feels hope, and the polarities 'meaninglessness' and 'death' go to the background.

Summary

In this chapter, we have shown how gestalt therapists and supervisors work with polarities. The term is defined and elaborated in light of polarities and needs, fear and desire, detecting opposite poles, developing flexible poles, the polarity pair 'topdog–underdog', and finally in a section on polarities as an existential theme.

Process and movement are created by contradictions, polarities, and the tension that exists between these contradictions or poles. The therapist is interested in both stagnation and movement because this in itself may be a polarity pair, but also because the client must first be aware of her own position. It is the client's recognition of herself in her situation that leads to change and further movement. The therapist's sensitivity along the way is support for the client's process towards new discovery. 'The client must be guided through contact with both poles to the point where polarities work together in a unified manner' (Ingersoll, 2005, p. 147).

Many of the examples of therapeutic practices outlined later in this book are based on the theory of polarities, in particular the classic experiments and chair work (Chapters 11–17) and contact forms (Part 3).

References

Clarkson, P., & Mackewn, J. (1993). *Fritz Perls*. London: Sage Publications.

Dyrkorn, R., & Dyrkorn, R. (2010). *Innføring i gestaltveiledning: Teori, metode, praktiske eksempler* [Introduction to gestalt supervision: Theory, method, practical examples]. Oslo: Universitetsforlaget.

Frambach, L. (2003). The weighty world of nothingness: Salomo Friedlaender's "Creative indifference". In M. Spagnuolo Lobb & N. Amendt-Lyon (Eds.), *Creative license: The art of gestalt therapy*. Wien: Springer Verlag.

Ingersoll, R. E. (2005). Gestalt therapy and spirituality. In A. L. Woldt & S. M. Toman (Eds.), *Gestalt therapy, history, theory and practice*. Thousand Oaks, CA: Sage.

Joyce, P., & Sills, C. (2014). *Skills in gestalt counselling & psychotherapy* (3rd ed.). London: Sage.

Latner, J. (1986). *The gestalt therapy book*. Gouldsboro, ME: Gestalt Journal Press.

Masquelier, G. (2002). *Gestalt therapy: Living creatively today* (K. Griffin & S. Reeder, Trans.). Paris: Author.

Perls, F. S. (1947/1969). *Ego, hunger and aggression*. London: Vintage Books.

Perls, F. S. (1969). *Gestalt therapy verbatim*. Highland, NY: The Gestalt Journal Press.

Polster, E., & Polster, M. (1974). *Gestalt therapy integrated*. New York: Vintage Books.

Zinker, J. (1977). *Creative process in gestalt therapy*. New York: Random House.

Chapter 11

Experiments

The experiment's place in therapy

In gestalt therapy, we have an open attitude toward the client. We believe that as therapists we cannot know what a person really needs or predict how our presence and interventions will affect her. This attitude helps us to be mindful of the client's response from moment to moment and to focus on our most important task: the ongoing exploration of the client's attention to her own experiences. This exploration occurs frequently in the conversation between the therapist and the client without the therapist proposing an experiment. It could just as easily occur via the spoken and body language with which the therapist addresses the client. As Fritz Perls himself says in Perls et al. (1951):

> the therapeutic interview is experimental from moment to moment in the sense of 'try it out and see what happens'. The patient is taught to *experience himself.* 'Experience' derives from the same Latin source—*experiri*, to try—as does the word 'experiment', and the dictionary gives for it precisely the sense that we intend here, namely, 'the actual living through an event or events'.
>
> (p. 262)

Perls often used experiments with his clients as part of the therapeutic conversation, and claimed that these experiments made it possible for the client to experience something new. The experiment is one of the cornerstones of experiential learning; by experimenting, we move from talking about something to doing or experiencing. Rather than explain and theorise, the client can use her imagination to immerse herself in situations and be present here and now with new experiences. The experiment makes it possible for the client to take an active part in the exploration of herself and to take ownership of her own learning process. Anything can manifest itself here and now in a therapy session, and transform dreams, imaginings, memories, and hopes into a lively and dynamic process between client and therapist (Zinker, 1977).

DOI: 10.4324/9781003153856-13

An experiment is the search for phenomenological data. It is an intervention and active technique that can increase the cooperation between the therapist and client and increase client awareness and attention. In an experiment, the therapist and client work together in order for the client to have a new and better understanding of her situation. Therapist and client do something new and different together. They might get up and move around in the room, imagine a situation, role-play, or even simply be silent together. The experiment itself is not intended to show a new and better way of doing things, but rather to be a tool for exploration of how the client lives her life in the world (Yontef & Schulz, 2016). When the therapist experiments, she has an open attitude almost like a scientist in a laboratory. Sometimes she forms a clear hypothesis or problem, and other times she examines a phenomenon that she feels is important without quite knowing where it will lead and without a clear hypothesis. This investigative and open attitude can be seen in qualitative research and the phenomenological method (Evans, 2016). An experiment often results in answer that are very different from those the therapist imagined. The information that comes up by experimenting is important to address and use in further therapeutic work.

In this chapter, we describe a model for how the therapist can design experiments and implement them together with the client, and we show various forms of experiments and how these can be applied in practice.

Phases in experimentation

Experimentation is often a gradual and natural part of a therapeutic conversation. It is, however, important that the therapist is aware of how she designs an experiment and that she invites the client to participate in the process. In Part 4 of this book, you will find several therapeutic process models where the experiment's place in the course of therapy is described in various ways. In this chapter, we focus on the design of one or more experiments, based on a revised version of Kurt Lewin's action research model.

Action research

Kurt Lewin, who developed field theory (Chapters 1 and 4), advocated that research on practical issues could be carried out as social experiments, or what he called 'action research'. Here we leave the scientific laboratory and relinquish control of all variables. In doing so, we can benefit by experiencing real life and may also contribute to reforming it. Lewin believed, for example, that most people know too little about how they affect each other. He therefore developed a model to study how group participants interact (Teigen, 2004/2015). Later, the action research model became one of the main methods in qualitative research and is also used for training and education. The model Lewin developed also helps therapists become more aware of the effect of the experiments they propose and carry out together with clients in the therapy room, how they can extend the experiment, and when it is appropriate to end it (van Baalen, 2014).

Lewin's action research model describes a helical stepwise process in which each step is part of a circle containing five elements (van Baalen, 2014). Later theorists developed a number of variants of this model, which we also have done in this book.

We have replaced some of Lewin's concepts in the model with concepts from gestalt theory. Our discussion includes the following points:

1   Identify a problem: identify a *figure*.
2   Make a plan: have an *idea* or *hypothesis* about a figure that can be explored.
3   Act—execute the plan by suggesting/doing an experiment.
4   Observe and collect data on the outcome of the suggestion of an experiment or of the experiment itself.
5   Reflect on the observations.

In Figure 11.1, we show a circular plan of this model. In Figure 11.2, we show a drawing of the model in the form of a spiral where the experiment is expanded, and the therapist and client continue in new circles.

It is useful for the therapist to have action research model points in mind as a reminder of the steps involved in facilitating an experiment and the process of

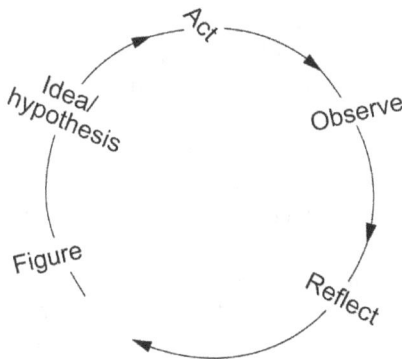

Figure 11.1

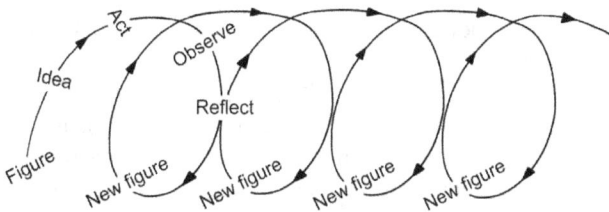

Figure 11.2

doing the experiment together with the client. It is especially important for the therapist to observe the client's responses to interventions and experiments. In this way, she can adjust the pace of the session to allow for reflection and new experiments. By observation, we mean that the therapist notices everything from slight changes in the client's facial expression, tightening of muscles in the jaw and neck, breathing, movements of parts of the body, pitch and tone of voice both in conversation and during the experiment, to verbal statements expressing spontaneous insight or resistance to the experiment. The therapist also notices her sensations, thoughts, and feelings in this part of the therapy. The outcome of the proposal for an experiment or the experiment itself can be completely different than what the therapist had imagined. It is important that the therapist captures what happens between herself and the client and does not view the experiment as a failure. The therapist can use everything that happens in the therapy room to increase the client's attention and create new experiences (Zinker, 1977).

The following is an example in which the therapist takes the time to observe and reflect.

Bill has been to a few therapy sessions. In this particular session, he sits with his head bowed as he talks about the relationship with his partner Gina, which he finds difficult. As the therapist listens, she becomes aware that he speaks in a monotone without looking at her, and she wonders about what is going on with him as he speaks. She thinks that he might not be aware of this himself, and that he is mostly concerned with what he tells her.

THERAPIST: 'When I listen to you, I see that you're looking down at the floor while talking, and I wonder how you feel'.

BILL: 'I'm sitting here telling you about the problems I'm having with Gina'.

THERAPIST: 'Yes, I hear that you're telling me about how difficult the relationship is. Can you sense the difficulty anywhere in your body?'

BILL: 'Yes, it's like a knot in my stomach, as if I'm very excited, and it almost feels like there's a big lump in there'. Bill rests his hand on his stomach while he looks up at the therapist with a sad smile.

The first figure that captures the therapist's interest is built on her observations of how Bill sits. He does not look at her and speaks in a monotone as he describes a difficult situation with his girlfriend. The therapist's idea or hypothesis is that Bill can get more in touch with his feelings by noticing what is going on in his body. She thinks that contact with both his emotions and physical sensations can give him a greater and more comprehensive understanding of how the situation is for him as he sits together with the therapist, and that this can possibly lead to a change in how he sees himself and his problems (see Chapter 5). The intention with the first experiment the therapist suggests is to help Bill notice his bodily sensations. The therapist observes that Bill responds by explaining what he notices as he rests his hand on his stomach and looks at her. She will then have confirmation that he understands what she means, and that they have a common understanding without the need for discussion.

THERAPIST: 'Can you describe the lump for me? How big is it?'
BILL: 'It's not so big, but very hard, almost like a fist in my stomach. It's really uncomfortable'.
THERAPIST: 'Does the lump have a colour?'
BILL: 'I think it's slightly greyish or maybe brown, it's hard to say. I don't know, but it's like I can see it'.

Here, the therapist proposes a new experiment. This new experiment builds on the previous intervention, which led to Bill being aware for the first time of the tension and of what he called a lump in his stomach. The therapist observes that Bill answers her questions about the lump and reflects that it might be possible for him to become better acquainted with the phenomenon of 'lump' without her knowing exactly what this exploration may lead to, beyond a heightened awareness. Here, the therapist employs a form of experimentation that we call visualisation; in other words, Bill imagines something that he notices in his body. The lump in his stomach is the figure that the therapist chooses to explore, and she expands the experiment according to this.

THERAPIST: 'Do you think you can draw the lump as you see it and feel it in your body?'
BILL: 'I don't know, I'm not good at drawing, but I can try. I have a clear image of the lump'.

The therapist gives Bill paper and coloured pencils. He draws in silence as the therapist watches.

THERAPIST: 'I see you've drawn the lump with several dark colours. Do these colours and this shape represent the lump as you see and feel it now?'
BILL: 'Not completely. The shape is always changing, and in a way there's even more colour in it than I can manage to draw. When I look at my drawing, it's as if the lump gets smaller and harder, very strange. I can feel it and see it'.

Here, Bill draws what he visualises in order to reinforce his attention on the lump in his stomach. Because he agrees to the therapist's suggestions to both visualise and draw, and immediately has new insight or a new experience (observation), the therapist chooses (reflection) to continue the experimentation. The therapist feels that continuing to work with the figure of 'lump' might lead to yet a new experience (new plan).

Grading experiments

By grading experiments, we mean that the therapist can increase or decrease the challenge inherent in the experiment (Zinker, 1977; Joyce & Sills, 2014). Laura Perls (1992) was interested in the relationship between challenging and supporting the client:

> So we start with the obvious, with what is immediately available to the awareness of therapist as well as client, and we proceed from there in small steps which are immediately experienced and thus are more easily assimilable. This is a time-consuming process which sometimes is misunderstood by people who are out for easy excitement and magical results. But miracles are a result not only of intuition, but of timing.
>
> (p. 156)

For example, the intervention in which the therapist asks Bill what he notices in his stomach is less of a challenge than when she asks him to visualise or draw. The therapist chooses to follow the same figure, the lump, in the next experiment, where she upgrades the experiment even more in the hope that the figure will become clearer, and perhaps give him insight or a new experience in terms of the feeling in his stomach.

THERAPIST: 'It's good that you're so aware of what you know and imagine. Do you want to explore more of what you feel and see?'

BILL: 'I don't know, how can I do that?'

THERAPIST: 'For example, you can pretend that you are the lump'.

BILL: 'Yes, I can do that, it's like I've already gotten to know it'.

The therapist then asks Bill to imagine that he is the lump, and to describe himself.

BILL: 'I'm hard, I'm round, and have dark colours. I'm not very big, and right now I'm a little smaller. I think I'm pretty impenetrable'.

THERAPIST: 'How does it feel when you say that you're round, have dark colours, and are small and impenetrable?'

BILL: 'Mmm, it's weird, but in a way that seems right, even though I can't really explain why. What I'd really like is to get rid of the whole lump and all the tension I feel. But right now I don't know how to do it'. As he speaks, he looks dejectedly at the therapist, and his body seems to fall into itself.

In this sequence, the therapist observes that Bill can identify with the lump and that he has a greater awareness of the sensations in his stomach.

The therapist hears Bill say (observation) that he would like to get rid of the lump and the tension he feels. The therapist has an idea (reflection) that the lump is an expression of his life situation, and that it is important for him to be aware of this connection. Bill himself is not aware of this. The therapist chooses not to tell him about her thoughts because it can easily lead them both back to his situation, rather than to explore and experience. The therapist feels she knows Bill well and thinks that it might be important for him to become acquainted with how his inner conflicts affect him physically and emotionally. She chooses therefore to invite him to experiment further, where the figure of the lump changes to internal conflict that manifests itself in his stomach.

THERAPIST: 'Can you go a step further in this experiment and let you-as-lump talk to yourself?'

BILL: 'What do you mean? I don't follow. I'm the lump in my stomach, talking to myself?'

THERAPIST: 'The idea is that you can initially be the lump, and afterwards you can be yourself. If you think it is easier to understand, we can use two chairs, so that when you're the lump, you sit in one chair, and when you're yourself, you can sit in another chair. I think there's an inner tension between you and the lump you feel, and that it might be useful to explore this. Does that make sense?'

Bill hesitates, but says he is willing to try. Together they decide which chair represents the lump and which represents Bill. He starts by siting in the chair that represents himself.

Turning to the therapist, he says: 'I want to start in this chair because I want to see how I can get rid of this lump and the tension in my stomach'.

THERAPIST: 'Can you say what you just said to me, to the chair where the lump is sitting?'

BILL AS HIMSELF: 'I don't know who or what's in the other chair'.

THERAPIST: 'You may want to put the drawing in the chair. Maybe that'll make it easier to imagine the lump sitting there?'

The therapist observes that Bill did not immediately say the same thing to the empty chair that he said to her. She reflects on what she can do. Her suggestion that he can put the drawing in the empty chair is an adaptation of the experiment. The therapist could also have asked Bill to tell the chair that he did not see the lump—that would have been yet another way to adapt the experiment.

The therapist could have stopped the experiment when Bill was not able imagine the lump in the other chair. He has already understood that the discomfort in his stomach is part of himself, and the therapist could have reflected together with him over this insight. Since they still have plenty of time left in the therapy session, however, the therapist suggests that they continue.

Bill, to the drawing in the empty chair: 'I don't like you, you're so hard and dark, and it's painful to have this tension in my stomach'.

THERAPIST: 'What's it like to say that to the drawing?'

BILL: 'Actually, it's really nice, it's the truth after all. What I'd really like to do is to throw the drawing in the trash'.

THERAPIST: 'Yes, I understand that. At the same time, you won't get rid of the unease and tension you feel in your stomach by getting rid of the drawing. It's just a drawing or a picture of what you feel in your stomach. Can you just for a moment put yourself in the chair where the drawing is, and pretend that you're the lump?'

Bill sits in the other chair.

THERAPIST: 'What do you notice in that chair?'

BILL: 'I'm not sure, my body's a little tense and maybe I feel a little sad. Yes, I feel sad, and it's uncomfortable to sit here'. He sits uneasily in his chair. 'I think I'll move back to the other chair'.

THERAPIST: 'Yes, do so. How is it to sit there and look at the other chair?'

BILL: 'It's much better to sit here. It's almost like I'm looking at another version of myself, who I am when I'm with Gina. I don't feel good at all in that situation'.

The therapist brings Bill out of the experiment and asks him to sit in the original chair. She thinks the time is right to end the experiment and integrate new insights. They talk about the fact that he recognised himself in how he is when he is together with his girlfriend, and that the tension and the lump he feels in his stomach is a result of the turmoil he feels when he is together with Gina. As they talk, it becomes clearer to Bill that he needs a break in his relationship with Gina.

When the therapist hears Bill say that he does not feel good together with Gina (observation), it becomes clear that he has a new understanding of their relationship as well as a new awareness about his bodily signals in the form of tension and unrest in his stomach. In this part of the conversation, Bill integrates what he has learned during the experiment and reflection afterwards.

In this example, we have shown several ways to experiment—from simple awareness questions to visualisation, drawing, and chair work. We have also shown how the therapist has moved between selecting a figure as she explores with Bill in the form of experimentation, observation, and reflection on the outcome, either alone or together with Bill. The therapist's choices along the way reflected that she wanted Bill to have a new experience through bodily and visual experiments and to integrate these experiences and insights through reflection. The choices were also based on the fact that he had a certain sensitivity to bodily sensations, and that he was open to experimenting and trying out a new way to gain insight. With another client, the therapist probably would have chosen a different approach.

Let us briefly see how the same principle could have been handled in a different way with the client Nina.

Nina is slumped over and speaks in a monotone about her partner. The therapist notices that Nina does not look at her.

THERAPIST: 'I see you sit slumped over when you talk about your partner. Can you sit even more slumped?'

NINA: 'Why should I do that? I'm sitting perfectly fine'. She looks up at the therapist.

THERAPIST: 'Yes, you can sit however you like. I was just curious if you were aware of how you were sitting'.

NINA: 'Actually, I wasn't. I'm more interested in telling you how I feel than in how I'm sitting'.

In this sequence, the therapist chooses Nina's position as the figure she wants to explore. She thinks (hypothesis) that there is a correlation between how Nina sits and what she says. When the therapist hears Nina's response to her proposal to sit even more slumped over (experiment), she realises that she has to adjust the level of risk in the experiment and explains the reason behind her proposal. Nina's response shows that she is aware that she is more concerned with telling her story than with how she sits. It is possible that Nina is now ready to explore the relationship between sitting and telling her story. We now look at a third alternative for experimentation.

Beth looks down at the floor as she speaks in a monotone about her problems with her partner. She barely breathes as she speaks.

The therapist has a feeling that Beth is upset and uneasy, and says quietly: 'It sounds like you're in a very difficult situation. As I listen to you, I notice I'm sad; I'd like to hear more about you and your partner'.

Beth looks up at the therapist with tears in his eyes: 'Yes, I'm very sad, I don't know what to do'.

In this situation, the therapist notices her sadness and unease when she hears and sees Beth (observation) and decides to use this observation in the conversation. She thinks that Beth needs support for her feelings, which she feels are just below the surface (hypothesis). She therefore chooses to describe her own experience (experiment). She gets an immediate response from Beth (observation), and her hypothesis is confirmed (reflection) when she observes Beth's tears. The therapist will likely choose a supportive and exploratory form of therapy in future sessions with Beth.

In these examples, the therapist uses many different types of experiment, depending on what she chooses to explore together with the client. The next section presents an overview of the various forms of experiments from which a therapist can choose in different situations.

Various forms of experiments

- Classical awareness experiments
- Role-playing
- Chair work
- Visualisation, metaphor, dream work
- Creative aids such as drawing, painting, plasticine, photos, cards, blankets, pillows, balls, and other objects in the therapy room
- Movement in various forms

Classical awareness experiments

Many clients pay little attention to what they say, how they speak, or the feelings and bodily sensations they have. They can learn to increase their attention by trying out simple awareness experiments together with the therapist. The three classic awareness experiments are:

- *Mirroring*: copying, pointing out or repeating movements, tones of voice, tempo, or words and phrases that are said. For example: 'I see that you move your hands when you speak'. As the therapist says these words, she copies the client's movements and asks the client to repeat them. The therapist can also repeat verbatim what the client says, or she can ask the client to repeat her own words, often several times.
- *Amplify*: exaggerate movements, tones of voice, tempo, or words and phrases. For example: 'I hear that you speak softly. Can you speak even more softly?' 'Can you say that even louder?' 'I see that you move your hands when you speak. Can you move them even more?' 'I can see you sitting forward in your chair. Can you bend even more forward?'
- *Do the opposite*: make opposite movements, speak with an opposite volume or tempo, or look for opposites to what is said. For example: 'When you sit bent forward, can you see how it would be to sit in the opposite way?' 'When

you speak so softly, can you say the same in a loud voice?' 'Can you speak the opposite of fast?'

All these proposed forms of experiments can be combined and can build on each other. In the example of Bill, we see that the therapist repeats his description of the lump in his stomach before she asks him to go further in the experiment. Awareness experiments are often used together with awareness questions, such as: 'What happens to you when I copy your movements? What happens to you when you exaggerate your movements?'

Role-playing

Role-playing is a technique taken from the theatre world where actors 'gestalt' a person (a role or character) and immerse themselves in the person's life and behaviour. By portraying another person, actors become acquainted not only with the characters they gestalt, but also with sides of themselves they make use of in the process of gestalting. The idea of playing roles in the therapy room was introduced by Fritz Perls as a method to help clients learn more about themselves and important people in their lives (Perls et al., 1951). The method was further developed for use in supervision, where therapists can act out situations from the therapy room in order to gain new insight about the observations they made during therapy sessions. As in all acting, it is the actor—or in our case, the therapist or supervisor—who creates the role or character based on her experience of that person. The role or character is never identical with the person being portrayed.

You will find different examples of role-playing experiments in this book, and especially in the chapter on projection, because role-playing is a way to work with projection (Chapter 14).

Chair work

Perhaps the most familiar form of experimentation in gestalt therapy is chair work. The earlier example with Bill includes some chair work. Perls developed chair work on the basis of his interest in and knowledge of theatre and psychodrama (Clarkson & Mackewn, 1993). Psychodrama is a form of therapy that uses techniques inspired by the craft of acting (Kolmannskog, 2018). More research has been done on chair work than on any other technique in gestalt therapy. This research shows that chair work has a good therapeutic effect on various types of clients (Strümpfel, 2013; Kellogg, 2015).

The definition of chair work varies in the gestalt literature. Various authors refer to the 'empty chair', the 'projection chair', or 'two-chair work' (Joyce & Sills, 2014; Kolmannskog, 2018). We choose to use the term 'projection chair' when working with client's projections or assumptions the client has about other people, and 'two-chair work' when working with the client's inner polarities and conflicts (Yontef & Schulz, 2016). All forms of chair work are either about contradictory needs that are expressed as internal conflicts in the client or conflicts or contradictions between the client and the people around her. In gestalt therapy, we call this 'polarity work', regardless of whether there is polarisation between the client and another person or an internal polarisation between the client's conflicting needs (see Chapter 10 on polarities and Chapter 14 on projection).

The purpose of work with the projection chair is to create a situation in which the client can gain new insight into herself and the assumptions she has about the other person. You can see an illustration of this type of chair work in the example with Magnus in the chapter on projection. It is important to emphasise that projection work is always centred on the client and her experience of the other person, and to a lesser extent on how the other person really is. That means that work in the projection chair cannot be automatically transferred to a conversation a client may have with the real person.

When the therapist and the client use chair work, it means that the client experiments by playing different roles in terms of both internal and external polarisation work. Experimenting with the help of chair work can take many forms—from situations where the actual chairs are barely used, to situations where multiple chairs represent different aspects of the client or of people in the client's environment.

Projection chair

The best-known way of working with assumptions we have about others in gestalt therapy is the use of the so-called projection chair.

Laura Perls (1992) stressed that working with the projection chair or an empty chair only can be done with comparatively healthy people. Fritz Perls also used this method for the most part on professional people already trained in gestalt therapy. For gestalt therapists and coaches, it is therefore important first to develop the client's awareness before experimenting with chair work.

In working with this method, Fritz Perls first emphasised that the client make clear who she would imagine in the other chair. He then set up two chairs that faced each other, appropriately spaced. The client placed herself in one of the chairs and Perls urged her to visualise the other sitting in the chair across from her, which was called the 'projection chair'. His idea was that the person the client placed in the other chair was simply her own projection of a person with whom she was in conflict. When the projection of the other was identified, the stage was set to ensure that the client could gestalt the other by sitting in the other's chair (the projection chair) and act out different poses that reflected the image she had of the other. When the time was ripe, the client was asked

(Continued)

to put herself back in her own chair and notice any changes in her picture, or projection, of the other. In some relationships several rounds in the two chairs were necessary before they felt they were finished, while at other times the process progressed faster and more freely.

Experiences the client had in this work helped her to take her projections back and acknowledge that what she experienced was as much about herself as about the person with whom she was in conflict. By seeing her own role in the conflict and not just blaming the other, work in the projection chair allowed the client to recognise the responsibility she had for the conflict.

This way of working was developed by Perls. Today the emphasis is on the client being able to explore how she puts her own projections on others, while Perls was more concerned with the recipient of the projection. When the client sits in the other chair, she has the opportunity to sort through her projections via a dialogue between the different 'people'. This allows her to acknowledge her projections and thus be able to recognise her own part in the conflict.

Chair work and field boundaries

In carrying out chair work, it is important that the therapist is aware of which field she and the client are working in: *the client's inner field*, her inner polarisations or contradictions, or *the field that exists between the client and another imaginary person*, representing projections the client has in relation to key people in her life. (See pp. 53–54 for field boundaries and field in the field.) During chair work there are also several possible fields the therapist can make clear to the client through experimentation. The purpose of limiting the field is that the excitement or tension in field becomes greater, which may increase the client's attention and pave the way for new experiences and spontaneous insight. First, we show a stepwise model for how the therapist and client can experiment together using chairs based on refinements of the field.

Overview of possible steps in chair work with a client, based on field boundaries

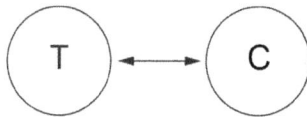

Figure 11.3 The field is between therapist and client prior to chair work.

The therapist explains the purpose of role-playing in the form of chair work, and how they can create the experiment together.

By projection: Clarify with the client a person with whom she has a challenging relationship that she would like to explore further in chair work.

By internal polarisation: Make the client aware of how conflicting needs can be seen as polarities. Explore both poles. Formulate conflicting statements for both poles, for example: 'I want to leave my husband' and 'I will stay with my husband'. The client can try out the statements by moving her hands or other body movement while she says: 'On the one hand I will . . . and on the other hand, I will . . . '

Therapist and client choose two chairs and set them up in the room. Via projection, the chair called C1 represents the client herself. Chair C1 represents one of the poles. Chair C2 represents the person the client projects on or has assumptions about. In internal conflicts or polarities, C2 is the other pole or side of the inner conflict.

Projection: The client looks at the representative in the projection chair and describes to the therapist what she sees, such as hair colour, clothing, posture, as well as what she perceives in her own body.

Inner polarisation: The client sits in the first chair (C1) and describes the sensations and thoughts she becomes aware of.

The client describes the sensations and feelings she is aware of by being the representative or the other side of herself.

The therapist facilitates a conversation between C1 and C2 depending on the client's response and understanding of the conversation, and ensures that the client swaps chairs and that C1 and C2 talk directly to each other and not to her.

Therapist and client reflect together over the chair work—what the client has experienced and the meaning this has for the situation she brought into the therapy session.

It is important that the therapist only sees these field boundaries as guidelines for how to carry out chair work and that this is not a recipe to be followed

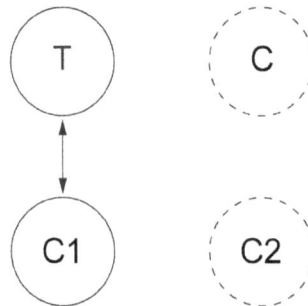

Figure 11.4 The field is between the therapist and a side of the client, or—in the case of projection work—the client herself (C1).

slavishly. If this is the first time the client participates in chair work, the therapist will naturally spend more time explaining and perhaps let the client linger
longer in each chair before she is asked to move to the other chair. In many
cases, the therapist will choose to terminate chair work without the client having been involved in a dialogue between the chairs, or perhaps there have been
several dialogues with reflection rounds between each dialogue. It is the therapist, in cooperation with the client, who directs and selects the next step in the
chair work.

Imagination and visualisation

Most people are familiar with visualising or imagining situations. We daydream
when we imagine ourselves far away from reality. Sometimes we recreate events
and situations from the past or prepare ourselves for what may come in the near
or distant future. In therapy, we use imagination journeys and visualisation so

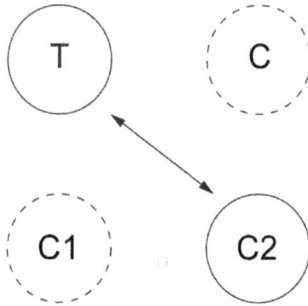

Figure 11.5 The field is between the therapist and another side of the client or the representative via projection work (C2). C1's chair is placed on the floor, but not
used.

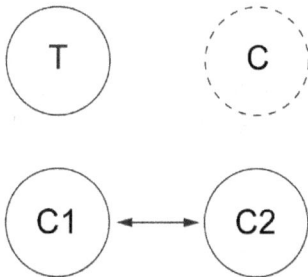

Figure 11.6 The field is between the two sides of the client (C1 and C2) or between the
client (C1) and the representative (C2). The therapist is outside the field.

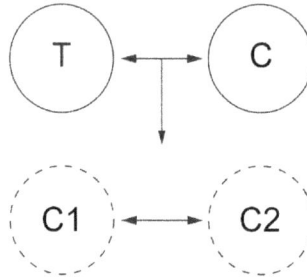

Figure 11.7 The field is between the therapist and client as they observe and reflect on the progress of the conversation and the relationship between C1 and C2.

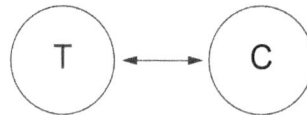

Figure 11.8 The field is between therapist and client, and chair work is completed.

that clients can become aware of the beliefs they have about the past or the future (Kolmannskog, 2018, p. 13). Another form of this type of work is to visualise bodily phenomena, such as Bill did in the example above. Clients can also imagine the person they put in the projection chair before they identify with them. In Chapter 14 on projection, we describe how visualisation can be used in therapy.

Metaphor

Metaphor is often used in gestalt therapy to clarify an idea or image that occurs to the therapist or client during the session (Kolmannskog, 2018). In the example of Bill earlier in this chapter, the therapist chooses Bill's image of a lump as a metaphor for the tension he felt in his stomach, and on p. 111 the therapist uses the metaphor of a boat and life preserver as an image of where the client is in her life. Such metaphors can in many cases provide a spontaneous insight for the client that would not have occurred to her otherwise (Zinker, 1977; Saxlund, 2014).

Dream work

Perls viewed a dream as a condensed reflection of our existence in which the therapist's task is to point out the obvious, without interpretation. In gestalt therapy we see dreams as aspects of the client that can be explored phenomenologically. The important thing is not the dream as it was experienced, but rather as it is during the process that takes place in the therapy room. This process can bring the client to new insight, provide her with an understanding of her situation today, or spark a new understanding of past events (Jørstad, 2006). This exploration can be done in several ways, depending on the dream's content and character. The most familiar form is dream projection, where the client plays out the parts of the dream. It is also possible to use the creative methods described below to experience parts of the dream. Another variation is to visualise or continue dreaming while awake; this is especially useful when the dream has ended abruptly or feels unfinished. For more about dreams, see Synnøve Jørstad's article 'Working with dreams in Gestalt Therapy' (2006).

Creative aids

Many creative aids can be used in therapy as a means to increase the client's awareness and attention to feelings, sensations, and experiences that are unfamiliar or difficult to put into words. The therapist may ask the client to express feelings by drawing, as Bill did, painting, or modelling in plasticine. Looking at pictures or objects can provide the client with associations and bodily reactions that can be explored and gradually put into words. Therapist and client can throw a ball back and forth to each other and explore poles such as spontaneity and control or hold onto a ball as they move together in different ways. The therapist can wrap the client in blankets if she's cold or in need of care. Pillows can be used behind the back and neck to see how support in various places affects the client's position and increases her awareness of bodily sensations.

Movement and bodily expression in therapy

Experimentation with the body and movement often begins with attention to how the therapist and client sit together in the room, how they breathe, how they look at each other, if they sense tension or unrest, and the influences they are aware of (Staemmler, 2011). Based on what catches the therapist's attention—that is, the figure she chooses—she can suggest, for example, that the client amplifies small gestures that one or both are aware of, or that they move in an opposite way. Perhaps the therapist chooses to mirror the client's movements. In other words, they use classic experiments as they expand or increase the degree of risk by for example standing up and moving around the room. The therapist might allow the client to move according to her needs in the situation, while the therapist looks on. Bodily unrest and tension become easier to perceive and recognise through movement than when we are seated, and experience gained through movement and the use of bodily expression can increase the client's attention to how she uses her body. It is she who tightens her muscles, holds her breath, tightens her jaw, or collapses (Kepner, 1987/2001). The client can also become more aware of the relationship between thoughts, feelings, and bodily sensations. In many of the examples in this book, we show how the therapist uses movement and attention to bodily expression in her work with clients.

Summary

In this chapter, we have presented Lewin's model for action research and shown how the model can be used in practice. The therapist can become aware of the effect of the experiments she proposes and carries out together with clients, how an experiment can be extended, and when it is appropriate to end it. Furthermore, we have described various kinds of experiments, including how to carry out chair work, with a basis in field theory. The various forms of experimentation have in common that they can contribute to the client's increased awareness of herself. She may be more aware of how she affects and is affected by the environment, and how she can adapt creatively to the situation she is in at any given time (Perls, 1992).

It is not possible to plan how being with a client in the therapy room will be. It is in itself an experiment, in which the therapist seeks to strike a balance between creating a safe space for the client while challenging the client and facilitating a process in which she can have new experiences. Experiments must be adapted to the situation the client and therapist create together. With the help of imagination and creativity, only fear and resistance can limit the opportunities that the situation provides.

We will end this chapter with a quote from Laura Perls (1992):

> A good therapist does not use techniques, he applies himself in and to the situation with whatever knowledge, skills, and total life experience have become integrated into his own background and whatever awareness he has at any given moment.

(p. 155)

References

Clarkson, P., & Mackewn, J. (1993). *Fritz Perls*. London: Sage Publications.

Evans, K. (2016). Research from a relational gestalt perspective. In J. Roubal (Ed.), *Towards a research tradition in gestalt therapy* (pp. 64–78). Cambridge: Cambridge Scholars Publishing.

Jørstad, S. (2006). Å arbeide med drømmer i gestaltterapi [Working with dreams in gestalt therapy]. In S. Jørstad & Å. Krüger (Eds.), *Gestaltterapi i praksis* [Gestalt therapy in practice] (pp. 129–152). Oslo: NGI.

Joyce, P., & Sills, C. (2014). *Skills in gestalt counselling & psychotherapy* (3rd ed.). London: Sage.

Kellogg, S. H. (2015). *Transformational chairwork: Using psychotherapeutic dialogues in clinical practice*. USA, New York, London: Bowman & Littlefield.

Kepner, J. I. (1987/2001). *Body process*. Cambridge, MA: Gestalt Press.

Kolmannskog, V. (2018). *The empty chair*. London: Routledge.

Perls, L. (1992). *Living at the boundary*. Gouldsboro, ME: The Gestalt Journal Press.

Perls, F. S., Hefferline, R. F., & Goodman, P. (1951). *Gestalt therapy: Excitement and growth in the human personality*. London: Souvenir Press.

Saxlund, A. M. (2014). To sider av samme sak: Hvordan bruke metaforer i arbeidet med polariteter? [Two sides of the same issue: How to use metaphor in polarity work?]. *Norsk Gestalttidsskrift*, *2*(11), 47–57.

Staemmler, F. M. (2011). Kontakt som første virkelighet: Gestaltterapi som en intersubjektiv tilnærming [Contact as a first reality: Gestalt therapy as an intersubjective approach]. *Norsk Gestalttidsskrift*, *8*(1), 7–20.

Strümpfel, U. (2013). Forskning på gestaltterapi—del 2 [Research on gestalt therapy: Part 2]. *Norsk Gestalttidsskrift*, *13*(1), 7–30.

Teigen, K. H. (2004/2015). *En psykologihistorie* [A history of psychology]. Bergen: Fagbokforlaget.

van Baalen, D. (2014). *An introduction to action research*. Unpublished, from gestalt therapy study programme compendium. Oslo: NGI.

Yontef, G., & Schulz, F. (2016). Dialogue and experiment. *British Gestalt Journal*, *25*(1), 9–21.

Zinker, J. (1977). *Creative process in gestalt therapy*. New York: Random House.

Part 3

Contact forms

The ways in which people are together varies; there are many examples of this from everyday life. Sometimes silence is intrusive, and at other times it can be life-giving and comforting. Speaking loudly to convince others is different from being low key, nodding, and listening to what others have to say. The content of what we want to convey is important, but the way in which we convey it—the form we use—is at least as crucial to the contact between us.

Gestalt therapy emphasises both describing the process of how contact between people develops over time and the form contact takes in a given situation. We have previously described what we mean by the terms 'contact' and 'contact functions' (Chapter 9). In this part, we describe several theoretical models that explain the forms contact can take in different situations, and how the therapist can use these models in therapy with clients. In the chapter on contact process (Chapter 19) we describe how contact can change over time and what the therapist can do to influence this change in the therapy room.

Form and creative adjustment

Form is a core concept in gestalt therapy theory and is derived from gestalt psychology. The term 'to gestalt' explains how something takes shape and becomes apparent—how it becomes a figure and something else goes to the background (Chapter 1). On p. 92 we describe how the client gestalts and gives life to and forms her roles in the therapy room, how her creative adjustment can be seen as a gestalting process, and how she forms contact together with the therapist. The types of contact created in a situation also depend on the dynamics of the field, the needs they each have at any given time, and how they seek to meet those needs (see Chapter 6 on creative adaptation and Chapter 4 on field theory in practice).

Initially, Fritz Perls and his colleagues were interested in the negative aspects of contact. They used words such as 'contact disorders' and 'healthy' and 'unhealthy' forms of contact. This was justified by their medical backgrounds, in which they were focused on illness and how to cure it (see the box on p. 92). Although they saw contact disruption as a survival strategy in difficult and challenging situations and as a form of creative adjustment, they paid little attention to the qualities the

DOI: 10.4324/9781003153856-14

patients developed in this adjustment. Today we look at both the qualities of different forms of adjustment and when these forms may be inappropriate for the individual, without labelling either as unhealthy or negative.

Contact disturbance

The founders of gestalt therapy thought there were different ways of avoiding or interrupting contact. They used various terms for this, including 'resistance' and 'contact breaks' or 'interruptions'. Initially, they referred to these as 'defence mechanisms', because they viewed them as the ways in which we defend ourselves in difficult and painful situations. They believed that these defence mechanisms were the expression of human resistance to experiencing pain or anxiety (Clarkson & Mackewn, 1993).

Fritz Perls came from a psychoanalytic tradition where Freud claimed that patients had resistance to the therapist. Perls believed, however, that they had resistance to contact. He was therefore interested in seeing how this resistance manifested itself in various situations. Like his predecessor, he was interested in illness and non-functioning aspects of his patients in order to understand how people could be cured (Wheeler, 1998).

Wheeler disagreed with Perls; he argued that we are always in contact and that resistance is itself a form of contact. He used the terms Perlas gave to the various defence mechanisms but chose to call them 'contact functions'. He did not regard contact as a defence, but rather as a way to adapt to different situations. He was interested in polarity thinking in gestalt therapy and devised a model in which all contact functions have one or more possible polarities (Wheeler, 1998). Other theorists look at contact disruption as the best possible creative adjustment in the situation and refer to these adaptations as contact styles (Mann, 2010). In this way, the therapist is more interested in how the person adapts to her surroundings than in seeing the adaptation as personal disturbance. We prefer to call these *contact forms* because this is nearer to the idea of gestalting and forming the contact together (Hostrup, 2010).

It was Perls (1969/1992) who first described various defence mechanisms within gestalt theory. He called the first three of these introjection, projection, and retroflection. Later, Perls et al. (1951) added confluence and egotism, and Polster and Polster (1974) deflection (Jørstad, 2002/2008).

In our view, we are only out of contact in very specific situations, such as when we are completely numb and without attention (coma or death). There can be instances where we do not feel a need to experience any contact or pay attention to the other, but this is not the same as no contact. In gestalt therapeutic work we are interested in what kind of contact we have, how it is experienced, what form it has, and how it can change (Wheeler, 1998).

Contact forms and their polarities

The possible forms of contact are unlimited. Perls chose five main forms of what he called contact disruptions or defence mechanisms, which he believed could be categorised to some extent. We have kept the designations Perls gave to what he called defence mechanisms but have chosen to refer to these as contact forms in order to emphasise that these are ways to be in contact (Hostrup, 2010). These five forms of contact are confluence, introjection, projection, retroreflection and self-monitoring. The sixth form of contact we describe is deflection, taken from Polster and Polster (1974).

According to Wheeler (1998), all forms of contact (or contact functions, as he chose to call them) may have one or more polarities. We have found this way of viewing polarity both useful and appropriate in therapeutic practice. In polarity work, the therapist and client explore contradictory needs between the client and other persons, or within the client herself (Chapter 10). On p. 171 we describe the span between the polarity, or needs, and that the therapist can work either with one or both polarities or with the span between them.

In the illustration, we show how a contact form's polarity only emerges (becomes figure) because it is one of the polarities of that contact form. The polarity is formed by the original contact form and helps to create the span between the polarity (see Chapter 10).

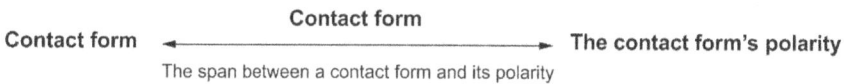

Contact form   **Contact form**   ⟵————————————————⟶   The contact form's polarity

The span between a contact form and its polarity

The span between the polarites, like it says in the drawing

When a therapist explores a contact form with a client, the polarity of the contact form or the span between the poles depends on the original contact form. For example, if we work with the contact form confluence (Chapter 12), we can explore how we flow together or distance ourselves from each other in the therapy room, and both phenomena are part of confluence.

In practice, it can be confusing for therapists to know which contact form is prominent, or becomes figure, in the conversation with the client. In many situations the different ways of being in contact will naturally flow into each other, and the therapist will be interested in figures that are completely different than the contact forms that might manifest themselves. It is only when a contact form hinders development, creates challenges between the therapist and the client, or creates challenges in the client's life that the therapist chooses to explore that contact form with the client. We will show examples of this in the coming chapters.

In gestalt therapy, there is no obvious theoretical model for how we humans develop and grow in relation to our surroundings beyond the theory of creative adjustment (Chapter 6; Gillie, 1999). Many gestalt theorists are interested in how contact forms can be understood and described theoretically as part of human development from birth to adulthood (Hostrup, 2010; Spagnuolo Lobb, 2013; Kokkersvold & Mjelve, 2003). We do not disagree with this way of understanding contact forms, but rather choose to emphasise the theory's practical application in this book. A gestalt therapist is interested in exploring the client's experiences here and now and less so in analysing the developmental understanding of the problems the client brings to therapy.

However, in our descriptions of individual contact forms, we comment in several places on the relationship between the current form of contact and how the form has been developed in interaction with parents and others during childhood. We feel it is important that the therapist has an understanding that there is a developmental connection between the client's way of contacting others today and how she was met as a child.

Because clients seek therapy when the form in which they contact the outside world leads to problems, pain, and suffering, it can often give the impression that contact forms are negative or wrong. In these cases, however, the client's way of being in contact is a form that has become rigid and inappropriate in the client's life situation. Clients in therapy often need to be aware of how they interact with the environment, and how the form they use can hinder them from achieving what they want. By increasing awareness of how clients use contact functions, how they sense the environment and themselves, and how they see, hear, and sense others, the therapist works with the very basis of the client's attention to herself and her surroundings, which is necessary in a situation that has become rigid. This increased awareness can lead to a greater degree of awareness in the client when she interacts with others and give her the flexibility to choose a way of contacting her surroundings that may be more satisfactory.

References

Clarkson, P., & Mackewn, J. (1993). *Fritz Perls*. London: Sage Publications.

Gillie, M. (1999). Daniel Stern: A developmental theory for gestalt? *British Gestalt Journal, 8*(2), 107–117.

Hostrup, H. (2010). *Gestalt therapy: An introduction to the basic concepts of gestalt therapy* (D. H. Silver, Trans.). Copenhagen: Hans Reitzlers Forlag. (Original work published 1999)

Jørstad, S. (2002/2008). Oversikt over kontaktformer [Overview of contact forms]. In S. Jørstad & Å. Krüger (Eds.), *Den flyvende hollender* [The flying Dutchman] (pp. 128–139). Oslo: NGI.

Kokkersvold, E., & Mjelve, H. (2003). *Mellom oss* [Between us]. Oslo: Gyldendal Akademisk.

Mann, D. (2010). *Gestalt therapy: 100 key points and techniques*. New York: Routledge.

Perls, F. S. (1969/1992). *Gestalt therapy verbatim*. Highland, NY: The Gestalt Journal Press.

Perls, F. S., Hefferline, R. F., & Goodman, P. (1951). *Gestalt therapy: Excitement and growth in the human personality*. Great Britain: Souvenir Press.

Polster, E., & Polster, M. (1974). *Gestalt therapy integrated*. New York: Vintage Books.

Spagnuolo Lobb, S. M. (2013). *The now-for-next in psychotherapy: Gestalt therapy recounted in post-modern society*. Siracusa: Istituto di Gestalt HCC Italy.

Wheeler, G. (1998). *Gestalt reconsidered* (2nd ed.). Cambridge, MA: CIGPress.

Chapter 12

Confluence

The first form of contact we examine is confluence, which can be described thus: 'one person and another . . . are confluent when there is no appreciation of a boundary between them, *when there is no discrimination of the points of difference or otherness that distinguish them*' (Perls et al., 1951, p. 365).

Most of us can recognise the feeling of flowing together as the 'we' at a football game, festival, or concert; when we sing together; when we share a meal; or when we work especially well with others. We can also recognise confluence as participants at a demonstration, at political or religious meetings, or when we fight together with others for a cause that is important to us. Other more pervasive examples of confluence are the strong relationships between parents and children and in love and friendship.

Flowing together

> Martha meets her best friend, Camilla, at a cafe after work. They hug each other, and Martha immediately starts talking enthusiastically. She tells her friend about her new boyfriend, how amazing he is, about the time they spend together, and how in love she is. She is so busy telling all this to Camilla that she barely manages to order anything to eat or drink. As Camilla listens to Martha, she leans forward and sits close to her friend as she nods, smiles, and repeats: 'That's wonderful, you're so lucky!'

Martha is completely engulfed by what she is feeling—it is the only thing on her mind when she gets together with Camilla. Camilla flows along with the story as Martha speaks. She forgets herself and immerses herself in Martha's world as she listens, nods, and smiles. While she listens, it is almost as if she becomes part of Martha's story.

This is an example that shows how nice it can be to flow together—how much care and warmth can be expressed in this form of contact. Confluence is often characterised by speaking softly; the person listening confirms the other

DOI: 10.4324/9781003153856-15

by nodding, saying 'mmm' and interjecting phrases such as 'Yes, I understand', 'Poor you', 'Exactly'. It can, however, also be characterised by speaking quickly with loud and eager voices, barely taking time to breathe, completely engaged with and engrossed by those with whom we are together and by the subject matter. In very close relationships we often use we-formulations, such as 'We fit well together, we can do it if we stick together'. This feeling that we belong together is often crucial for nurturing and developing relationships with others. This way of being in contact, of being confluent, is thus necessary for people to experience belonging and unity. Our ability to be confluent is related to the extent to and manner in which our caregivers flowed with us when we were children, and how they understood us, met our need for closeness and care, and showed us empathy.

Confluence and empathy

The ability to empathise with other people's situations is related to being confluent (Staemmler, 2012). This view of confluence has gradually grown within the gestalt therapy milieu. Perls considered confluence to be negative and warned of the danger of flowing with the client and losing oneself as a therapist (Perls et al., 1951). However, later theorists have renounced this one-sided negative attitude towards confluence and emphasised a dialogic and relational approach (Chapter 4) and the ability to imagine and empathise with the client's life (Kolmannskog, 2018).

The term 'empathy' originally comes from Greek, and means to understand and share another person's emotional life. Having empathy with someone means that we use our experiences of our own and others' feelings to understand how someone else is feeling, and that we can differentiate between our own and others' experiences (Chapter 4). The concept of empathy in psychotherapy is often associated with the psychologist Carl Rogers (1967). Rogers was one of the pioneers of humanistic psychotherapy, and even developed a type of therapy he called 'client-centred counselling'. The basis of his therapy form was that the therapist was empathetic, that she did not analyse the client, and that she had a non-judgemental attitude (Clarkson & Mackewn, 1993).

Empathy, mirror neurons, and resonance

Frank Staemmler has had a great deal of influence on the development of how empathy is viewed by gestalt therapists. He has published the book *Empathy in Psychotherapy* (2012) and countless articles in which he describes trends from new psychoanalysis, phenomenological philosophy, the latest brain research, including mirror neurons, and the implications this research has for psychotherapy. Staemmler (2007) describes how knowledge about mirror neurons confirms what we experience with young children: that

(Continued)

children naturally mirror and imitate adults, and adults often reflect back. Research has shown that everyone has reflexes to mirror others, but that the reflexes are controlled and are less visible the older we become. Staemmler describes how this new research shows that people can understand the experiences of others to a greater extent than previously assumed, and that this experience is as much a bodily and emotional experience as it is cognitive. Staemmler associates confluence with empathy, as a necessary prerequisite for empathy. He also talks about body alignment in empathy, a bodily resonance between the parties in a situation. This bodily resonance in a therapy process occurs both ways between client and therapist, which means that empathy is a reciprocal process. This view replaces the traditional notion that it is the therapist who attempts to understand the client. Staemmler further developed the understanding of empathy as a two-way process to what he calls a shared situation between therapist and client (see field, p. 179), where he emphasises the value of the physical and sensory in the field between therapist and client, and how they create the therapy situation together (Krüger, 2012).

Ruella Frank (2016) shares Staemmler's view of the mutual bodily influence that occurs between the client and therapist in the therapy room and calls it kinaesthetic resonance. Frank is particularly interested in how this kinaesthetic resonance is expressed in both the client's and the therapist's bodily expressions and movements, and how the therapist can use this knowledge in her work with clients.

In gestalt therapy today, the knowledge of brain research, mirror neurons, and research into factors affecting the therapy process has meant that the therapist can be both empathic and confluent in the therapy room, and be more interested in what is happening at the sensory and physical level than previously. Confluence is not just about flowing together, but also about how we separate ourselves from the outside world (Møklebust, 2016). Wheeler (1998) believes that resistance is a polarity of confluence, and that it is man's inherent ability to flow with the environment, provide resistance, and regulate the relationship between herself and others in proximity and distance in the field that creates and forms the contact between us.

Polarities to 'flowing together'

There are three polarities to 'flowing together' that we find appropriate to use in therapy: resisting, isolation, and differentiation (Wheeler, 1998). The span in the contact form confluence can thus be illustrated as shown in Figure 12.1.

	Confluence	– to resist
– to flow together	←————————————————→	– to isolate
	the span between the poles	– to differentiate

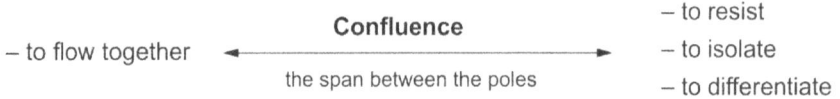

Figure 12.1 The span between polarities

In the illustration, we have placed the polarities of flowing together and resisting as the first and basic polarity pair inherent in confluence. Using gestalt terminology, we can say that the organism seeks a different form, and in contrast to 'flowing with', the need arises for a form of separation where we resist flowing together with the surroundings in the field. This resistance can cause us to either isolate or differentiate ourselves from the environment (Wheeler, 1998). To isolate oneself is described as feeling alone, introverted, or isolated when with others. The feeling of being on the outside is dominant, and the experience of belonging is gone. Differentiating means distinguishing between what is 'mine' and what belongs to others in a field—without feeling isolated (Wheeler, 1998).

To resist or flow together

In some relationships, for example, between mothers and children or between romantic partners, it is sometimes natural to flow with the other while at other times it is natural to resist or introduce differentiation into the field (Wheeler, 1998). Resistance is necessary in order not to flow completely with the other or eradicate oneself. However, too much resistance complicates the matter when it comes to being a 'we'. In some cases, these contradictions can be extreme, and create challenges in regulating the contact between us, as shown in the following short example.

> Martha and Camilla have been talking for a while when Camilla says: 'I'm really jealous of you. Terry broke up with me just a few days ago and I don't know what to do. I'm so upset'. 'Oh, poor you', Martha says in a low, comforting voice and puts her arm around Camilla. At this point, Camilla starts to cry.

Here, we see that there is differentiation when Camilla initially tells about herself and her relationship with Terry. Martha and Camilla move in the continuum between confluence and resistance. Perhaps Camilla feels especially lonely as a response to Martha's confluence with her boyfriend. When Martha hears how unhappy Camilla is, she flows with her friend. She understands and comforts Camilla by putting her arm around her, saying 'poor you' and speaking in a low, comforting voice. Confluence again appears between them.

Often, we are not aware that we flow together and are a 'we'. It can happen without being noticed and is difficult to spot before we are in the process of moving away from confluence. It is only when we begin to feel resistance that we can differ-entiate, which can lead to both guilt and anger in one or both parties in a relationship (Kokkersvold & Mjelve, 2003). It is an unpleasant feeling to break a close and good contact, and those who are abandoned and exposed to the lack of confluence often feel that there is good reason to be hurt, upset, and maybe furious, as we show in the example where Camilla meets her boyfriend, who has ended their relationship.

TERRY: 'I can't take all the hassle of not understanding you and how you think I should be. I've found a place I can stay for a while. I'm moving out now'.

CAMILLA: 'You can't mean that. I'll do everything I can to avoid hassling you. Of course you can have your own opinions'.

TERRY: 'I don't believe you—you've said that many times before. It's over'.

CAMILLA screams angrily: 'Yeah, just get as far away as you can, get out right away'.

Terry shows resistance to Camilla's nagging about him understanding her, which he experiences as an implicit demand to have the same opinion she has. Camilla initially tries to appease Terry, which in turn can be considered an attempt to flow with him, and which could have made Terry feel guilty. However, Terry insists on moving out, which we can see as both resistance to Camilla's expecta-tions and as differentiation, in which he distinguishes between them by disagree-ing with her. Camilla, in her last reply, shows both confluence and resistance when she becomes furious and asks Terry to move as far away as he can get, right away. We sense her despair and anger and that she feels betrayed by Terry and places the blame on him. She becomes overwhelmed by her own emotions and flows with them as she isolates herself from Terry.

Borgen (2014) uses the phrase 'healing and stifling confluence'. She describes how necessary it is to be understood and experience that others flow along with us but also how stifling a lack of differentiation can be. Expressing a 'we' empha-sises the positive aspect of flowing with others, but this experience also has its challenges. It is possible to become so engulfed in something or someone else that it can bring about an unpleasant experience of losing oneself. For many, dis-agreeing with another or having needs or desires that are not the same as those we are with is difficult, as the example of Camilla and Terry shows. Both at work and in private life we can see how some people constantly try to smooth over disagreement, make sure everyone is happy, take care of others, invite others to have a good time, and are generally the 'glue' between colleagues or family mem-bers. On the other hand, there are those who solve tasks on their own, who travel around the world for work or on their own, and who are content in their own company. Most of us can recognise ourselves in both these examples, and often it is the life situation we find ourselves in that helps shape how we make contact with our surroundings, as the example below with Oscar and his mother shows.

To flow together or differentiate

Oscar is eighteen and lives with his mother. They have had a very close relationship where Oscar has felt supported and loved. This is also true of the times he has chosen to be with his father and his new family. However, he now feels that his mother is controlling and pesters him at all hours. She wants to know where he is in the evenings, whether he does his homework, who he is with, whether he is eating well, and so on. Oscar becomes more and more annoyed at his mother, until one day he loses it. He screams at her that he is moving out to live for a year in Africa to work with refugees. His mother tries to stop him, but he is determined to leave. He is over eighteen and makes decisions about his own life.

This is an example of how 'flowing together', as Oscar and his mother have done for many years, can lead to the opposite, namely a lack of understanding and distance. If we take this example further, we see several possibilities:

Option 1:

Oscar's mother eventually realises that her concerns have been unfounded and that she has tried to control Oscar, and tells him so. She adds that he can of course travel to work in a refugee camp. She thinks it sounds like a good idea. She asks him to tell her if he needs anything before he leaves. Oscar is very relieved; there are tears in her eyes when he hears his mother's understanding words and that she offers to help him.

Here, his mother chooses to differentiate by saying that Oscar can leave, which leads to Oscar being able to approach his mother in a different and new way. They can differentiate rather than flow together, and this differentiation leads to a different kind of closeness between them.

Option 2:

Oscar's mother becomes despondent and very angry when she hears what Oscar is thinking of doing. She screams at him and says that he can leave right away and that she is very disappointed with his lack of gratitude.

Here, the resistance results in isolation. When neither of them feels understood, it may feel better not to see each other at all in order to avoid being constantly reminded of the disagreement between them.

This example shows how intense the experience of confluence can be, that this experience becomes too demanding for Oscar and his mother, and that they need to find other ways—forms—in which to be together.

To flow with one's own thoughts and feelings

How we feel about ourselves and whether we are aware of feelings and thoughts also affects how we are with our surroundings. When we flow with our own thoughts and feelings there is little room for our surroundings, and others can easily perceive us as differentiated or isolated. These are forms of contact that can be recognised in retroflection and self-monitoring, which are addressed in Chapters 15 and 16.

The examples of Camilla and Terry and of Oscar and his mother describe the contact relationship, but we have not yet described what happens in and with the individual. We have an idea of how Camilla feels; she is distraught and sad that Terry has ended the relationship, and it is easy to imagine that her emotions overwhelm her both when she is alone and when she is with Terry. Camilla's need for closeness and security is threatened when Terry leaves her. The fear of being alone, no longer with Terry, and the uncertainty of what the future might bring overwhelms her, and she fails to see the world around her clearly. All the feelings she identifies with prevent her from being aware of how she is when she is with Terry, and how he responds to her form of contact. Terry is also full of emotions such as anger and irritation. He is aware of these emotions to some extent, but perhaps it is just as much his own thoughts that control him—thoughts about how he can solve the unpleasant situation he is in. His thoughts continue to occupy him, causing him to pay little attention to the feelings that are the reason for the thoughts, for his own behaviour, or for Camilla's reactions.

In the example of Oscar and mother, both are affected by having inner and conflicting feelings, which are expressions of conflicting needs. The fact that they are happy with each other and need to flow together, while Oscar has an ever-growing need for distance from his mother, to be independent and to live his own life, creates great tension both within each of them and between them. Oscar's mother has a certain understanding of and draws attention to Oscar's needs in the first version of the conversation between them. This attention means that she can differentiate from her own need to flow with Oscar, and thus also differentiate when she talks to him. This means that Oscar does not flow as much with (confluence) his own emotions and can listen to his mother and change his behaviour. He can also differentiate. In the second version of the conversation, Oscar's mother flows completely with her own feelings of fear of losing Oscar and of being separated from him. Her confluence with her own feelings results in her screaming at Oscar, who isolates himself. They both become confluent with their own emotions and, as a result, distant from one another.

Confluence in therapy

The interest among gestalt therapists to use the theoretical model of the contact form confluence and its polarities in practice has led to a greater awareness and knowledge of the approaches and techniques therapists can use in the therapy room (Frydenberg in interview with Møklebust, 2016). In therapy, the therapist is aware whether she flows with the client or differentiates, how the client expresses herself verbally and nonverbally, and which aspects of the contact form become dominant or less flexible between them. For example, on the basis of these observations, the therapist can explore how she and the client are constantly intertwined, or perhaps the client's constant resistance to the therapist's interventions and suggestions for experiments (see Chapter 10 on polarities).

Here we show an example from therapy where the therapist both flows with and differentiates when Camilla, at the request of her friend Martha, is in her first therapy session.

Camilla tells the therapist about how awful things are and how angry she is at Terry. The therapist listens to Camilla and 'flows with' her by nodding, smiling, and saying that she understands that it must be difficult for her that Terry has moved out after living together with him for several years.

CAMILLA: 'I have no idea what I've done to make him leave me. He says I'm always on his case, but that's not true. I'm really very patient and do a lot to make things good between us. I keep a nice home, make good food that he likes, invite him to the movies and out to cafes and do things with him that he likes to do'.

THE THERAPIST nods and says with conviction: 'I'm sure what you're saying is correct, and I understand you're sorry he doesn't see everything you do to make things good between the two of you'.

CAMILLA: 'It's good to hear you say that. When I tried to talk to Terry he was annoyed and said he didn't have time to talk'.

THERAPIST: 'Hmm . . . what did you want to talk to him about?'

CAMILLA: 'I was trying to talk about my job, plan when we were going to renovate the bathroom, if we could invite guests, and when we were going on vacation this summer, but it didn't work . . . '

THERAPIST: 'And Terry wasn't interested . . . '

CAMILLA: 'No, that's when he thought I was on his case. He didn't seem to care about my job, our apartment, or doing anything together, just about working, going to the gym, and being with friends'.

> THERAPIST: 'Hmm, it sounds like you had very different interests. It sounds like it was hard for you that he didn't want the same things as you did?'
> CAMILLA: 'Yes, but it wasn't like that at first'.
> THE THERAPIST nods: 'I'm sure it wasn't. What did you do when he didn't want to talk to you about the things you wanted to talk about?'
> CAMILLA: 'Argh . . . That's when I started to mumble and wanted to talk about it anyway. Maybe that was part of what he meant . . . I don't handle it well that he doesn't listen to me, or that he doesn't want the same things as I do . . . And I think it's hard for him to handle it when I bug him about these things . . . '

The therapist first chooses to support the side or pole of Camilla that is afraid of losing Terry, something she does by nodding, listening to her, and saying she understands. When Camilla feels understood, it becomes easier for her to hear and reflect on the therapist's questions and to differentiate from her own overwhelming feelings. By asking questions, the therapist differentiates from Camilla, which helps Camilla to see herself and her actions, and also to differentiate from Terry.

To flow along with in therapy

In the beginning of a therapy process it is natural for the therapist to spend time getting to know the client. It is usual thing is to 'flow' with the conversation by listening to the client's narrative, confirming what is said with words, nodding, or repeating to make sure what was said is understood. The therapist is often restrained in regard to her own opinions or assessment; rather, she listens actively to the client's narrative. This is where the foundation is laid for a belief in the good intent of the other and is thus the basis for further therapy. This is especially important for clients who have a history of heavy traumatic experiences, where it is necessary that the therapist be alert and supportive and take her time in establishing contact between herself and the client.

At this stage, in the very beginning of the therapeutic collaboration, there is no doubt that the contact form confluence is both obvious and necessary. It is about getting to know each other and establishing a sense of community and supporting a 'we' experience in the therapy collaboration. We see how the therapist uses this theory in practice with Eleanor.

> Eleanor's family doctor has recommended that she contact a gestalt therapist to talk about a rape she was recently subjected to. Eleanor sits in the therapist's office and talks about the rape, and how difficult she finds things now, afterwards. Eleanor talks with tears in her eyes and in a subdued voice; the therapist is touched and is drawn into the story.

> THERAPIST: 'I'm touched when I listen to you, and I understand that this has been and still is very difficult'.
> ELEANOR: 'Yes, I'm so sorry, my whole life has been turned upside down. I feel dirty and ashamed. I feel so stupid . . . '
> THERAPIST: 'I understand that it's possible to feel that way, even though what happened wasn't your fault. It's the fault of the man who raped you'.
> ELEANOR: 'It's easy to say it's his fault, but I drank too much and was out on the town, I was an easy mark'. Eleanor sits bent forward and cries quietly as she talks.
>
> The therapist senses that her body feels heavy and that she is barely breathing. It is as if she is in unison with Eleanor and does not know what to say or do.

Here, the therapist becomes aware that Eleanor is sad and that her own body feels heavy. She would like to help, but at the same time she feels helpless. This is a sign that there is confluence between the therapist and Eleanor. As she becomes aware that she is not only flowing with Eleanor because it is useful in the first session but that she is caught up in Eleanor's story, she strives to differentiate. This is already the beginning of a separation from Eleanor. With increased awareness of how she involuntarily flows with Eleanor, she can articulate how she feels, and hear that Eleanor's experience is not quite the same—they differentiate. We also hear that Eleanor flows in her own story, that is, she is confluent with her own experience. The therapist thinks that it will be useful for Eleanor to say out loud what she senses in her body and the emotions she experiences in order to distinguish between the experience there and then and the situation now in the therapy room.

> THE THERAPIST says in a gentle voice: 'I see that there are tears in your eyes. I'm also sorry and feel tears in my eyes.
> ELEANOR: 'I don't know what to do now. I can't bear to go to work and don't know how to be with my partner . . . ' She continues to cry.
> THERAPIST: 'Yes, I can understand that you don't know what the future holds . . . and that you cry now . . . At least I'll be with you when you cry . . . would you like me to put a blanket around you? . . . sometimes that can feel good'.
> ELEANOR looks at her quickly and says with a small smile: 'Yeah . . . I think that would be nice'.

The therapist continues to flow with Eleanor, both because she thinks Eleanor needs it and because she has no other thoughts or impulses. It is only when she hears Eleanor's words and sees her tears, observes how she has slumped in her chair, and senses that she herself is heavy and cold that she has an impulse to put a blanket around Eleanor—and differentiate. She asks Eleanor if she wants a blanket around her, something Eleanor answers in the affirmative. When Eleanor is wrapped in the blanket, she feels the therapist's caring attitude. This makes it easier for her to flow with her own emotions.

It may be that Eleanor, by being wrapped up in this way, becomes more aware of the sensations she has in her body and more aware of her needs in the situation. She probably has several needs together with the therapist. We can imagine that *one need* is to be taken care of and continue to flow with feelings of sadness and shame, and *another need* may be to move on, leave the painful experiences behind and differentiate from the pain and discomfort. The therapist is aware that she also has conflicting needs: a need to help and care for Eleanor where she can flow along with her, and another need to make Eleanor stand on her own so she is not so helpless.

Feeling helpless as a therapist

It is important for the therapist to be aware when she wants to help and when she feels helpless, and see that there may be signs that there is confluence between them. In the need for help we can also recognise warmth, care, and empathy, and it is only when these feelings take over and the therapist cannot distinguish between her own need for help and the client's need for help that she should be on guard that she can lose herself as a therapist. When the therapist becomes aware of this confluence, she can regulate the relationship between herself and the client, depending on what she thinks they each need in the situation. In the example of Eleanor, we see how the therapist waits to say and do something other than flow along with the client before she receives an impulse based on her contact functions (see Chapter 5), that is, what she sees, hears, and feels with Eleanor.

We follow Eleanor further into therapy and have come to the fourth session.

Eleanor and the therapist have become better acquainted with each other. The therapist gradually begins to notice that Eleanor continues to talk about the rape and her feeling of shame as if it is the first time she tells it. Eleanor's voice has more of a complaining tone, her body seems to be stiffer, and the therapist begins to feel a growing irritation. It dawns on her that Eleanor is afraid to leave the security she experiences by flowing along with being helpless and feeling sorry for herself. She thinks that Eleanor is unaware of this fear, and that it can be helpful for her to realise that she is scared and how her fear affects her.

THERAPIST: 'Eleanor, as I sit with you now, I notice that I'm barely breathing and that my body feels stiff. I wonder how you experience your own breathing, and what you feel in your body'.

ELEANOR looks at the therapist and straightens up in her chair: 'I'm not breathing very much . . . and my body is probably stiff, I think I've been like that ever since this man attacked me'. She then begins to tell the same story she has already told several times.

THE THERAPIST, with a gentle voice where she chooses to 'put aside' her irritation: 'I understand that your body stiffened when that man attacked you. At the same time, I notice that you now continue to tell me about what happened, something you've already told me several times. It's almost as if you don't remember telling me you were raped . . .'

ELEANOR: 'It's not like I don't remember telling you, but it's as if I can't get the incident out of my head, as if the same pictures of what happened return again and again. It's just awful . . .'

THERAPIST: 'I see . . . the pictures come again and again, and you can't stop them . . . It sounds bad . . . At the same time, I notice that when you tell me these things, you talk very fast, you don't look at me, and it's like you're lost in these pictures . . .'

ELEANOR: 'I haven't thought about that . . . maybe I get lost . . . in the pictures I see . . . and the emotions . . .'

Here, the therapist tries to help Eleanor be present here and now by mentioning breathing and bodily sensations, and by helping her differentiate instead of flowing into her own story. However, when Eleanor continues to talk about the rape, the therapist points out that she has heard the story before, and asks if Eleanor remembers, which Eleanor confirms. The therapist understands that Eleanor is not ready to explore the breath and stiffness she feels in her body, and therefore downgrades the intervention. When Eleanor talks about the images she has in her head, it is as if she realises how it is for her to be here and now with the therapist. This touches the therapist, who again flows with Eleanor before stating that she has noticed that Eleanor speaks quickly, and that it is as if she is lost in the pictures she envisions. Eleanor follows the therapist in what she says. She differentiates, and it is as if she has a moment of insight about herself.

To confront with the heart

When the therapist points out that she has heard Eleanor's story before, she creates a cautious confrontation in hope that Eleanor can become aware of how she repeats herself and gets lost in the pictures. Perhaps increased attention may lead to a change in Eleanor. In vulnerable relationships, such as between Eleanor and the therapist, the therapist must be careful so that the client does not feel rejected or misunderstood. We call such confrontations 'carefrontations' (Greenberg, 2016), or confronting with the heart (Skottun, 2002/2008). It is important that the therapist does not let her irritation become prominent. She has to put it aside, as she did in the example of Eleanor, and instead choose to feel the warmth she has for the client. She chooses to follow her heart. The therapist differentiates from her irritation and chooses to flow with the goodness she feels for Eleanor. She chooses which feelings and thoughts she follows (Skottun, 2002/2008).

Differentiation through movement

The therapy process between Eleanor and the therapist continues.

Together with Eleanor, the therapist explores how it feels for her to repeatedly envision pictures of the rape, and whether she wants to think of something else. Eleanor says she would like to think about something else but does not know how to get rid of the pictures or what she can think about instead. She says that the rape fills her life and that she does not talk about anything else with her partner or friends. Eleanor still talks very quickly, cries a lot, and is stiff in her body. The therapist continues to support Eleanor by saying that seeing pictures and thus reliving the rape is a common reaction when a person has been subjected to such a trauma. She asks if Eleanor wants to try an experiment, which Eleanor says yes to.

THERAPIST: 'I'd like us to get up and walk around the room a little bit. My own body feels heavy and I'm almost out of breath . . . Maybe it might be good to move instead of sitting still thinking and talking . . . Does that sound okay?'

ELEANOR nods and says at the same time: 'I don't know what the point is, but yes, I can try . . . '

The therapist gets up and starts moving slowly around the room, and Eleanor follows as she talks about how strange she thinks it is to walk around the room with the therapist.

THERAPIST: 'Yes, it's a little unusual . . . It's probably more common to sit in two chairs and talk like we usually do . . . As you walk, you can feel your feet hitting the floor with every step . . . I can't feel it very well myself'.

ELEANOR: 'No, I don't know, I'm wearing thick shoes . . . By the way, it feels good to move . . . '

THERAPIST: 'Can we take our shoes off and see if there's a difference?'

Eleanor nods, and they walk around without shoes. Together they try out what it is like to walk heavily and lightly, and how the surface feels where there is carpet and on the wooden floor. They walk towards each other and then apart as they look at each other. Both breathe more deeply, and colour returns to their faces. After a while, they sit down and talk about what it was like to do this experiment.

Eleanor says that she feels calmer and that it was nice to walk around with the therapist. The therapist feels less heavy and breathes more easily and says that she noticed that Eleanor looks at her more and spoke more quietly. Eleanor says that all the pictures are gone and that she is now more interested in what it is like to be with her therapist.

In this sequence, the therapist chooses to involve Eleanor in an experiment by walking around the room. The intention is that Eleanor can turn her attention from her mind to her body and become aware of the therapist and the room they are in. This is a way to differentiate from the images and thoughts Eleanor has. By walking around in the room, they also emerged from the trapped physical situation they experienced, where Eleanor was heavy and stiff and the therapist felt heavy and short of breath. This is a way of mobilising energy that we saw in the example of Simon on p. 186. In this experiment we can see how the therapist and Eleanor flow together and differentiate. For example, Eleanor joins the experiment, but comments that she thinks it is odd to walk around the room with the therapist. They walk together, trying out proximity and distance by walking towards and away from each other. On the one hand, they flow together in the experiment, and on the other, they move independently and separately from each other where the therapist leads and Eleanor follows.

Being confluent can sometimes feel like being 'stuck in the body', as if all thoughts and feelings are being withheld and the body controls the chaos of emotions and thoughts by stiffening. When the therapist becomes aware of this confluent lock, it can sometimes be useful to invite the client to get up from the chair and move, as the therapist does in the example of Eleanor. Movement increases awareness of bodily sensation, and thoughts retreat to the background. Moving out of the chair can also be an experiment, to explore how confluence is experienced here and now. What is it like to sit in the chair, what is it like to get up, what is felt in the body, and how is the relationship between therapist and client affected when they walk together instead of sitting in two chairs?

Summary

In working with confluence and its polarities resistance, differentiation, and isolation, it is important that the therapist is aware of how she and the client regulate the relationship between them. The therapist is interested in when they flow together, when there is resistance in the form of unpleasant feelings, and how they differentiate or are 'far apart' in the therapy room. When the therapist becomes aware of unpleasant sensations or feelings, she can explore with the client how the distance is experienced. In this way, the client can become aware of bodily sensations, whether the contact has become too close, and if there is a need for distance. It is important that the therapist teaches the client to become aware of how associations and unclear thoughts can create chaos and misunderstanding for her in situations she finds herself in and make it difficult for her to make choices. In this work, it is important for the client to experience how the therapist can flow with her in therapy and for the client to feel understood and heard, while at the same time experiencing how the therapist's resistance can be liberating as she confronts her and holds her in a theme or issue.

References

Borgen, K. (2014). Konfluens—kvelende eller helende? [Confluence: Stifling or healing?]. *Norsk Gestalttidsskrift, 11*(2), 58–67.

Clarkson, P., & Mackewn, J. (1993). *Fritz Perls*. London: Sage Publications.

Frank, R. (2016). Self in motion. In J.-M. Robine (Ed.), *Self: A polyphony of contemporary gestalt therapists* (pp. 371–386). St. Romain la Virvée, France: L'Exprimerie.

Greenberg, E. (2016). *Borderline, narcissistic and schizoid adaptions: The pursuit of love, admiration and safety*. New York: Greenberg Press.

Kokkersvold, E., & Mjelve, H. (2003). *Mellom oss* [Between us]. Oslo: Gyldendal Akademisk.

Kolmannskog, V. (2018). *The empty chair*. London: Routledge.

Krüger, Å. (2012). Bokomtale [Book review]. *Norsk Gestalttidsskrift, 9*(2), 65–71.

Møklebust, L. (2016). Konfluens—teori eller metode? En samtale med Hans Petter Frydenberg [Confluence: Theory or method? A conversation with Hans Petter Frydenberg]. *Norsk Gestalttidsskrift, 13*(2), 44–55.

Perls, F. S., Hefferline, R. F., & Goodman, P. (1951). *Gestalt therapy: Excitement and growth in the human personality*. London: Souvenir Press.

Rogers, C. (1967). *On becoming a person: A therapist view of psychotherapy*. London: Constable.

Skottun, G. (2002/2008). Reisebrev. Essay om kontaktformer og figurdannelser [Travelogue: Essay on contact forms and figure formation]. In S. Jørstad & Å. Krüger (Eds.), *Den flyvende hollender* [The flying Dutchman] (pp. 105–127). Oslo: NGI.

Staemmler, F. M. (2007). On Macaque monkeys, players, and clairvoyants: Some new ideas for a gestalt therapeutic concept of empathy. *Studies in Gestalt Therapy, 1*(2), 43–63.

Staemmler, F. M. (2012). *Empathy in psychotherapy: How therapists and clients understand each other*. (E. J. Hamilton & D. Winter, Trans.). New York: Springer.

Wheeler, G. (1998). *Gestalt reconsidered* (2nd ed.). Cambridge, MA: CIGPress.

Chapter 13

Introjection

> Daniel impatiently calls out to his partner as he puts on his jacket in the hallway: 'Hurry up, Ellen, or we'll be late for dinner with Hilde and Tom!' He continues: 'You know how I hate to be late'. 'I'm almost ready, I just have to find another sweater. I want to look nice when we finally go out for a change', Ellen replies irritably. 'There's no rush, they won't be ready when we get there anyway'.

Contact between the couple is characterised by Daniel thinking they need to be on time to meet their friends, while this is not so important to Ellen. She is more concerned about what to wear, which is more important to her in this situation than being on time. We get the feeling this might be a source of conflict between them if being on time truly is important for Daniel and he continues nag Ellen. Failing to be on time may irritate Ellen even more, causing her to be stressed, with the result that she is not able to find a sweater she thinks is appropriate for the occasion.

Another scenario we can imagine that would affect Ellen and Daniel's contact is if Daniel agrees with Ellen about it not being so important to be on time when meeting their friends. Maybe he sees instead how nice Ellen looks in another sweater, compliments her, and appreciates that she takes the time to dress up to go out with him. Maybe Ellen likes this, feels flattered, and hurries to get ready to be with Daniel.

Ellen and Daniel's relationship to expectations, rules, and norms characterises the contact between them in this short conversation, which many of us can likely recognise from our own lives. Everyday life consists of many such moments in which people have opinions and attitudes about how they or others should be, such as being on time or dressing appropriately. Many people have a more or less conscious attitude that they should be good and act appropriately. They try to have a healthy diet, exercise, study, get a good education, make a lot of money, and have a house, a car, and a stable financial situation. They are conscientious

DOI: 10.4324/9781003153856-16

and work hard to fulfil the demands they place on themselves or that others have of them. They must finish what they do, they must not make mistakes, and they must have complete control over themselves and their lives. When people try to be good and do what is right, it is because they need to live up to the expectations, rules, and norms in their environment that dictate how to live and that they have more or less consciously accepted.

To some, these expectations, rules, and norms may feel like injunctions and compulsions. There are also examples of people who rebel against expectations and demands, who postpone what they should do, act on impulse, are creative, and live in chaos and clutter. These two cases are the extremes in the contact form called introjection.

Integrating feedback

The word 'introjection' originates from the Latin *intrō-* and *-iectiō*, which can be translated 'to throw in'. In gestalt theory, introjection is understood as to receive or ingest one or more messages from others without reflection. In practice, this means that the opinions, attitudes, injunctions, and rules that are given are accepted unreservedly by recipients and transformed into their own opinions and attitudes, which they then pass on to their surroundings.

In all learning and education, the ability to receive is important. During childhood we learn norms and rules for right and wrong, how to behave in the family, at school, and in society in general. How this learning process has been will affect our ability to receive and learn in adulthood. We take our childhood values and norms into adulthood, where reflection and adaptation are usually necessary. This is because many of the values and norms we were given as children were either pushed on us uncritically, without reflection, or do not fit into our lives today (Hostrup, 2010). We are not always aware of the norms and rules we have integrated in ourselves.

In this chapter, we describe various forms of introjection and how introjection affects human contact. Through examples from clinical practice we show how the therapist explores and increases awareness of introjection in the therapy room and in the client's life.

Instructions, demands, and expectations from others are called *introjects* in the gestalt theory literature. We often find introjects in sentences where words such as should, ought to, and must occur (Jørstad, 2002/2008).

In this book, we choose for the most part to use non-theoretical words such as 'message', 'injunction', or 'expectation' instead of the theoretical concept introject. It is the content of the expectation and how it is delivered and received that affects the contact between people, as seen in the example of Ellen and Daniel.

In the gestalt literature the term 'introjection' is also used to describe how we internalise, uncritically 'swallow', or incorporate these expectations into our own attitudes and behaviour.

Fritz Perls used metaphors derived from eating in his discussion of introjection (Perls, 1947/1969). He argued that many people simply 'swallow' the expectations they are served without first considering, or 'chewing' them, and that they therefore later in life need to learn to 'spit out' and can experience anger in the process. Perls looked at introjection as the fundamental resistance to contact, and he believed chewing or oral aggression was its opposite. The challenge of the concept of introjection, as Perls introduced it, is that we easily associate it with physical and physiological processes for swallowing, chewing, and digestion. We are critical of this use of this particular metaphor and feel that Perls was overly concerned with the physical process, especially as it relates to assimilation and aggression. We believe it is important that the concepts surrounding introjection are not taken literally, but rather are only used as images or metaphors for psychological processes.

Introjection and Perls' concept of aggression

Fritz Perls' use of metaphor in the form of swallowing, spitting, and chewing is based on his knowledge of Freud's understanding of *oral aggression*. According to psychoanalysis, strong aggression has its origin in the oral phase of psychosexual development during the first two years of a child's life. The oral phase is often associated with feeding and the ways in which the infant has contact with the parents.

To show strong aggression as an adult is a powerful expression of frustration over a lack of satisfaction in life's first two years. Although Perls broke with psychoanalysis in most areas, he continued to agree with Freud's theory that oral aggression is related to anger. Perls was particularly concerned with what he called *dental aggression*, and how humans can learn to use their teeth to chew all the expectations, or introjects, that they receive. He was very critical of the uncritical, complete swallowing of other people's opinions, which he had seen in Nazi Germany before and during World War II. He also believed that swallowing one's own opinions rather than expressing them ('spitting them out') or 'chewing them' in order to digest them caused an accumulation of anger in people. He wrote an entire book on the theme, entitled *Ego, hunger and aggression* (1947/1969). Perls believed that this anger had to be worked on in therapy, and he used forceful means to get clients to express and therefore let go of their anger. Perls and his successors are known to have provoked a client's unexpressed anger, encouraging her to scream or trample and hit pillows. In some cases, client and therapist even fought physically (Yontef, 1993). In this view of introjection, it is clear that Perls and his close followers viewed introjection and 'swallowed' expectations as something negative that clients

(*Continued*)

needed to get rid of or stop doing. This view can still be seen in some gestalt therapists today, in how the therapist meets clients who come to therapy in order to rid themselves of expectations from their childhood and upbringing (Clarkson & Mackewn, 1993).

In today's gestalt therapy practice, this explosive form of expression that Perls became so well known for has less emphasis. Anger still has a place as a phenomenon in therapy, but emphasis is now placed on helping the client to recognise her anger in the same way as other emotions need to be recognised, and thus their place in the process of change in general receives more emphasis (Staemmler, 2009). Metaphors are no longer direct expressions of aggression, but merely meant to be what they are, a symbolic help in exploring experiences.

Swallowing, spitting out, or processing

We can respond in several ways to expectations from those around us. We can for example do what is asked of us, thereby accepting the expectation without conscious reflection. An example of this might be that we pay for public transportation when we are asked to. A polar reaction to this acceptance of an expectation could be to react with resistance and refuse to pay, or 'spit out' the expectation, such as when we feel the ticket is too expensive when we only plan to travel two stops. Another and more moderate form of resistance to an expectation is what we call reflection, or 'chewing'. In the example of the public transportation ticket, we would consider the issue, and then come to the realisation that it is natural that we pay to travel, even if we disagree with the price.

Wheeler (1998) found Perls' metaphorical formulations useful and significant for processes in which introjection is figure, and devised a model for the contact form and its polarities that can be used by therapists (see p. 170). For example, when exploring the introjection 'I have to get along with others', it is illustrative and helpful to ask the client to reflect on or 'chew' what this statement means to her. When the experience is 'tasted' long enough, it may be possible for the client to know what she wants to keep and what she wants to spit out.

In Figure 13.1, we show the three forms of introjection mentioned above that we find helpful in therapy. One side of the polarity is to accept or swallow, and on the other side we find rejecting or spitting out, or a milder form in which the expectation is processed and becomes our own (Wheeler, 1998).

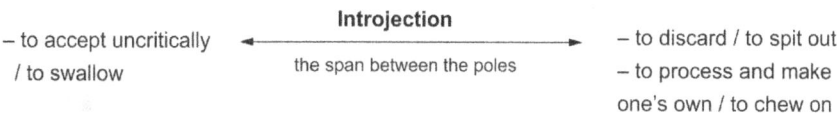

Introjection

– to accept uncritically / to swallow   ◄————————►   – to discard / to spit out

the span between the poles   – to process and make one's own / to chew on

Figure 13.1 Three forms of introjection.

The tension between these poles is an expression of the tension that may exist in the choice between accepting or rejecting the expectation. In this continuum from rejection to acceptance, the client is often helped by the therapist to explore, reflect over, and chew the expectations, rules, assumptions, or attitudes she has. In a therapy session, the pole to integrate/chew on one side often becomes either to accept/swallow or reject/spit out on the other.

Giving and receiving expectations: a field phenomenon

As in all forms of contact, introjection is a phenomenon that occurs in a field with others. In the model of introjection shown in Figure 13.1, based on Wheeler, the field between the recipient and the expectation is not included, which gives a simplified picture of the complex interaction between people that characterises introjection.

In Figure 13.2 we show a new model, in which a person or group communicates expectations, needs, or demands, and a recipient of the communication. Giving and receiving expectations are interconnected, and there is a continuum and a tension between them. We have designed the illustration in Figure 13.2 based on Wheeler's (1998) discussion of contact and polarities.

In the model, there is a connection between how an expectation is communicated and how it is received; both are called 'introjection'. However, the gap between accepting and rejecting is not visible in Figure 13.2, because both forms can be ways of receiving an expectation. Both Fritz Perls and Wheeler believed that the content of expectations and how they are expressed affects the recipient, but this relationship is not reflected in Wheeler's model (Figure 13.1).

The model shown in Figure 13.2 is particularly useful in therapy, where the therapist is always part of the field with the client and is the one who both gives and receives expectations and has her own needs. The therapist is interested in the field in which the client experiences an expectation, whether it is the field between the therapist and the client or the field between the client and people in her surroundings (see Chapter 1, 'Field Theory', and Chapter 4, 'The Field in Practice').

The gestalt therapist and introjection

The gestalt therapist's work is influenced by her therapist training and previous education. It is important that the therapist is aware of her relationship to norms and rules, how she herself has swallowed, accepted, spit out, and processed the expectations she has experienced while growing up and while studying to become

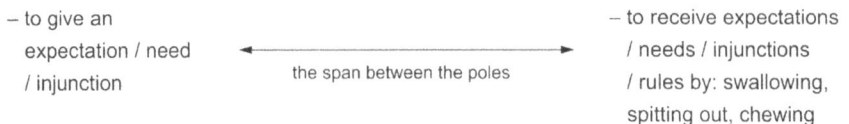

– to give an
expectation / need
/ injunction

the span between the poles

– to receive expectations
/ needs / injunctions
/ rules by: swallowing,
spitting out, chewing

Figure 13.2 Introjection as a figure in the field.

a gestalt therapist, and how she meets the client in the therapy room. Therapy is also a form of teaching where clients learn new ways of living with themselves and their surroundings; the therapist's approach to this teaching will influence the meeting between them. The therapist's values, ethics, and morals, her ideas about what good therapy consists of, and her expectations of herself and the client will shape the relationship between them (Joyce & Sills, 2014).

Introjection in the therapy room

The therapist is aware of how the client expresses herself, moves, and approaches the therapist. When the therapist hears the client refer to rules or ideas about how she should be, she may experience introjection in the field. If the client continues to talk about expectations, the therapist may experience that introjection has become the most prominent form of contact between them. She comes to this hypothesis by noticing what the client talks about, observing different degrees of control and stiffness in the client's body and movements, and she may even be concerned about being good enough herself or doing good therapy. There can be many expectations in the room, and spontaneity and impulsivity can go to the background. The client may be looking for advice and solutions to her problems, and expect the therapist, whom she thinks is the expert, to know what is right and wrong. When the therapist asks her a question, the client may be concerned with giving the correct answer or what she thinks the therapist wants to hear. If the therapist intervenes in relation to the body, movement, or breathing, the client can easily become focused on how to breathe properly. Such experiments can often lead to more introjection (Skottun, 2002/2008). Therefore, when the client participates in experiments, it is important that she be extra mindful of whether the experiment is being done to satisfy the therapist's expectations or whether it is something she, the client, wants. One way to do this can be to explore the client's norms and expectations by thinking aloud and sharing one's own reflections.

Introjection, body movement, and anger

Some clients have learned to live with expectations and requirements, and in some cases these become so intrusive and strict that they cause clients to feel abandoned and depressed. Expectations about what the client 'should' do, both from the client herself and from her surroundings, can become so intrusive that the client feels paralysed and does not know what to do. Energy diminishes and tasks remain undone. This is the case for Tanya when she comes to therapy.

> Tanya is eighteen and in her last year of upper secondary education. She tells the therapist how difficult she thinks life is. She sleeps poorly at night and often lies awake worrying about everything she has to do. In her free time, she plays soccer and participates in a school drama production. Her parents complain that she has to spend more time on homework, and her

boyfriend has repeatedly complained that she doesn't seem to have time for him. As Tanya speaks, her upper body is caved inward, her breathing is shallow, and she look straight ahead.

TANYA says in a defeated voice: 'It's as if all my energy is gone. The thought of everything I need to get done stresses me and makes me feel desperate. And sometimes I just panic'.

THERAPIST: 'It sounds like all these demands are quite a burden. And I think that must really be difficult'.

TANYA: 'Yes. My father says I have to play soccer, my mother says I should start medical school, and my boyfriend says I have to spend more time with him. (sighs) Ugh, I've always been so happy, but now I just feel tired'.

As the session progresses, the therapist becomes aware that she has an impression that there are many expectations and demands in Tanya's surroundings. She shares these thoughts with Tanya. She chooses to listen to Tanya, confirm what she hears her say, and flow along with her story. All of this characterises the form of contact called 'confluence' (Chapter 12). The therapist is careful not to say anything that might give Tanya a feeling that she expects something from her, as she thinks there is enough introjection in the field between them already.

Tanya continues to talk about how frustrated she is with her parents, who expect so much from her.

THERAPIST: 'When I listen to your voice and look at your body, you look and sound annoyed, maybe almost a little angry. Do you notice that your foot moves back and forth as you speak? What if you try to exaggerate the movement?'

Tanya joins the experiment. The therapist is initially a little unsure if Tanya joined the experiment because she was asked to, that is, because the therapist had introduced a new introject into the field, but is reassured when she sees Tanya's engagement and how she moves her foot even faster as she speaks louder and more clearly.

As Tanya experiments, she realises that she is angry with both her mother and father, and that an impulse to kick them arises. Tanya's voice has more power when she tells the therapist about this. The therapist notices that she is affected by Tanya's movements and voice. She suggests that they both get up and walk around the room a bit to increase their awareness of movement and of what is happening in their feet. As Tanya joins the therapist in walking around, she feels her feet against the floor and begins to step more forcefully while repeating that she is angry. The therapist walks alongside her while saying that it is okay to be angry.

After a while, Tanya stops and says that she feels much calmer. She says that it has been liberating to express the anger she had been holding back, and that she now feels stronger rather than tired.

Here, the therapist chooses to focus on Tanya's facial expressions and body movements rather than the content of what she says (see Chapter 11 on experiments). She believes that these are spontaneous expressions of what Tanya is feeling in the situation. This provides a different kind of contact between them than if they had talked about what Tanya must and should do, and is therefore another opportunity for Tanya to become aware of feelings and emotions. At this point in the session the therapist decides not to ask Tanya questions, because she thinks that questions too early in a conversation involving introjection can easily be perceived by the client as an expectation (Skottun, 2002/2008).

The therapist supports Tanya by copying the movement of her foot and by walking around and stomping on the floor with her. She also confirms Tanya's experience by saying it is okay to be angry.

She thinks that Tanya has an old expectation that anger is not allowed, and therefore has little attention to her feelings. The therapist chooses to stop the experiment when Tanya stops walking, because she thinks that Tanya has become aware of her anger. The therapist could have provoked her even more by reinforcing the negative image she had of her parents, but since she did not see any signs that she had pent-up anger she needed to express, she chose another route.

By discovering her anger through her body and emotions together with the therapist, Tanya experiences what we have previously described as a paradoxical change (Chapter 5). As Tanya realises that she is tired of expectations and demands, the expectations go to the background, and change can occur.

In the following, we see how the last part of the therapy session develops.

As the end of the session draws nears, the therapist and Tanya sit on their chairs opposite each other and reflect over the experiment they just did.

TANYA: 'I really didn't know I was so mad at my parents. It's a bit strange, because I think they've always been so kind to me and given me generous boundaries. But now I realise that they have very high expectations of me since I am their only child . . . And they have always taken really good care of me and been afraid that something would happen to me . . . there's been a lot of control, and there still is. Oh . . . I can't handle all that control and all the demands . . . ' Her voice starts to get louder again, and she becomes angry again.

THERAPIST: 'I think it's natural that you're angry and that you don't need to be controlled. After all, you're practically an adult, obviously you want to make decisions about your own life. At the same time, it's no wonder your parents are afraid something would happen to you'.

TANYA: 'Yes, I understand that too, and it's easier now for me to be angry and at the same time love them. I think maybe I'm not going to move out right away, like I'd planned. But my parents act they like know everything and are on my case about everything I should and shouldn't do and . . . '

In the course of the sessions, as she reflects together with the therapist, Tanya becomes more aware of her conflicting feelings towards her parents. The therapist thinks that Tanya needs to explore these conflicting thoughts and feelings even more, but chooses to end the session here. She thinks it might be good for Tanya to have time alone in this process of reflection, so that she as a therapist does not become a new adult who starts to direct, decide, or give advice, as Tanya's parents have done. It is easy for the therapist to recognise introjection in the field with Tanya, and she is aware that the reflections she shares with Tanya are not expectations or advice. Instead, she emphasises that it is natural for Tanya to be in the situation she is in as an eighteen-year-old with parents who love her.

Exploring choices

The therapist can also choose to work with Tanya's introjection by paying attention to the content of what is being said, which she does at a later session.

The therapist asks Tanya to tell her some of the demands she feels, starting her sentences with 'I'.

TANYA: 'I have to spend time with my boyfriend'.

THE THERAPIST asks: 'Do you have to?'

TANYA: 'It feels like that, he expects it from me.' Tanya speaks in a loud and thin voice and seems to barely be breathing. The therapist senses that she herself is also barely breathing.

THERAPIST: 'Do you have to, even if he expects it?'

TANYA: 'No, I want to . . . It's just that I almost don't have the space to know what I want when I'm with him . . . ' She speaks more softly and becomes sad.

THERAPIST: 'It's as if you breathe a little more when you say you want to spend time with him . . . at the same time it looks like you're getting sad . . . '

> TANYA: 'Yes, I'm sad . . . and I haven't thought about how I breathe . . .
> Maybe I should breathe a little more . . . '
> THERAPIST: 'I don't know if you should breathe more . . . I said it looked
> like you were breathing more when you said you wanted to be with
> your boyfriend'.

Here the therapist points out how Tanya's breathing is different when she says has to spend time with her boyfriend compared with when she says wants to spend time with him. Tanya hears that she should breathe more, something other than what the therapist said. The therapist repeats what she had said. Here, the therapist realises that she herself did in fact automatically think it would be better for Tanya to breathe more, and that Tanya heard this implication since she is very receptive to messages that have to do with how she should be.

> THERAPIST: 'First of all, could you see what it's like to say: I have to spend
> time with my boyfriend?'
> TANYA: 'I have to spend time with my boyfriend . . . It feels heavy . . . and
> I'm probably not breathing that much . . . '
> THERAPIST: 'Okay. Now you can try saying: I want to spend time with my
> boyfriend'.
> TANYA: 'I want to spend time with my boyfriend . . . maybe I'm breathing
> a little bit better . . . '
> THERAPIST: 'Where in your body do you feel you are breathing?'
> TANYA: 'Mmm . . . in my chest . . . Yes, I can feel myself breathing . . . '
> THERAPIST: 'So, do I understand you right when you say you want to spend
> time with your boyfriend?'
> TANYA nods and smiles: 'Yes, of course I want to, it was good to be aware
> of that . . . Now I feel much more relaxed . . . and yes, I'm breathing
> more'.
> THERAPIST: 'It can be wonderful to discover what you want. I know that I
> breathe easier too; it was almost as if I were holding my breath when
> you said you have to spend time with your boyfriend'.

When Tanya experiments with changing from 'have to' to 'want to' in the first sentence the therapist gives her, she becomes aware that she wants to spend time with her boyfriend—that it is something she chooses herself, not something that is imposed on her. By chewing the expectation she has for herself, she becomes aware of the choice she has in the situation. She feels joy and relief, and we see an example of how she gains spontaneous insight. The therapist's intervention of pointing out what she sees in Tanya's breathing along the way, and the experiment she suggests with the phrases 'have to' and 'want to', make Tanya aware of feelings she has without the idea that she should breathe differently. At the end, the therapist shares her experience of her own breathing to reinforce Tanya's awareness of her own sensations and to help her understand that it is permissible to breathe in different ways. The therapist thinks that in the long run it will be important for Tanya to become aware of the relationship between introjection and breathing. This example illustrates how expectations and demands tend to settle in the body, whether in the breath or in tight muscles (Kepner, 1987/2001).

In the examples with Tanya, we see that she becomes more aware of conflicting needs and expectations she receives from her surroundings and herself. In adulthood, it is important for Tanya and indeed all of us to be able to understand the difference between what we want to spend time and effort on, and what we choose to do, and we need to be aware of the price that comes with choosing one option over another, such as a guilty conscience or the fact that someone else may be disappointed in us. Experience shows us that it is easier to be disciplined and to carry out projects and tasks that are based on our own wishes and needs than when these are based on expectations and demands from others. The ability to endure difficult and challenging situations is also closely linked to the awareness of choices we have made, and to be able to check whether these choices still apply by noticing bodily sensations such as breath and tension as well as the expectations we experience. The motivation, willingness, and ability to perform tasks are related, and can be recognised in situations such as when training for important competitions, practicing difficult pieces of music, or when accidents and crises occur.

Expectations in the coaching room

In coaching as in therapy, it is not uncommon for clients to come to a session with expectations of getting good advice or a solution to their problems. This expectation is often expressed in the form of a client seeking help or waiting for the coach to solve the problems for her. In this expectation there is often an implied requirement that the client must behave correctly so that she can get the help she needs.

Steven is in his first coaching session. He sits opposite the coach and looks at her awkwardly with his eyes wide open. He says he has a conflict at work that he hopes the coach can help him with. The coach senses tension in her body, notices that she sits uneasily in her chair, and that it is difficult to meet Steven's gaze. She says nothing about this in the beginning and instead lets Steven talk a bit about the difficulties he has at work.

After a while, however, she says: 'When I listen to what you're saying, I have an idea that you expect me to find a solution to the problem for you. Is that so?'

STEVEN: 'Yes, of course, that's why I'm here. I'm at the end of my rope with all these problems and you have to advise me'. He looks hopefully at the coach, who meets his gaze.

COACH: 'I understand that you're frustrated with having so many problems and that you're asking for advice. It's natural to want advice in a difficult situation. At the same time, I'm afraid that advice from me can lead you to feel that you have to follow my advice, and in that case, you'll have even more demands to meet than you already have . . . Can we first look at what you expect help with? Then maybe we can find out which expectations I can fulfil, and if there are some I have to say no to'.

STEVEN: 'Oh, do you think my expectations of you are too high? . . . Of course I don't expect you to tell me what to do, but some advice would be nice . . . Or maybe you think I shouldn't expect advice from you . . . '

COACH: 'I think it's good that you expect something from me. Why else would you come here? I just want us to look at what it is you want so that you don't go away feeling rejected. I'd love to listen to you and explore and sort out the issues you have at work. I have a lot of experience coaching others who have been in difficult work situations'.

STEVEN: 'That's good to hear. I need to talk to someone who has experience . . . '

In this situation, the coach chooses not to share her bodily unease. Her hypothesis is that introjection is the form of contact between them, and that it is better to reflect together Steven. Experientially, saying something about what the coach herself feels or pointing out observations about the client can easily lead to uncertainty and more introjection for the client (Skottun, 2002/2008). Instead, the coach chooses to support Steven by repeating what he says about his problems and his expectation of help. Here she flows with him; confluence is thus the form of contact between them (Chapter 12). The coach emphasises that she would like to explore Steven's problems and expectations so that he does not feel rejected and think that he should not have expectations. In addition, the coach wants to reassure Steven that she has experience even if she does not provide advice, as she thinks that Steven is concerned about what is right and wrong. In further work, the coach continues to explore Steven's problems so that he can become more aware of his situation at work.

Expectations and creativity

Having expectations of oneself and others is important and necessary as part of having ideas about the future, as we see in Steven's expectations of the coach. Expectations are often the hopes, desires, and dreams that help shape our ideas of how something should or can be. These expectations and ideas can give us motivation, which leads us to invest time and energy in accomplishing what we want. We can become creative in our search for solutions and ways to fulfil our dreams (Zinker, 1977). However, our ability to be creative is limited when we have many rules for how we should, must, or ought to act. In those cases, we can become more concerned with how to do something right rather than looking for a good solution to our problem.

Steven has an idea that coaching is a place he can get advice and help, which may be in line with what some coaches offer. However, a gestalt coach does not offer advice, and has a more exploratory approach than Steven expects. The coach is aware that Steven's expectations do not match what she offers, that she may disappoint him, and that Steven can quickly become uncertain as to whether his expectations are wrong. The challenge of having high expectations of others is that we can be disappointed if they are not fulfilled. Lack of expectations can mean that we have nothing to look forward to, that we lack motivation, and do not prepare and mobilise to achieve what we want. At the same time, we are not disappointed, and it is possible to be pleasantly surprised when something unexpected happens.

Introjection and learning

In all training and teaching, the contact between us will be characterised by how we receive the knowledge that is communicated to us. Are we open and willing to listen to what others say and want to teach us, or would we rather find the answers on our own? Our attitude in a learning situation is, of course, crucial to how we receive new knowledge. It is also important to be aware of how the training takes place, what form it has, and whether it is appropriate in relation to what is to be learned. In some contexts it is important to be able to listen and receive orders and instructions or follow recipes and guidelines. In other situations it is necessary to have time to reflect, try things out, and learn by experience. Furthermore, it is important that the person who imparts knowledge, injunctions, and rules is aware that different situations need different forms of training and teaching.

Summary

In this chapter, we first described the contact form introjection as information in the form of expectations, rules, and norms, and how these are received. Introjection is expressed between us in the form of assumptions and information we carry from our childhood and upbringing. In introjection, contact between people is easily characterised by ideas and assumptions about how other people or oneself should be or act, which can lead to challenges and conflicts. With increased attention to and awareness of the content of messages and how they affect contact, it becomes possible to change fixed ideas and ways of responding.

Therapy, coaching, and counselling are situations in which clients want to learn and experience something new. Clients usually seek help because they have an experience of being stuck in life. They have expectations of the therapist and can easily fall into the trap of accepting the therapist's opinions and suggestions uncritically. This means that introjection is usually present in the therapy room and is something the therapist is aware of, especially when this contact form inhibits the client's own exploration and discovery.

Change can occur by increasing clients' awareness of how introjection affects the relationship between therapist and client, and that it is also prominent in important situations in the clients' lives. The goal is not to get rid of introjection or even to swallow or spit out introjections, but rather to become aware of what we choose to take in from the environment, to reflect before we take something in, and to be aware that we can discard introjects.

References

Clarkson, P., & Mackewn, J. (1993). *Fritz Perls*. London: Sage Publications.

Hostrup, H. (2010). *Gestalt therapy: An introduction to the basic concepts of gestalt therapy* (D. H. Silver, Trans.). Copenhagen: Hans Reitzlers Forlag. (Original work published 1999)

Jørstad, S. (2002/2008). Oversikt over kontaktformer [Overview of contact forms]. In S. Jørstad & Å. Krüger (Eds.), *Den flyvende hollender* [The flying Dutchman] (pp. 128–139). Oslo: NGI.

Joyce, P., & Sills, C. (2014). *Skills in gestalt counselling & psychotherapy* (3rd ed.). London: Sage.

Kepner, J. I. (1987/2001). *Body process*. Cambridge, MA: Gestalt Press.

Perls, F. S. (1947/1969). *Ego, hunger and aggression*. New York: Vintage Books.

Skottun, G. (2002/2008). Reisebrev: Essay om kontaktformer og figurdannelser [Travelogue: Essay on contact forms and figure creation]. In S. Jørstad & Å. Krüger (Eds.), *Den flyvende hollender* [The flying Dutchman] (pp. 105–127). Oslo: NGI.

Staemmler, F. M. (2009). *Aggression, time and understanding*. Santa Cruz, CA: Gestalt Press.

Wheeler, G. (1998). *Gestalt reconsidered* (2nd ed.). Cambridge, MA: CIGPress.

Yontef, G. M. (1993). *Awareness, dialogue & process*. New York: The Gestalt Journal Press.

Zinker, J. (1977). *Creative process in gestalt therapy*. New York: Random House.

Chapter 14

Projection

People are curious about others. They ask questions and travel around the world seeking new experiences. They want to understand and see what others think and do; they compare themselves to others and consider how new ideas and the unknown fit into their lives. Others are the opposite; they measure or consider others in relation to their own ideas, rather than exploring their surroundings. They wonder what others think about them, become suspicious of their surroundings, and pay attention to what others say and do to see if it matches with their previous experience. In both cases, attention is turned outwards toward the surroundings. These two ways of relating to others are the two extremes, or poles, of the contact form projection.

When we assign ideas or perceptions about ourselves to others, we no longer see others as they actually are, but rather through a lens coloured by our own ideas. We relate to thoughts, feelings, and opinions as if they were the other person's thoughts, feelings, and opinions. We become each other's 'projection screen', where we transfer our understanding of ourselves to the other (Hostrup, 2010). Projection affects the contact between us in that someone in the situation assigns opinions and attitudes to someone else, and that person's response is then based on the projection. How the contact evolves depends largely on the type of projections we assign to each other and the extent to which we are aware that these are projections.

This chapter describes various forms of projection and how they are expressed in everyday life, where we can experience our own projections on others and receive projections from others. We show how we work in therapy, coaching, and supervision to explore and recognise these forms of projection in different situations.

Definition of projection

The word 'project' originates from the Latin *prōicere* (*prō*: 'from, in the place of; for') + *iaciō*: 'throw, hurl'), which can be freely translated as 'to throw from', a formulation that describes one of the polarities of the contact form: 'putting [one's] own attitude into the other person' (Perls et al., 1951, p. 348). Attention is thus turned from one's self to one's surroundings. Instead of seeing something

DOI: 10.4324/9781003153856-17

with openness and attention, we are biased, and transmit our own ideas of ourselves to those around us, which gives us assumptions about people whom we may not really know. Ideas about what we see and hear thus determine how we perceive and understand ourselves and our surroundings, as the following example with Martin and Adam shows.

Martin has asked his colleague Adam for help with a computer program he is developing. Adam explains what Martin can do and the reason for the problem. At a certain point, Martin starts to feel agitated and irritated, and says to Adam: 'It's great that you're willing explain what I can do, but you don't have to give a lecture on everything you know about programming'.

ADAM stops in surprise and says: 'But Martin, you asked me for help, I'm just explaining'.

MARTIN, in an accusatory voice: 'But you're not just explaining, you're telling me everything you know about programming. It's like you want to show me everything you know and how good you are . . . '

ADAM responds in a loud, annoyed voice: 'You'd rather tell everyone how much *you* know . . . You're describing yourself, not me'.

Here, Martin becomes annoyed with Adam and accuses him of lecturing and Adam defends himself and then accuses Martin. The contact between the two colleagues gradually becomes irritated and distrustful. This conversation can continue in several ways. Here is an example where Martin has self-insight:

MARTIN breathes for a moment and says: 'Ah, I'm afraid you're right, Adam, I like to talk about how much I know. It's not a part of me that I'm particularly proud of. Maybe that's why I got so annoyed with you when you started explaining more than was necessary'.

ADAM looks at Martin and smiles: 'I'm relieved to hear you say that. Sometimes I also talk about how much I know about programming, but it was the situation and the way you said it that made me angry . . . '

In another version of the conversation, Martin is not aware that his irritation can have something to do with himself, and might sound like this:

MARTIN: 'Cut it out. You're the one lecturing *me* about everything you know about programming. This isn't about me . . . '

In this example, Martin is initially unaware that the feelings he has about Adam's behaviour are related to ways of being that he recognises in himself. We see how different the conversations can be between the two if Martin is aware of how he influences Adam. Unconscious projections on others often create strong emotional reactions on both sides of a field and contribute to a form of contact that can be challenging.

From us to you and me

The chapter on confluence (Chapter 12) describes how children and parents flow together, and that it can be difficult to distinguish between the needs of each. Children gradually learn how they should act through introjection (Chapter 13). When the child starts to protest and does not want to do as her parents instruct, she stands apart from the parents by saying no, by saying that father or mother is stupid, that her parents are unjust, or that they do not understand. In this way, the child imposes feelings and characteristics on the parents because it becomes too difficult to handle these herself. In the eyes of the child, that which is stupid, unjust, or causes anger does not have anything to do with her, but rather with everyone else. This is understandable and recognisable when we encounter this behaviour in children but can be more difficult to handle when we encounter it in adults (Hostrup, 2010).

We start experimenting early in life with trying out our projections on others, and in this way learn about ourselves and the environment around us. Children mimic their parents' movements, facial expressions, and speech as they attempt to become familiar with who their parents are and who they themselves are. Curiosity about others as well as an interest in and the ability to understand another person's situation develops as part of this process (Hostrup, 2010). As adults, we continue this process of experience where we sort, check out, accept, and reject our assumptions about and perceptions of others, our surroundings, and ourselves in ever-changing situations. Gradually, we form images of the world and reality that we believe are true and that characterise our encounters with others.

Projection gives us an opportunity to get to know our surroundings and ourselves. When I project that the other is happy when she smiles, I can acknowledge what being smiling and happy means to me. When I imagine that someone is angry with me, I can wonder if I am also angry without being aware of it. An example of this phenomenon is where one person says to another: 'I think you're angry', and the other replies: 'I'm not the one who's angry, you're the one who's angry!' The first person can then respond: 'Yes, maybe I am . . . ', as we see in the example of Martin and Adam, where Martin is able to recognise that he also lectures others about his knowledge of programming.

Exploring our own projections also leads us to discover less useful aspects of ourselves, as we saw in the example above with Martin. We all have assumptions and prejudices about others, which becomes evident when we meet people from foreign cultures. It is easy to be blinded by the strange and unfamiliar and to view others as strange or different instead of having a positive attitude towards and becoming acquainted with things we experience as strange or unfamiliar. Information about and increased knowledge of other cultures can make foreign ideas less daunting. This is important in working with assumptions, prejudice, and projection.

Projection and its opposing polarity

When we project our ideas on to others, we are only concerned with the other and pay little attention to ourselves. However, it is I who projects, it is I who has an assumption about the other. The moment I realise that I am introducing projection into the field, the opportunity arises to become acquainted with my own understanding of the situation. I can look in the mirror and ask myself, 'What is it about what I've attributed to others that really belongs to me?' (Wheeler, 1998; Wollants, 2012). The person who receives the projection is in a similar situation, and can ask herself, 'Do I recognise this projection in myself?'

In both situations, the person is in a so-called polarity gap between conflicting needs. In this span lies the opportunity to move towards the other pole. The person can return the attention from the other to herself by exploring conflicting needs, and thus move into the projection's other pole (Hostrup, 2010). Both parties in this process are thus moving in the span between the two poles: *to project, to be projected on* and *to accept, to take back and look into or reject.*

Projection is therefore the process that occurs within the polarity span *from* projecting or being projected on *to* accepting the projections, taking them back, looking at them more closely, or rejecting them. Contact between people is influenced by how attentive they are to their own conflicting needs when it comes to receiving and projecting, and how they move in the polarity span. This extended definition of projection is ours, but is based on Wheeler's (1998) discussion of contact and polarities.

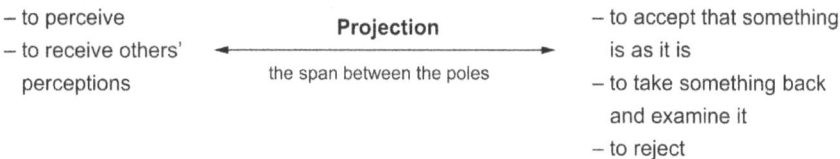

– to perceive – to receive others' perceptions	**Projection** ◄─────────────────► the span between the poles	– to accept that something is as it is – to take something back and examine it – to reject

Figure 14.1 Projection and its opposite pole.

Projection: a historical view

The term 'projection' was originally coined and used by Freud in psychoanalysis. He believed that the patient often unconsciously tried to defend herself against

(*Continued*)

unacceptable motivations and ideas in herself by passing or projecting them on to the analyst. The analyst was seen as a projection screen for the patient, who strived to be as neutral or blank as possible in order to ensure that the patient could freely pass her projections on. None of the analyst's own thoughts or feelings should affect the patient in this transfer process. The analyst then used these transfers as a basis for further analysis of the patient (Clarkson & Mackewn, 1993).

Fritz Perls included the concept of projection from psychoanalysis in his own theory, but gave it phenomenological content. Projection was no longer simply regarded as a tool for the analysis of the patient, but now became a description of a practical, everyday way of being with others. Nor did Perls think that the therapist was a blank projection screen, but rather a person who showed herself in the course of therapy. This meant that she was given projections that were also based on how she met the client (Clarkson & Mackewn, 1993). Despite this new thinking, Perls nevertheless believed that patients' projections were a sign of illness and should be treated in therapy so that they could become aware of their projections and, at best, stop projecting (Wheeler, 1998).

Exploring projection in therapy

In the therapeutic situation between client and therapist, the therapist assists the client in exploring the span between projecting and looking at herself and thus gaining increased awareness of the content of the projections. The situation becomes a kind of framework for exploration of the opportunities that lie within the projections. Exploration of the projections themselves is also the method used by the therapist in her work with clients where the figure is projection. As the therapist and client explore how they make assumptions about the other's opinions and attitudes, or how the client projects or is projected on, this exploration is part of a process in which the client takes back or acknowledges her projections. The therapist uses her own assumptions about the client in the therapy room deliberately, as a starting point for choosing interventions and experiments. As mentioned earlier, projection is necessary in order to be able to understand how someone else experiences the world and is therefore necessary for a therapist.

The therapist makes phenomenological observations about the client and herself in the therapy room so that the projections are as consistent as possible with the client's experience. The therapist makes sure to check out these projections both directly and indirectly. For example, she might say: 'I see you look sad. Is that right?', 'When you talk about your mom, you smile, and I get the idea that you're very fond of her', or 'I notice that I stop breathing. I think you're talking about something that's hard for you, is that correct?' Therefore, when projection is a figure in the field, it is useful and necessary to ask questions based on the contact functions of sight and hearing and on our assumptions.

Projection and introjection

In projection, we often use the 'you' form when we speak to others. We might for example characterise the person we are talking to by saying, 'You're always so happy, you're much nicer than I am . . . you look like a good person, it seems like you really like children'. In other cases, we might say,

'You probably think I should . . . you don't think I'm pretty . . . I think you should . . . ',

and so on. In these examples, projections are often ideas about what others 'should' or 'must' be or do (see Chapter 13). There is therefore a close connection between the contact forms projection and introjection (Hostrup, 2010).

In many situations, projections can include considerable aspects of attack, defence, and opinion about what the other should do differently, as in the following statements: 'You never clean up after yourself in the kitchen', 'You were the one who was supposed to take care of the children today', 'You don't understand me', 'Why can't you see how tired I am?', and so on. In these examples, it is clear that introjection lies behind the projection; it is as if the speaker's words contain implicit rules: one should clean up, one should take care of the children, and so on. Other examples of implicit introjection are placing blame for what went wrong on the other. Not infrequently, such annoyance over aspects that are perceived as lacking in others lead to frustration and anger, such as the driver who rages over other people's driving skills and the passenger who is annoyed at the driver's emotional outburst. Here, an accelerating spiral of mutual projections and messages between the two is wrapped up in our ideas of right and wrong. The challenge is to learn to speak for oneself using 'I' language, as we show in the example of Rachel and the management team she is part of.

'You' language and 'I' language

Rachel is a member of a group of department heads in middle management, led by a gestalt coach. At a meeting, they talk about the assumptions they have about each other. Rachel says she thinks the others are very cautious, and that they do not dare to express themselves clearly.

The leader asks her to be more specific and say this directly to one of the participants. Rachel looks at Jan and says: 'Jan, I think you beat around the bush when you have something to say to the others in the group. You don't dare to say what you really mean. I wish you were more direct'. Rachel turns red when she says this, and adds: 'Oh, that probably sounded very negative. It's not wrong that you choose your words carefully, and you probably have your reasons for saying things that way'. Jan looks at her and says: 'I think I'm pretty forthright most of the time. But I don't want to hurt people's feelings'.

The coach stops them and says to Rachel: 'What's going on with you right now, Rachel? Do you recognise anything about yourself in what you said to Jan? I heard that you weren't direct about what you were thinking when you first talked to the whole group. It wasn't until I asked you to look at one of the group members that you turned to Jan. I also heard that you tried to gloss over what you said, afterwards'.

Rachel nods and says that that is probably why she is annoyed that Jan and the others are so careful about what they say. She feels a little cowardly when she realises that she can also be unclear. Then Jan says that she also recognises herself in what Rachel says, although she still thinks she is one of those in the group who has also addressed others directly.

Here, Rachel speaks in 'you' language, and attributes something she does not like about herself to Jan. She dares to say what she thinks directly to her, even if it is unpleasant. After a new confrontation from the coach, she acknowledges how she strives to be as direct as she wants Jan to be. Jan accepts only parts of the projection, and dares to disagree with Rachel. Both move in the span between the need to project/be projected on and to see themselves and each other as they actually are.

Seeing things as they are

Monica sought out a therapist after she became aware of how she projected on her boss. In the first session she tells the therapist about how difficult it is for her to have a relationship with a man, and that she has come to understand that this is because she constantly sees traits in other men that remind her of her father. The therapist asks Monica to talk a little about what her father was like, and Monica describes a stern father who could explode with anger over little things and whom she was always afraid of. Monica speaks with a rather low and monotonous voice, and it is as if she is crawling into her chair.

THERAPIST: 'I notice you're speaking in a low voice and it's like you're trying to make yourself smaller than you are. What's it like for you when I say that?'

Here, the therapist first expresses her own projection when she says that it looks like Monica is trying to make herself smaller than she is, and then checks with her what it is like for her to receive that projection.

MONICA looks up at the therapist: 'I didn't realise that. Maybe I feel like my father is here when I talk about him. I might be a little scared that he sees me now and feel that he'd be angry that I'm talk about him like this'.

THERAPIST: 'That makes sense. So you imagine he is here now . . . '

MONICA replies hesitantly: 'I know he's not here now, but still . . . '

THERAPIST: 'Can you look around the room for a bit?'

Monica does as the therapist suggests, taking time to look at the pictures on the walls, furniture, curtains, and carpet before she shakes her head.

MONICA: 'No, he's not here. It was good to actually look around and see that. It's amazing how quickly I imagine he's around when I think about him'.

Here, Monica gets help from the therapist to look around and make sure the danger she feels is not in the room. By using the contact function of sight, she becomes aware of the room she sits in. She sees 'what is' and can put her idea of danger to rest. Moreover, it becomes clear to Monica how the fantasy of her father prevents her from seeing reality.

Projection and seeing what is

Opening up to something new is often about taking a chance. The challenge in the situation is to dare to take off the metaphorical glasses through which we view the situation and move into the span of the unknown polarity. Hearing the other's opinion gives no guarantee as to how what is conveyed is interpreted by the other. In other words, hearing another's ideas and projections can be both daunting and unpleasant. The reciprocity, tension, and vulnerability of such confrontations are familiar to most of us.

The following example shows how the therapist facilitates a discussion in such a way that participants can discover and become acquainted with projection and the opposite pole, 'seeing what is'.

This therapy group has met over a period of time, and at the group leader's request, Harold finally finds the courage to talk about the difficulties he has with his girlfriend. He tells the others about loud arguments and his subsequent despair. But after he has finished, he suddenly becomes quiet and introverted. He looks down at the floor and mutters: 'Damn! Now I feel ashamed. I can't look at you. I think I've taken too much of the group's time and that what I say is totally uninteresting'. He turns on his chair and blushes.

In this meeting with the group, Harold imagines that he has taken too much space. He does not dare to look at the other members because he assumes that they are accusatory and disinterested, and he would now prefer to stay in the background. Harold projects on the group members without being aware of it, while also criticising himself. He has a message to himself that he is unaware of: 'I'm not going to take up the group's time' and 'I have to say something interesting'. He imagines the group members think the same about him as he himself thinks.

THE THERAPIST notices that Harold holds back, and says: 'It sounds to me like you were scared you were spending too much of our time on your own issues. But today I'm the one who gave you the time, and who encouraged you to talk. You did what I asked you to do'. Harald looks up at the group leader and nods weakly before turning his gaze downward again.

THERAPIST: 'It was nice that you looked at me and nodded. When you do that, I get the feeling that you agree with me. At the same time, I notice that you're not looking at the others in the group who are here with you. You might be afraid to look at them because you think they think you've taken up too much of their time'.

HAROLD looks up and nods again, and says: 'Yes, it's so hard. I'm so afraid of what they think of me'.

THERAPIST: 'Mmm, I can understand that. At the same time, you can't figure it out without looking around. What if you start by looking at just one person in the group?'

HAROLD: 'Yes, I can do that, I can start with John, who's sitting next to me'.

HAROLD turns to John and tells the therapist 'John looks like someone who thinks it's ok for me to take up the group's time'.

THE THERAPIST answers: 'Yes, I think so too! Do you want to hear from him about your assumption?'

HAROLD to John: 'Do you think it was okay that I used up so much of the group's time with my issues?'

JOHN smiles and nods to Harold: 'I'm so glad you asked me. I recognise myself very much in being afraid of taking up others' time and people getting bored when I talk . . . I wasn't bored and I thought it was good that you shared what was going on with you'.

HAROLD exhales, smiles at John, and says: 'That was good to hear. I'm really relieved'.

THE THERAPIST asks Harold to look at several of the group participants, which he does, and he eventually becomes aware that the others are smiling and nodding at him.

This example shows how Harold, with ample help from the therapist, becomes aware of the projections 'They think I take up too much time' and 'They're not interested in what I have to say'. The therapist in turn checks out her projections that Harold is scared and does not dare to look at the others by asking him if this is what he thinks. When the therapist confirms her projections, she asks Harold to explore his own assumption by looking at one of the participants. The therapist thinks that it is easier for Harold to look at each participant individually, and in this way downgrades the experiment (see Chapter 11 on experiments).

When John smiles and answers Harold's questions, Harold understands that his assumptions about John were incorrect. In the further process, Harold examines whether his assumption about the other group members is true, and thus sorts his projections. This means that Harold can see the others smile and nod, which he interprets as interest on the part of the others. This changes the contact he has with them. Both Harold and the others in the group have taken the chance of being rejected, have known the excitement and discomfort of being projected on, and have experienced the relief that can come from checking out assumptions. The experience they have when they are able to see each other in a new way is one of relief and happiness, and they now have the opportunity to bring this new experience to their next meeting.

In this example, Harold becomes aware that his ideas about the others are incorrect. His projections might also be messages he has to himself, in which he says: 'Don't take up the others' time' and 'I have to be interesting'. He can explore this further in therapy. John becomes aware that he recognises himself in Harold's projection and experiences it as a support that he is not the only one who thinks about how he should act in the group. It is likely that John also has thoughts about how others in the group should act, although in this situation he did not think that Harold took up too much of the group's time.

When the therapist believes that there are many assumptions in the group, she may ask the members how they think they should act and what they think she and other group members think about the rules in the group. This can be an awareness-raising process for participants where there is less focus on a single member's projections and more on their own assumptions about others, which means that they can see both themselves and others as they actually are and not as they imagine them to be.

The projection chair

One of the most well-known ways to explore projections in gestalt therapy is chair work. In Chapter 11 on experiments, we described the purpose of chair work and the different ways in which the therapist can use chair work with a client. In the following, we show an example.

Magnus in the projection chair

Magnus comes to therapy because he is afraid that his wife, Hilda, is unfaithful. He says that he has long been unsure of what she does when she is traveling for work, or worse, when she comes home late at night. The therapist suggests that he explore the situation in chair work. Magnus is a bit doubtful and is not immediately willing to try, but after the therapist explains more about the experiment he agrees to try. The therapist asks Magnus to place two chairs, which he positions facing each other with some distance between.

THERAPIST: 'Imagine that one chair is yours and the other represents Hilda. How would you sit if you were talking at home?'

MAGNUS says that they might have sat next to each other on the couch, and the therapist urges him to put the chairs next to each other. Magnus moves back and forth between the chairs before sitting down on one in such a way that he looks sideways at 'Hilda'. The therapist asks him to describe what he imagines when he looks at his wife, which Magnus does.

MAGNUS: 'She's looking out into the air. I think she feels insecure'. At the therapist's request, he continues to describe what he sees.

MAGNUS: 'She's wearing a green sweater, blue pants, and she's sitting a little sunk together'.

THERAPIST: 'What do you feel in your body when you look at Hilda?'

MAGNUS: 'I'm getting a little sad and uneasy'. Magnus moves his legs and arms; the unease shows in his bodily movements.

THE THERAPIST asks him to move to the other chair. Magnus gets up slowly and spends some time sitting in the chair that represents Hilda.

MAGNUS, AS 'HILDA': 'When I sit here looking off to the side, I have an experience of being distant and unconcentrated'.

After spending some time in 'Hilda's' chair, the therapist asks him to move back to his own. Here, Magnus is surprised at how much easier he feels in his body and how much more attentive he is to the surroundings than he was when he sat in the other chair. The therapist chooses to stop the chair work to make room for reflection.

Spontaneously, Magnus says he did not realise that 'Hilda' felt so sunken and sad: 'I don't think I've looked at her properly lately. Maybe she's tired, and tired of working so much. Maybe she doesn't have a lover after all! I think I should go home and ask her how she's doing'.

Here, the therapist challenges Magnus to play the part of Hilda in order to experience his own projections. The therapist imagines that Magnus is resistant to exploring his suspicion of his wife's infidelity because he is scared of what he might discover, and as a result, the therapist sticks to her chair-work proposal. In his own chair, Magnus first describes what he sees; then the projection 'she is inse-cure' emerges, which he explores further by sitting in 'Hilda's' chair. The therapist supports Magnus in becoming aware of both bodily and emotional changes he experiences when sitting in the various chairs. Magnus dares to confront what he is most afraid of: the possibility that his wife might leave him. He could have said no to the experiment and held on to his assumptions, but instead he moves into the span between the poles in order to imagine and to see things as they might be. In doing so, he gains new insight into his wife's behaviour. He sees new opportuni-ties in what was previously frightening and fixed.

The therapist could have continued the chair work where Magnus and 'Hilda' talked to each other in the therapy room. However, the therapist thinks that Mag-nus' discovery through this work is sufficient for him to continue sorting the pro-jections himself, together with Hilda. We can see here that the therapist builds her choices on the assumptions, or projections, she has of Magnus, and allows these to guide what she chooses to do.

Projection as a creative method

Artistic and creative activities are also expressions of projection. We use our abil-ity to imagine situations when painting or drawing—we recreate what we see on the paper or canvas. When we write books or create theatre or dance, we also use our imagination, which is based on past experiences that we project. Many of these creative expressions are used in gestalt therapy and other therapeutic direc-tions such as psychodrama, dance therapy, art, and expressive therapy. The most well-known methods in gestalt therapy are working with the 'projection chair' or 'empty chair', projection in dream work, and forms of visualisation and fantasy journeys (see Chapter 11 on experiments).

'Playing the client' in supervision

In supervision of gestalt therapists, the supervisor often uses creative methods to facilitate the therapist's awareness of the challenges she brings to supervision. One common method is to let the therapist explore her own projections on the client. This is often called 'playing the client'. When the supervisor encourages the thera-pist to, for example, 'walk as if you were the client', she does so in order to allow the therapist to explore her own perceptions—her projections—of how the client walks. It is of course not possible for us to 'be' the other. The closest we can come is to investigate and thus become acquainted with our own assumptions of the other, which develop gradually as we become better acquainted. It is this assumption that the therapist is encouraged to explore in supervision (Gilbert & Evans, 2000).

Gestalt therapist Trine is in supervision because she thinks she is stuck in her work with a client. The supervisor first asks her to say a little about what she experiences as difficult. After some clarification, the supervisor asks her to 'play the client' in order to further explore her own perceptions of the client. Trine is familiar with this way of exploring. She gets up and walks around the room while imagining that she is the client. After a little hesitation, she starts talking and associates freely: 'I'm a woman about forty years old. I'm busy and have a lot to do. I'm married and have children'. As she speaks, she speeds up and speaks in a louder voice. At one point, the supervisor asks her to stop, and asks: 'What do you become aware of when you walk around as your client?' Trine says she notices that as the client, she walks and talks quickly. She feels breathless, and this gives her a feeling of constantly having to do something, like she needs to catch up with something, as if there is always someone who expects something from her. The supervisor then asks Trine to reflect on how this information fits into the therapy process. Trine says that she has become particularly aware of the phenomenon of expectation, and that this phenomenon is something she recognises from the situation with the client.

By stepping into the role of the client, Trine embodies what she has noticed in the client and becomes aware of it in her own body. When she becomes aware of her breathing and movements, she recognises that she has seen this in the client without realising it. It had already occurred to her that the client has many expectations both of herself and of the therapist. This awareness leads Trine to see herself and the client in a new way, which she brings with her to the next session with the client.

Visualisation

Visualisation is a projection method that can support clients in situations where they are preparing for something they dread in the future or for processing previously unpleasant or traumatic experiences (see Chapter 11 on experiments). It is important for the therapist to pay extra attention to how such a guided visualisation into past experience can be retraumatising in some situations.

It is important that the therapist ensure that the client constantly tells her what she sees and what happens to her. The therapist can also repeat parts of what the client says, so that the client hears what she herself has said and becomes aware that the therapist is present and hears her. We also use this method when dealing with different types of dreams, especially nightmares or dreams that suddenly stop (Chapter 11).

Cecilie has been in coaching for a while. She is offered a new job and does not know if she wants to keep her current job or switch to the new one. Cecilie tells the coach about the current and potential jobs. After a while, the coach asks Cecilie to close her eyes and imagine herself five years in the future. The coach guides her in this visualisation so that Cecilie can 'see' where she is and what she does in her imagination. In this way, Cecilie becomes aware of what she wants, which was difficult when she thought about it alone. She sees herself in completely different and unfamiliar surroundings, something she experiences as a good situation, and that makes her want to explore the new job offer further.

Here, we show how Cecilie is able to direct more attention to what she wants, and what she was not aware of in regard to her projections about the future. The coach and client can further explore this discovery and connect it even more to the client's life. It would also be possible to ask Cecilie to visualise being in her current job, in order to give her an experience of the emotions and bodily sensations it creates in her.

Summary

In this chapter, we have defined the contact form projection and discussed projection's various aspects through theory and practical examples. Projection, whether conscious or not, helps us to orient ourselves in the world. We mirror ourselves in our surroundings and learn to know ourselves through others' reactions to us and by taking back our projections. Receiving others' projections can be a gift when we become aware of them, making it possible to become acquainted with unknown sides of ourselves. In therapy, coaching, and supervision we explore the range of projections: those we have, those we are the recipients of in the therapy room, and in society in general.

References

Clarkson, P., & Mackewn, J. (1993). *Fritz Perls*. London: Sage Publications.
Gilbert, M., & Evans, K. (2000). *Psychotherapy supervision: An integrative relational approach to psychotherapy supervision*. Buckingham: Open University Press.
Hostrup, H. (2010). *Gestalt therapy: An introduction to the basic concepts of gestalt therapy* (D. H. Silver, Trans.). Copenhagen: Hans Reitzlers Forlag. (Original work published 1999)
Perls, F. S., Hefferline, R. F., & Goodman, P. (1951). *Gestalt therapy: Excitement and growth in the human personality*. London: Souvenir Press.
Wheeler, G. (1998). *Gestalt reconsidered* (2nd ed.). Cambridge, MA: CIGPress.
Wollants, G. (2012). *Gestalt therapy: Therapy of the situation*. London: Sage.

Chapter 15

Retroflection

Retroflection is defined as 'the act or condition of bending or being bent backwards'. The word comes from the Latin *retrōflectere*, to bend back. The gestalt-theoretic definition of the term is to 'hold myself back, stop myself; to do to myself what I wish to do to others, or to do something to myself instead of receiving it from others or asking others for it' (Jørstad, 2002/2008, p. 130, our translation). This affects our contact with the outside world; we are more concerned with ourselves than with our surroundings. When retroflection is present in the field, the ability to be actor, audience, and the one who is exposed to the action in the situation is made clear (Polster & Polster, 1974).

In this chapter, we define the contact form retroflection. We describe different forms of retroflection, how the contact form is expressed in everyday life, and the polarities of the contact form. Through examples from therapy, we show ways to increase clients' awareness in situations where retroflection is evident between therapist and client.

Inner conversations turned outwards

Turning thoughts and actions towards ourselves means that we have inner dialogues in which we evaluate and reflect on what we have done and want to do, and to a lesser extent allow ourselves to be influenced by the opinions of those around us. This is a process in which we are self-critical and try to develop and change ourselves and our ways of being, often without being conscious of the process.

It may also be that parts of the conversations we have with ourselves are spoken aloud, as shown in this example with Marianne:

A group of friends sits around the dining room table when Marianne brings in dinner. She says apologetically: 'I think the fish might have been fried too long, and now I see that maybe there are too many vegetables'. One of her friends says: 'But Marianne, you don't have to apologise, I'm sure it will be great'. Marianne replies: 'You're right, I shouldn't be so self-critical. I

DOI: 10.4324/9781003153856-18

really should be a little more confident'. Another friend says: 'I think you're just fine the way you are'. Marianne laughs with the others and does not pursue the issue, but the atmosphere around the table is a little tense. The friends are unsure if Marianne fully understands that they like her as she is and are enjoying themselves.

Here we can see that Marianne criticises herself out loud and not only in her thoughts. She has spent a lot of time preparing dinner for her friends and wants them to be satisfied with what she makes. The friends gathered around the table may not be aware that they have expectations of Marianne's cooking, and that their expectations influence Marianne and make her more self-critical. We can imagine that Marianne has talked to herself as she prepared for the visit and that the self-critical comments she says aloud are part of a longer inner conversation. The contact between her and the guests becomes tenser when it seems that Marianne does not fully believe her friends' assurances. It may be that Marianne continues the conversation in her thoughts instead of taking in what her friends are saying to her. In that way, she shuts them out. A friend might be upset by Marianne's self-criticism and another might be annoyed, but they hold this back, and the room becomes quiet for a while. In this situation, retroflection becomes figure.

In that same situation, Marianne could listen to what her friends say and believe that they are right, that she is actually doing the best she can, and that they are friends who love her. In that case, she would have sorted out the self-criticism and could meet her friends in a different way, which would change the contact between them.

Retroflection—introjection and projection

Retroflection can be seen as the opposite of projection. Instead of turning the assumptions—introjections—out towards others, they are turned inward, often without our realising that this is what is happening, as in the example of Marianne. In retroflection we have unclear expectations of others because we are afraid of being disappointed. Instead, we expect something from ourselves, where we can control thoughts and act in such a way that things happen as we wish. Instead of meeting our needs by engaging creatively in the situation and directing our energy outwards to connect with the environment, we change the direction of our energy and activity within ourselves and meet our needs as best we can on our own. While focusing our attention on ourselves, we compare ourselves to others. We project our assumptions of what others think about us onto those around us, as we see Marianne do with her friends.

Coming out and holding back

Retroflection is both about coming out and holding back, and about how we evaluate ourselves and our actions. An example of this is when we consider whether to show emotion, and ask ourselves: 'Dare I cry here?', 'What happens if I get angry now?', or 'Maybe it's better if I don't say anything right now'. We evaluate and change inappropriate ways of being or make changes that lay the groundwork for further action. This can mean that we remember and compare what we have done previously, and rethink. Retroflection can often be a painful and demanding process, where we see both our weaknesses and strengths (Perls et al., 1951). In practice, this can be understood as withholding something, and is expressed as self-restraint, self-control, and impulse control (Hostrup, 2010). Often, this reflection and self-evaluation happens without our attention to how looking inwards in this way affects the contact between ourselves and others.

Retroflection can occur in three ways:

- By being aware of our thoughts, telling ourselves what we think, want, and feel instead of telling others. By turning the conversation around and talking to ourselves instead of our surroundings and by not hearing the opinions others have of us. Examples: criticising or praising ourselves and discussing with ourselves.
- By doing to ourselves what we want to do to others. Examples: rewarding ourselves when we are happy with ourselves by eating well, going to a spa, or taking a vacation. We can punish ourselves when we are unhappy or angry with ourselves by not eating, dieting, working a lot, not taking holidays, or tightening our muscles.
- Yet a third way is by doing to ourselves what we want others to do to us. We turn the action towards ourselves instead of asking others for advice and help. Examples: we buy flowers for ourselves, we stroke ourselves, we masturbate.

The inner critic

As we grew up, many of us experienced that we were punished or spoken to severely when we did not follow the rules and norms for how we should behave. As children we were often stopped when our actions did not fit into prevalent norms of what was safe or appropriate, and our needs and desires were not always taken seriously. Others experienced praise and support, room to make mistakes and try out new ways of being. How we were met by our environments as we grew up, and whether we were praised, rewarded, criticised, or punished, influences how we experience ourselves and our contact with the outside world later in life. We take in and absorb the norms and rules of the environment—the introjects— quite easily as children, as mentioned in Chapter 13. This also applies to the ways in which others reacted when we did not live up to their expectations and rules. In these cases, we adopt the norms and rules of others as our own.

Instead of someone in our environment scolding or praising us, we do it ourselves. We assess our actions and behaviours by talking to ourselves or treating ourselves in the same way others have treated us (Hostrup, 2010). It is as if we take the voices of important people around us and make them our own

(Staemmler, 2016). For example, we can say to ourselves: 'You did this really well' and remember that this is something our father often said to us. Likewise, we can say: 'You could have done this much better. What do others think about you now?' and recognise our mother's voice. We can hear other voices, such as the teacher who criticises and says: 'You have to work harder on your homework or you'll never learn' or 'You have a talent for this, this is an area where you can excel'. A coach might say: 'You have to run faster, get off your big butt'. The way these messages have been conveyed has a strong impact on how we remember their content and how our self-esteem develops. It is not important whether we know where these voices come from, only that we are aware that the way we speak to ourselves is something we have learned from others, and that this affects our self-image and how we are in contact with others.

Our own assessment of ourselves is more or less consistent with how our surroundings perceive us, and of course depends on the feedback we have received and how this fits into the situations in which we grew up. Some grow up in environments where they receive little or no correction or praise. There is a lack of feedback, which makes it difficult to reflect on one's own actions. In these cases, there are few 'voices in the head'. For example, a person might say: 'I don't know what to say now, maybe it's best that I . . . ' or 'It was just a whim. Maybe it wasn't a good idea to bring it up now?' For others, the feedback they received may have been general and not directly related to a situation. The praise or criticism was unmotivated, dependent on impulses in the environment, which also creates confusion about how to identify desirable behaviour. For example, a person may think that something went very well without that being the case. She thinks she is a world champion; she considers herself and the results of her actions in an excessively positive light and has an unrealistic picture of what she can achieve. In some situations, the person may hold back too little and take up a great deal of time and space in meetings or social encounters. Another person may struggle with the opposite, underestimating everything she does and never knowing if she herself or what she is doing is good enough for others (Hostrup, 2010).

Retroflection's opposing polarity

The polarity to retroflection is to exchange and meet, where exchange is understood as telling or showing others what we think and feel (Wheeler, 1998). Dialogue and action are directed towards the surroundings rather than turned inwards; we meet the others in the situation. At the same time, others in the field also consider whether they want to meet us or turn their attention inwards.

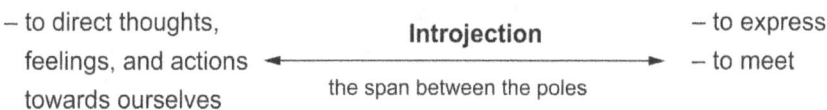

| – to direct thoughts, feelings, and actions towards ourselves | **Introjection** ⟵————————————⟶ the span between the poles | – to express – to meet |

We are constantly moving along the continuum that spans the need to hold back and the need to reach out and share with others. It is a challenge to be able to regulate these conflicting needs when it comes to how and when it is appropriate to hold back, and when we can meet others by showing what we feel and sharing what we think. When we manage to regulate our impulse to hold back and rather express ourselves in a flexible and appropriate manner, it can give us a sense of security in ourselves and our ability to regulate our need to emerge and stay in the situation (Spagnuolo Lobb, 2013).

The contact between us

When we turn the conversation inwards it affects the contact between us and our surroundings in many ways. If one or more people in a situation are reluctant to show emotion and say little about what they are thinking, it can create emotions such as calmness, irritation, or uncertainty. An example of the first might be a mother holding her crying child. She is unsure why the child is crying, whether it is her fault, whether she has done something wrong, and whether there is something she should do. She continues to cradle the child and does not show her uncertainty. Eventually, the child becomes calm and falls asleep. We can also imagine a couple who disagree, where one is accusatory and angry and the other is calm and holds back her own annoyance. The accuser may become angrier about her partner's calmness and insist that she say what she thinks and feels. The opposite can also happen: the fact that her partner holds back her annoyance might cause the accuser to be calmer.

Some situations require that we hold back our thoughts and feelings, such as during a lecture where the professor wants the students to wait with their questions and comments until after the lecture, in quiet areas of open office landscapes, and on trains or airports, so that those present can concentrate and be at ease. There are few situations where it is expected that we turn all thoughts, feelings, and actions outwards towards others. Even in couple relationships, some degree of restraint will be appropriate.

Doing to oneself rather than to the other

For many, it can be important to be independent, take care of themselves, and have control over their own lives. Some choose to live alone for this very reason. They are good at self-support, do not ask for advice, and rarely accept help when it is offered by the surroundings.

In many situations it can be safer to do to ourselves what we want to do to others. In challenging situations at home, at school, or at work, we might be afraid of our feelings being hurt or of hurting the feelings of others. In those cases, we often hold back what we want to say and direct our thoughts to ourselves instead. It feels safer to speak harshly to oneself, to be self-destructive, stop eating, or even vomit or hurt oneself than to do these things to those around us. It may also be helpful and necessary to hold back feelings by turning them inwards, as the example of Frederic shows.

Frederic has two young children aged two and four years. He is stressed and angry with them because they argue, yell, and fight. He can feel his anger growing and feels a temptation to yell back and hit them. Instead of doing so, he leaves the room for a moment. He boils with anger while saying to himself out loud: 'I can't handle this, I'm not cut out to be a father. I get angry too easily'. After a while he goes back to his children, is able to control his anger, and can be together with them in a different way.

Here, Frederic holds back his anger by talking critically to himself instead of to his children. It is uncomfortable for him, but he manages to prevent himself from hitting them and shouting at them, which is important to him in the situation.

Working with retroflection in the therapy room

In retroflection there are two conditions of which the therapist is aware and often explores:

- How the client self-assesses in regard to her actions, thoughts, and feelings, both in and outside the therapy room, and to what extent the therapist becomes self-assessing when together with the client.
- How the therapist and client hold back or emerge and share with each other, the form they have together in the therapy room, and how conscious they are of their form. Perhaps they sit together very quietly or perhaps the client talks a lot and shows her emotions; perhaps the therapist becomes cautious and considers what she can say.

To begin, we show an example of the first point, where the client self-assesses and is focused on how she is and should be, and what she thinks is right. She considers her actions against these introjects.

Exploring retroflection and introjection

Jenny is a college lecturer who has sought out a therapist because she is always nervous before giving lectures. The nervousness makes her unable to prepare as well as she thinks she should, and she has long, internal conversations with herself beforehand.

JENNY: 'I tell myself that I should've started preparing a long time ago, that I really don't know anything about this topic. I never get it right, I never learn, and the previous lecture was no good at all. This is going to be absolutely awful. This is how I criticise myself, and I can barely read or prepare the lecture'.

THERAPIST: 'It sounds tiring, I know I'm holding my breath while you talk'.

JENNY: 'Yes, it's very tiring. I spend my time talking about how bad I am at preparing instead of preparing. I'm just completely hopeless'.

The therapist notices that she is sad when she listens to Jenny and is unsure if she should say anything about it. She thinks that Jenny's insecurity is perhaps 'spreading' to her, and that something is happening between them.

THERAPIST: 'Mmm, I feel sad when I listen to you. I recognise myself in what you say—I can also have problems preparing and can speak critically to myself. At the same time, I've learned that in a way, these inner conversations are a way of preparing. Is that how it is for you, too?'

JENNY: 'I don't know, maybe sometimes. It doesn't feel like it now, but when you mention it . . . I don't think of anything else all day . . . it's a kind of preparation. It's just that I get so incredibly self-critical'.

THERAPIST: 'Yes, I understand, and it seems you're making it even harder for yourself when you say that you get so incredibly self-critical'.

JENNY exhales and looks at the therapist: 'Yes, exactly, it's so hard to accept that I'm self-critical as I prepare. I can't stop myself . . . and it's like I think I shouldn't be self-critical'.

THE THERAPIST repeats the last sentence: 'So you shouldn't be self-critical'.

JENNY smiles a little: 'I shouldn't be self-critical . . . and that's exactly what I am'.

Here. Jenny becomes aware that her inner conversation is about how hopeless she thinks she is and how she thinks she should be. As she and the therapist speak together, she gains spontaneous insight in which she acknowledges that she is self-critical, even though she thinks she should not be, leading to a paradoxical change.

The therapist thinks that retroflection is a figure between them, which leads her to share what happens to her, how she recognises herself in Jenny's situation, and what she thinks about being self-critical. The introjection that lies behind self-criticism becomes clear when Jenny says that she should not be self-critical, something the therapist repeats to reinforce and make clear to Jenny so that she can chew the introject and decide what she thinks about this herself (Chapter 13 on introjection).

The client and therapist can both feel vulnerable when many thoughts and feelings are held back in the therapy room. They do not know what the other is feeling and thinking, which can pave the way for assumptions. In such situations the therapist does not ask the client what she notices, feels, or needs. The client often does not know this herself and may feel ashamed of not being able to answer. Instead, the therapist becomes more predictable by telling the client what she is thinking and what is happening to her—the opposite of retroflection. This is illustrated in the example of Trudy.

Trudy is in her mid-thirties and in therapy for the first time. She has told the therapist that she sleeps poorly, has a lot of pain in her body, is ill and on sick leave. The therapist asks her to say a little more about what it is like to be on sick leave. Trudy replies that it is uncomfortable but that she is unable to go to work for the moment. She says no more, looks at the therapist, and turns on her chair. They sit together in silence for a while, and the therapist notices that she is beginning to be uncertain whether to ask Trudy to tell her more or wait for Trudy to say more on her own initiative.

Here, the therapist's hypothesis is that retroflection has become a figure between them and that it is difficult for Trudy to talk to her about what she is thinking. She feels that she herself is tense and thinks that it is better that she say something about herself instead of asking Trudy about her experience.

THERAPIST: 'I notice the silence between us, and I'm uncertain what to say. I'm thinking about the fact that this is your first time in therapy, and it may be difficult for you to know how I can help you'.

TRUDY, after some time: 'Yes, I don't know if there really is anything you can do for me. I tend to take care of myself, and now I'm here because someone said it might help me'.

THERAPIST: 'Mmm, I understand that you're wondering about that, and I don't really know either. But my experience is that it can be good to think out loud together rather than just letting the conversation keep going inside our own heads. It occurs to me that you might have many thoughts about why you're in pain and on sick leave'.

TRUDY: 'Yes, I think about it a lot, but I don't understand it, although I think it might be because I'm tired and feel like I never get anything done properly'.

THERAPIST: 'Mmm . . . and all these thoughts you have might make you tired too?'

TRUDY nods and exhales for a moment: 'Yes, they really do make me tired. I think and think about everything I do, that I should relax, that I have to accept help at work . . . '

Here, the therapist is interested in helping Trudy to share what she thinks without that leading to looking for a cause for the pain and sick leave. The therapist is aware of her own uncertainty and that she becomes cautious with Trudy, which leads to her share more of her own thoughts than she otherwise might do. She chooses to share in this way in order to create security in the therapy room. The therapist wants to support Trudy in doing the opposite of holding back, and thinks that in the long run this can help Trudy to relax and gain confidence in herself and her surroundings.

Working with bodily reactions in the therapy room

Like Trudy's therapist, many of us can acknowledge that we hold back. This can be expressed in many ways, such as by speaking very little and in a low voice, a loss of facial expression, and showing few impulses and emotions. The body might sink inwards in an attempt to be invisible, or the muscles might tighten so much that the body experiences stiffness and pain. We can hold back without being aware of it, for example by biting our lips, talking with our hand in front of our mouth, or not finishing what we started to say. We can become strict or judgemental with ourselves and have a sense of having no value, as the example of Tim shows.

Tim comes to therapy because he has been feeling depressed and scared since his wife left him. In the first session he says that he feels like a failure as a husband, that his wife often complained to him, and that it is as if she chose another man instead of him because he could not do anything right. The therapist gets the impression that Tim assumes all the blame for his wife leaving him and that he also appears as a victim in the situation. The therapist chooses to say something about what she feels. She feels sad and tight in her body and sees that Tim sits bent forward. Instead of asking Tim questions, she tells him what she sees and feels, which leads to Tim eventually experiencing his tension. The therapist follows up by telling him what she thinks: that she believes Tim is upset and angry, and she believes this because of the irritation she hears in his voice when he speaks and how he tightens his body. Tim admits that he is actually very angry with his wife. He straightens up in the chair, looks straight at the therapist, and with a loud and angry voice talks about all his trapped emotions and thoughts. Eventually he becomes calmer, and together they can reflect on the new insight he has gained about how he has withheld feelings without being aware of it.

The therapist has a hypothesis that Tim is scared to acknowledge and feel that he is annoyed and angry with his wife, and that it is safer for him to take all responsibility for the breakup. When the therapist says what she thinks and sees, Tim's attention to emotions other than sadness increases. He dares to open up to forbidden and previously unacknowledged feelings, such as anger and irritation, and can reflect on his actions in a new way. What makes a change in this situation is that Tim becomes aware of his conflicting feelings. The therapist can support him by making clear that it is reasonable to have such feelings in the situation he describes and that it is important for him to express them. Admitting to the anger he has for his wife does not mean that he has to tell his wife about it; it might be just as sensible to hold it back when he sees her.

The therapist could have chosen other ways to make Tim aware of his anger, for example by suggesting an experiment in which he bent forward in the chair even more while increasing the tension in his body. When Tim reinforces how he sits, he can become aware of how he holds himself back physically together with the therapist. This can lead to his awareness of the feelings he is holding back, such as anger and sadness.

Withheld emotions

When a person withholds emotions over time without having any safe places to express them, she can strive to regulate those feelings when she is with others. Withheld emotions, such as anger or sadness, can sometimes come to the surface and overwhelm both the person and the environment. The person appears polite and submissive while the mind rages beneath the surface and emotions come out in small jokes, comments, and looks. This can be experienced by others as threatening. The issues that trigger these unexpected outbursts of emotion can be unimportant. For example, this can happen when an employee at work is criticised by her manager or is informed that her work duties are being changed. This can result in the therapist feeling insecure and be cautious with the client. As she gets to know the client in these situations, she might find that there is no correspondence between what the client says and how she behaves. The therapist can work with this in different ways. For example, she can say in a friendly voice: 'When you talk about your boss, you smile, and at the same time you say you're mad at him. Did you notice that?' or 'I get the impression that you're pretty angry with your boss. Is there anyone else you're angry with?' or 'I notice that I get confused when you say on the one hand that you're angry with your boss, and on the other hand I see that you smile at me when you tell me this'.

Exploring retroflection and projection

Sometimes we believe that the surroundings judge us as strictly as we judge ourselves, as shown in the example of Marianne (p. 217). Such projections (Chapter 14) add fuel to the fire when we are self-critical and can thus help to strengthen our own self-criticism. In these situations, we sometimes do not trust our surroundings; we have a hard time believing that that they want the best for us. We continue the example with Jenny, to show how she is self-critical after the lecture.

Jenny has a therapy session after she holds the lecture. She sits with a bowed head and talks in low voice as she tells how bad the lecture was. She says that she did not cover all the points she had planned to and that she more or less fled the lecture hall when she had finished, for fear of hearing what the students thought. She was sure they did not like it. The therapist asks how she left the room and whether anyone had tried to talk to her.

Jenny says that a few students approached her while she was gathering her papers but that she did not hear what they said because she was so busy planning to leave as quickly as possible.

The therapist asks Jenny to visualise the situation, which she does. With her eyes closed, Jenny says that she can now (in her imagination) see the two students approaching her. It looks as if they are smiling, but she thinks this is only because they want to make her feel better about how badly it went. Together with the therapist, Jenny gradually becomes aware that she is breathing more and that she is less sad when she looks at the two students in her imagination than when she thinks about how badly the lecture went. She realises she has a choice: she can stay in her own ideas about how the lecture went and be sad or be present with the two students and breathe better.

In this example, the therapist wants to increase Jenny's attention to how critical thoughts prevent her from seeing and hearing the students around her. The therapist has a hypothesis that the contact between Jenny and her surroundings is characterised by retroflection and projection, and she chooses an experiment in which she lets Jenny imagine the situation she fled in order to take the projection back (see pp. 210–211). The experiment causes Jenny to 'see' the students' smiles and become aware of how she thought about what she saw, as well as what she feels bodily in the therapy room.

Guilt and shame

Guilt and shame are two important concepts when working as a therapist and are often part of the retroflection in the field between therapist and client or between the client and her immediate surroundings. We understand guilt as the feeling that arises when we have done something we think is wrong or failed to do something we should have done, and shame as the feeling of being wrong, which is a result of the attitudes to and actions towards us from our surroundings (Kolmannskog, 2018).

We see in the earlier example of Tanya (pp. 196–197) how she felt bad if she did not do what her parents expected of her. A bad conscience and guilt often arise when we do not follow the prevalent norms or rules and are a consequence of how we relate to introjection (Perls et al., 1951). Guilt is important and necessary for how we regulate impulses and reflect on what we believe to be right and wrong. In therapy we often meet clients who readily assume guilt for actions they have not performed themselves, as we have shown previously in the example of Tim (p. 224), or who on the other hand do not feel they have done anything wrong when they should have acknowledged their action or mistake. The therapist can then work on having the client reflect over and share experiences if there is in fact a basis for the guilt, and the extent to which the attitudes of the surroundings and the client's assessment of the situation are in agreement.

The client's poor self-esteem often has its background in the negative and critical attitudes of the environment as she grew up and can lead to a feeling of being wrong. She may feel a sense of shame about who she is, and the messages from her surroundings can introduce retroflection into the field, with the result that the client directs the messages inwards. The client imagines that this sense of being wrong is confirmed in her surroundings; that is, she projects the feeling of being wrong on her surroundings, which reinforces her feeling of shame. It is therefore important that the therapist be aware of how she is consciously and unconsciously critical of the client, and how this underlying criticism can lead to retroflection and shame in the client. The therapist also needs to be aware that clients often compare themselves to her, and the fact that clients believe the therapist to be more successful than they are can in and of itself lead to more retroflection in the field. We cannot avoid shame in lives or in the therapy room, since the feeling is related to our ability to judge ourselves, both positively and negatively. When we consider shame to be a form of retroflection, we can support our clients by sharing our own experience, as we do in other work where retroflection figures.

When retroflection is lacking

In many situations it can be useful to hold back, to stop ourselves from doing or saying something. The situation from earlier with Frederic and his children comes to mind, where he manages to hold back his anger by turning it towards himself rather than his children. At meetings in the workplace, in discussions, and in relationships, it can create considerable problems if one or more people are unable to keep themselves from speaking out or from controlling their impulses, emotions, or actions.

Some people have not learned how to hold back and are not able to be self-critical when the situation calls for it. The consequences can be serious for all involved; it can lead to violence, abuse, and much suffering. These individuals may need help learning how to handle strong emotions. This can be accomplished by raising their awareness of bodily and emotional signals and stopping impulses before they become actions (see Chapters 5, 7, and 20).

A lack of knowledge—a lack of awareness

Some people lack the ability to think self-critically because they have not learned what is expected of them and what is acceptable in a given situation. It is important for the therapist to understand that the client has a lack of knowledge of society's norms and rules, and to spend time exploring what the client understands the social codes to be. This information can help the therapist understand how to help the client reflect on her own actions. Clients with little ability for self-critical reflection often become scapegoats and lonely in social relationships. This can be expressed as unsocial behaviour or withdrawal and isolation (Hostrup, 2010; Spagnuolo Lobb, 2005).

Unrealistic beliefs about oneself

Another form of retroflection is expressed when someone boasts about herself and has unrealistic ideas about what she can do and accomplish. This often occurs in cases where there were unclear guidelines during childhood or where caregivers did not provide appropriate correction and praise, as the example with Johan shows.

Johan's boss has sent him to coaching. Johan doesn't understand why; he thinks everything at work is just fine. He tells the coach about how everything he does is successful and how everyone except his boss is happy with him. Initially, the coach gets annoyed; she thinks that Johan has little self-understanding and is simply boasting. Eventually, she notices that she is getting sad and feels compassion for Johan. She thinks that he might have a hard time at work without even knowing it. She holds this back and listens to him, nods, and smiles. She gets a picture of a small, vulnerable boy who wants to show his mother how good he is at everything he does. She chooses not to comment on the content of what Johan says, and simply says that she is listening and would like him to come to regular coaching sessions. Johan says that he has enjoyed telling her about himself, and that he may as well come, even if he does not fully understand the purpose.

Here, the coach is touched by Johan's way of being, and she lets this experience guide how she acts and speaks. She believes that Johan has lacked encouragement, loving criticism, and support during his upbringing, and that her restraint combined with her expression of genuine interest touches Johan and motivates him to come back.

In this example, it is the coach who holds back because the client's way of evaluating himself is not in accordance with how she and his boss see him. The coach thinks it is important that she withholds her assessments, and instead seeks ways to be with Johan that give him a sense of security and support. Perhaps, rather than the coach holding back and Johan talking, they can eventually find ways of being together in which the coach can gradually and cautiously comment on Johan's statements and behaviour.

Summary

Retroflection is a form of contact that is expressed when we self-critically reflect on our own actions and thoughts or withhold impulses and turn them inwards towards ourselves in various ways. Our challenge lies in the tension between the need to manage on our own, be self-sufficient and independent, and the need to meet, share with, and be accepted by others. These challenges are expressed through how much we hold back and how much we show and share of ourselves, something the therapist often explores with the client in the therapy room. Retroflection is closely linked to the contact forms introjection and projection, and can also be confused with the contact form self-monitoring, which you can read about in the next chapter.

References

Hostrup, H. (2010). *Gestalt therapy: An introduction to the basic concepts of gestalt therapy* (D. H. Silver, Trans.). Copenhagen: Hans Reitzlers Forlag. (Original work published 1999).

Jørstad, S. (2002/2008). Oversikt over kontaktformer [Overview of contact forms]. In S. Jørstad & Å. Krüger (Eds.), *Den flyvende hollender* [The flying Dutchman] (pp. 128–139). Oslo: NGI.

Kolmannskog, V. (2018). *The empty chair*. London: Routledge.

Perls, F. S., Hefferline, R. F., & Goodman, P. (1951). *Gestalt therapy: Excitement and growth in the human personality*. London: Souvenir Press.

Polster, E., & Polster, M. (1974). *Gestalt therapy integrated*. New York: Vintage Books.

Spagnuolo Lobb, S. M. (2005). Classical gestalt therapy theory. In A. L. Woldt & S. M. Toman (Eds.), *Gestalt therapy: History, theory, and practice* (Chapter 2). London: Sage.

Spagnuolo Lobb, S. M. (2013). *The now-for-next in psychotherapy: Gestalt therapy recounted in post-modern society*. Siracusa: Istituto di Gestalt HCC Italy.

Staemmler, F. M. (2016). Self as situated process. In J.-M. Robine (Ed.), *Self: A polyphony of contemporary gestalt therapy* (pp. 103–121). St. Romain la Virvée: L'Exprimerie.

Wheeler, G. (1998). *Gestalt reconsidered* (2nd ed.). Cambridge, MA: CIGPress.

Chapter 16

Self-monitoring

Vera is in a meeting at work with several colleagues. They are planning a seminar for which Vera is responsible and for which she has spent a lot of time and energy preparing. They have gotten to the point where they need to send out invitations to all employees. Vera summarises the programme they have agreed on and asks if anyone has comments before they send it out.

She asks because she has a running inner dialogue in which she goes back and forth about whether some parts of the seminar might be boring and whether there are things they should do differently. Her colleague Jason has some suggestions for what he believes are improvements to the programme. Vera hears what he says, but at the same time continues her inner conversation without taking in the content of what he says. She thinks that at this point the issue has been discussed enough; she wants to be the one who decides the programme content, even though she is in doubt about what is best. There is not much time left to make changes—they can't start over now. The others give their opinions, and the discussion goes back and forth until Vera stops them. She concludes that they will keep the programme as it is; the invitation should be sent out now.

In this example, Vera listens to the others' feedback without dealing with it. Instead, she continues her inner conversation about the original plans for the seminar. After all considerations for and against, she finally chooses to keep the original programme and is not affected by what her colleagues say. We do not know if this decision is good for the company or how the employees react to her way of making a decision, but we can imagine Jason getting annoyed at Vera because she asks for opinions without listening to them. Maybe the others are relieved that she made a decision; now they know what they have to deal with. Vera herself is not aware of how her manner affects her contact with her colleagues, and we can imagine that there might be an uncomfortable atmosphere at her workplace if she continues to make important decisions without listening to her co-workers.

DOI: 10.4324/9781003153856-19

This chapter describes what is meant by the contact form self-monitoring and how it affects the contact in the field. We illustrate self-monitoring with examples from everyday life and from clinical therapeutic work.

Self-monitoring and contact with the outside world

When we think back and forth about what we need, how to perform an action, or what we think is best to say in a situation, we become more concerned with ourselves and our trade-offs than with our surroundings, as we saw in the example with Vera. She barely heard or saw her colleagues, did not take in what they said, and did not share her inner dialogue. It was as if she were in a bubble. This way of being closed off can be described as 'nothing comes in and nothing goes out' (Jørstad, 2002/2008, our translation).

A definition of the contact form self-monitoring is the ability to make independent and autonomous choices after a process of deliberation and stick with choices once they are made. This is closely related to the others with whom we find ourselves in a situation, the ideas we have of ourselves, who we want to be, and how we evaluate ourselves and our decision-making process. Self-monitoring is normally 'indispensable in any process of elaborate complication and long maturation' (Perls et al., 1951, p. 237). In this contact form, we wait to act on our impulses: we postpone our actions, set down the pace, and assess the situation and who we are in it (Perls et al., 1951). Self-monitoring is about assessing and seeing oneself from the outside. It is characterised by 'self-talk' and brooding. In its most extreme form, awareness of the surroundings can fade into the background (Joyce & Sills, 2014).

When we are not aware that we are self-monitoring, contact with the outside world can be characterised by the fact that we have little spontaneity, feel depressed, or feel dead. It can feel as if there is no correlation between how we are, what we say, and the roles we play or masks we wear. We may not know what we want or need and have trouble making difficult choices. There can be a fear of losing control and lack of trust in ourselves and our surroundings (Spagnuolo Lobb, 2013).

The result of an inner process of back-and-forth discussion can be that we hold firmly onto our final decision. This contact form can also be seen in a teacher's conviction when she conveys her knowledge to her students or in the therapist's ability to hold her client firmly in what she thinks is best at the moment.

Self-monitoring, egotism, and egoism

Goodman and Perls (Perls et al., 1951) originally used the term 'egotism', for want of a better way of expressing this type of contact. They stressed that egotism is the 'slowing-down of spontaneity by further deliberate introspection and circumspection, to make sure that . . . there is no threat of danger or surprise—before he commits himself', in other words the ability to use caution to ensure that unfortunate and quick decisions are not made (p. 237). Instead of egotism, we have chosen to use the term 'self-monitoring', which we believe provides a more precise description of the contact form. In our opinion, the formulation egotism is not only misleading but also has a negative association to the term 'egoism', which is easily associated with selfishness and the individual's one-sided self-interest (Mann, 2010). The term 'self-monitoring' is used by the English theorists Joyce and Sills (2014) because they believe that the term 'egotism' is 'misleading' (p. 109).

Goodman and Perls believed that egotism could be compared to the 'neurosis' of a person who has been in psychoanalysis for a long time (Perls et al., 1951, p. 457). The Italian gestalt therapist and theorist Spagnuolo Lobb (2005) makes this comment on the challenges of being a client who has had a great deal of therapy:

> Isadore From was often heard saying that egotism is the illness that psychotherapists ('even Gestalt therapists', he would say humorously) communicate to their patients when they give them the capacity to know everything about themselves but cannot give them the trust necessary to plunge into life. The egotist can be the 'recovered' patient who has learned everything about his or her contact interruption, even how to avoid it, but who is still not able to be in the fullness of life, accepting the risk that is implied in trusting the environment to allow for true spontaneity of contact.
>
> (p. 35)

Many clients can thus become skilled at interpreting the environment and adapting to what those in their surroundings expect of them. This can become apparent in the client's relationship with the therapist. In that way, the conversation can be steered away from talking about themselves, such that their insecurity and anxiety about having their insecurity revealed remains hidden. Paradoxically, it may seem as if they are outgoing, social, capable of listening, and easy to communicate with, while they are in fact more concerned with reflecting on their own problems and are afraid to share what they really think and feel; afraid of being revealed as failures (Perls et al., 1951).

Self-monitoring and other forms of contact

In the same way as the contact form retroflection, self-monitoring develops gradually as we grow up. There is a close connection between self-monitoring and the contact forms introjection (Chapter 13) and projection (Chapter 14). The ability to consider, brood, and assess conflicting needs before we choose is a demanding process and assumes that we have language for and an experience of who we are and what we think our surroundings want from us. The messages we were given during adolescence, how they were given, how we received them, how we were met by others, what we imagined, the attitudes and opinions we projected onto our environment, and how we copied others has helped shape us and make us self-critical or self-monitoring in our relations with others today.

The contact forms retroflection (Chapter 15) and self-monitoring can be easily confused because both deal with the need to turn attention inwards by reflecting, assessing, and talking to ourselves. The differences lie in the fact that in retroflection we assess ourselves in terms of norms, rules, and what others think of us, which affect our feeling of self. In self-monitoring, however, we consider how to carry out our actions in the best way in regard to who we feel we are and what we believe in. In retroflection we are aware of the surroundings and attitudes and opinions about us, and much of our inner conversations revolve around our assumptions about what others think about what we do and how we are. In cases of self-monitoring, the surroundings are not really of interest. We are more concerned with finding out what we ourselves think and barely take in the fact that there are people around us. Naturally, in many situations we experience that our contact with our surroundings is characterised by both contact forms, because in our deliberations we are focused on who we are and what we believe in, and are self-critical in relation to the processes we are in with others.

Being in one's own bubble

The ability to hold onto what we believe in and the opinions and attitudes we have is fundamental in today's changing and fluid culture (Spagnuolo Lobb, 2013). It is also challenging when one's own view is on a collision course with the environment when it comes to being able to assess what to take in, what is of value, and which parts of the opinions of others to reject (Parlett, 2015). It is important to be able to withhold strong emotions when the environment cannot support them, such as in cases of sudden death, accidents, or long periods of illness. In extreme situations, this type of self-control is necessary in order to survive, something we know from the accounts of concentration camp survivors. Viktor Frankl (1947/1966) describes how he deliberately shut out his surroundings and went into his own bubble in order to hold onto his godliness, which was of paramount importance for his survival and the later development of his own method of psychotherapy, logotherapy. If, however, emotions and bodily reactions are held back for a long time, spontaneity and the ability to surrender to those around us can be lost.

Self-monitoring's opposing polarity

The opposite pole of self-monitoring—the continuation of internal deliberation—is the ability to surrender to others. Surrender in this sense is the spontaneous 'let[ting] go of the self' or '*giving of the self*' to something or someone (Wheeler, 1998, p. 82). In surrender, we sometimes even flow along with and give in in order to join with others, as in the contact form confluence.

– to make thorough	**Self-monitoring**	– to surrender impulsively
internal assessment	← ———————————— →	to others
– to hold a choice firmly	the span between the poles	– to be spontaneous

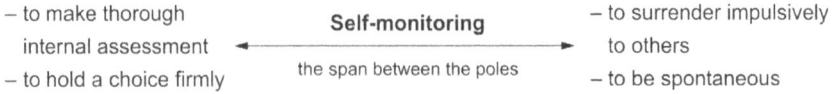

Working as a therapist, supervisor, or coach, we often meet clients who struggle with being locked into one of these poles. They experience a need and are not aware that they can have more than one need. Perhaps they incessantly consider, think, plan, and worry about the future and tasks to be solved, or constantly find themselves getting into trouble because their important life decisions are made quickly and impulsively. The therapist increases the client's awareness of both poles of the contact form, explores the needs, and works in the tension between the poles so that the client can become acquainted with more ways of being in contact in the field. When working on one of the poles or the relationship between poles with clients, we are working on the contact form self-monitoring.

With too much control, spontaneity can be lost, and it becomes difficult to make choices and act. With too little control, there can be too many impulses and too much spontaneity, which can cause us to make unfortunate actions and choices and brings little satisfaction. In adulthood, clients can become aware of how one form of contact has unilaterally characterised them and discover how they can find a more flexible way of being. By doing so, they become familiar with how and when they can be spontaneous and outgoing, and when consideration and deliberation is appropriate.

Self-monitoring and therapy

It is important that the therapist has the ability to hold onto what she thinks is good therapy, that she can reflect and consider various approaches for her client, and that she does not lose spontaneity and creativity in her process of deliberation. Providing good therapy lies not only in the therapist having faith in the method she uses, but also that she knows who she is and what she stands for and that she is simultaneously attentive and open to her client's beliefs and values. It is important that the therapist is aware that contact with the client can be characterised by the therapist becoming 'the one who knows best' and self-absorbed, and that she can then lose her focus on her client. The therapist is also aware of situations in which it becomes apparent that the client uses her insight and self-understanding as a way to avoid being present in the moment with the therapist and where the therapy itself becomes a support for the client's self-monitoring, as we discuss on p. 232. In such cases, the therapist can work to increase her client's attention to what she senses and experiences, in order to get her out of the cycle of brooding and looking for explanations. We see this in the example with James.

James has been to a few therapy sessions because his wife has threatened to divorce him if he does not do anything about the way he is. James tells the therapist that he has trouble being truly present when he is with his wife and children, and that he therefore also understands that his wife is frustrated with him. He has been trying for a long time to be the way his wife and children want him to be, but no matter how much he tries, it feels as if he is playing an unnatural role as a father and spouse. It is as if the person he wants to be cannot come out. He tells the therapist about his upbringing with an alcoholic and absent father and an unpredictable mother. He learned early on to be quiet and retreat when things became difficult at home. He can see why his wife complains that he 'doesn't seem genuine' or that he is not being himself. He has explained to her that this introspection is due to his childhood experiences, but this explanation does not help them in their relationship.

As James talks, the therapist becomes aware that it is as if he is talking to himself, without eye contact with her. He leans back in his chair, and when he talks, she notices that she herself becomes distant, starts thinking, and has trouble concentrating on what he says. She tells James about what she has become aware of, and suggests that they experiment with how he sits and where he directs his gaze, so that he can experience instead of simply talk about how his behaviour affects her. She asks him to move backwards and forwards while switching between looking at her and looking down as he speaks. James has a clear bodily reaction and becomes aware that he holds his breath, feels pressure in his chest, and becomes very upset when he looks at the therapist while sitting very close to her, and that these reactions are much less evident when he looks away and sits back.

When James and the therapist reflect together after the experiment, he becomes aware that it is almost impossible for him to look at the therapist while she looks at him, which confuses and upsets him. When he gets confused, he retreats and leaves the conversation, and he becomes aware that he is using his bodily movements and eyes when regulating the distance in his contact with the therapist. He elaborates on this discovery by explaining that he is not used to looking others in the eye when he speaks, and that this is related to his childhood. His mother never looked at him when she spoke, and since he never knew what kind of mood she was in, he just pulled away. As James continues in a monotone voice, the therapist becomes more inattentive.

After a short while, she says: 'As I hear you start to explain why you're struggling to look at me and that you're pulling back, it occurs to me that you're doing both of these things again. Are you aware of that? Can you feel it in your eyes and torso?'

> JAMES nods, and says: 'Yes, I can sense that I'm not looking at you, and I don't like pulling away from you. It's not intentional, and I should probably look at you when I talk, but it's because I'm not used to it, and it's hard to think about what I want to say to you while I'm looking at you'.
>
> THE THERAPIST responds quickly so that James cannot continue explaining: 'Yes, I can understand that. It's not easy to do something new. I also think that it might be a little uncomfortable for you, and that you might feel some fear without being fully aware of it'.
>
> JAMES: 'I don't know if I'm afraid, you're not someone I'm afraid of, but . . . and yes, it's a little uncomfortable'.

Here, the therapist wants to increase James's awareness of the quality of the contact between them in the therapy room. James becomes aware that he is doing something active with his body and eyes when he regulates the contact between them. Because James already understands the connection between his childhood and how he reacts with the therapist, the therapist looks at his explanations as 'detours' from the matter at hand and chooses instead to keep his attention on the relationship between them. The therapist has an idea that when James's attention turns to his bodily sensations and his relations, he will become less concerned with the ongoing self-observation that he easily disappears into. This attention to relation also affects the relationship between the therapist and James. The therapist becomes more engaged and present as they together explore the distance between them.

The therapist has an assumption that James is afraid, and chooses therefore to 'grade' her interventions. The challenge for James is to let go of explanations and dare to experience something new together with the therapist. By admitting that it is a little uncomfortable to sit with the therapist, he comes into contact with a new feeling that may be the gateway to further exploration of his emotions. He has come to therapy because he struggles to be present in the situation, so this is an important place to start.

Talking more with oneself than with the therapist

When there is much deliberation and evaluation in the field between therapist and client, the therapist will pay attention to the extent to which the client takes in what the therapist says and the extent to which the client is impulsive and spontaneous or deliberates in inner conversations. We illustrate this in the next example with Amy.

> Amy has been in therapy for a while and has told the therapist about a difficult childhood in a commune with several adults and children. She often felt that no one saw her; there was always so much going on and so many people with opinions about everything. She felt that she gave into everyone

else while she grew up and did as she was asked. The therapist lets Amy share stories of her upbringing. She follows along as she nods, smiles, and comments.

Amy has a lot on her mind. Among other things, she wonders if she should move in with her boyfriend Jake or if she should move abroad. As Amy talks, the therapist becomes aware that she is becoming confused and is unable to follow Amy's narrative. It sounds to her as if Amy is talking more to herself than with her. She wonders if she should make Amy aware of this or let her keep talking. She also becomes aware that she herself is starting to consider what to do when it comes to Amy, and decides to interrupt her client in her monologue.

THERAPIST: 'It sounds like you're talking more to yourself than with me. I hear you argue and weigh the pros and cons of moving in with Jake, without asking me what I'm thinking. Do you see this?'

AMY responds, and it's as if she is still in her own inner dialogue: 'Yes, you understand that I don't really think I can live with just one person. I'm used to living either with a lot of people or no one. So maybe it would be good for me to try to live with just Jake, even if it might not work out'.

Amy's monologue affects the therapist such that she also begins with an inner dialogue, to a greater extent than she normally would, about what to say or not say to Amy. The contact form between them is self-monitoring. The therapist becomes concerned about how she can make Amy aware of how the contact form affects her, without Amy thinking that it is wrong to talk more to herself than with her. We continue the example and see what the therapist chooses to do.

The therapist looks at Amy and repeats verbatim what she said: ' . . . So maybe it would be good for you to try to live with just Jake, even if it might not work out'.

Amy looks at her for a moment, nods, and keeps talking about how she thinks they can move in together. The therapist continues to repeat parts of what Amy says, and every time she does so, Amy stops a little and nods. Eventually, it is as if she becomes aware that the therapist is repeating her words and not stating her own opinion.

After a while, Amy says that it is nice that the therapist repeats what she says, because it makes her more aware of what she thinks. When Amy says this, the therapist stops repeating Amy's words. Instead, she tells her how much easier it was for her to understand what Amy meant when she repeated parts of what Amy said.

Then Amy says spontaneously: 'It's sort of crazy, but it was like I realised you were in the room too when you repeated what I said. I became more focused on you and wanted to make you understand what a hard time I'm having, and . . . Now I'm actually wondering what you think of me . . . '

The therapist laughs a little and looks at Amy: 'Right now I'm happy. Before, I felt like you were talking more to yourself than to me, and now I feel like I'm breathing more freely. I'm not so tense and worried, and I like being here with you'.

The therapist here chooses 'to flow along with' Amy by repeating what she says, without being confluent with her (see Chapter 13). The therapist's hypothesis is that Amy is not aware of how the contact between them is influenced by the fact that she is more concerned with her own inner conversation than with talking to the therapist. When the therapist repeats what Amy says, Amy hears and becomes more aware of the therapist, and takes in both her own words and the therapist's presence. Amy becomes more spontaneous and dares to ask the therapist what she thinks of her, at which point the therapist also becomes spontaneous, laughs, and becomes less tense.

Self-monitoring as a contact form in supervision

In therapy and supervision, we occasionally meet people who are too self-controlling or self-observing. They struggle to make choices or they choose based on what is safest and are not spontaneous, as we see with Sara in supervision.

Sara works as a gestalt coach, and therefore participates regularly in supervision. The supervisor sometimes finds it challenging to work with Sara, because it is as if Sara is in her own thoughts, and therefore it is hard for the supervisor to convey what she wants to say to Sara or get her to experiment. This is also what happens during this supervision session.

Sara talks eagerly about a challenge she has in her coaching practice. She uses many words and explains in detail what she thinks the problem is. The supervisor listens for a while, but eventually interrupts the stream of words. She suggests exploring Sara's problem in a different way than as a story. Sara nods anxiously at the proposal, but in the next moment she is again in the process of telling and explaining.

After a few minutes, the supervisor stops her again: 'Can you stop for a moment, Sara? I hear you say a lot about your client, and I understand that you are very engaged in this client. But it's as if we haven't started the supervision yet. What do you think?'

'Yes', Sara says, 'I'd like supervision on this case. It's just that I want you to know as much as possible about my client so you can understand the problem. I think this is a client who needs . . . ' Sara continues as before.

The supervisor is looking for a form that does not amplify Sara's self-talk, and notices that she herself becomes a little distant and more focused on her own thoughts. It is as if they are both introverted and not paying attention to each other. Against the backdrop of this discovery, the supervisor again tries to capture Sara's attention.

In as calm and clear voice as possible, she says: 'Hey! Now you're talking about the client again. I need to get to know the way you and your client work together'. She asks Sara to stand up and encourages her to walk around the room and imagine that she is her client. Sara does as the supervisor suggests. She gets up and starts walking while she talks: 'I don't know how she walks; she might hold her body erect, and I think she thinks a lot. That's because . . . '

The supervisor again becomes aware of all Sara's words. She thinks that all the words block the immediate experience of 'being the client'. She therefore asks Sara to try out what it is like not to talk while she walks around the room, which Sara does. The supervisor continues to support Sara in the experiment where she first is her client and then herself. Eventually, Sara notices the difference between when she imagines that she is her client, and when she is herself.

Reflecting after the experiment, Sara says that she found it very challenging to play her client. She was afraid that the supervisor would not understand what she meant, which she found uncomfortable. At the same time, it felt good to be practically commanded to get up, so that she no longer could consider for and against. In this way, she gained the experience of trying something new and being a little more spontaneous.

In this example, both Sara and the supervisor consider and hold on to their ideas. Sara is not at first aware of this phenomenon, and the supervisor eventually becomes aware of her own contribution to the process. The supervisor thus proposes an experiment for Sara, so that they can experience something new and become aware of bodily phenomena. The supervisor holds on to the idea that Sara should try to walk around the room as her client, even if Sara continues talking and is not aware of the purpose of the experiment. This is how she facilitates a process in which Sara can experience spontaneously here and now, which means that Sara also has a new experience of daring to yield to the supervisor's proposal. At the same time, the supervisor raises her own awareness of how she is with her client.

The supervisor believes that Sara becomes locked in her thoughts about her client because this is a phenomenon that also applies in the contact between Sara and her client. Without being aware of it, Sara brings her projections about her client and expresses these in supervision (see Chapter 14). This phenomenon is called a 'parallel process' and is taken from psychodynamic theory (Gilbert & Evans, 2000). The supervisor chooses to make Sara aware of this in a later supervision session. In gestalt therapy and supervision, parallel processes are a recognised phenomenon because emphasis is given to Lewin's field theory and the complexity of human interaction is taken into account (Mjelve, 2016).

There are people who change their minds from moment to moment, who have few views of their own, who reflect little over life's challenges and opportunities, and who spontaneously and impulsively dive into new relationships and situations. These individuals rarely come to therapy until confronted with the harsh reality of life in the form of an accident, illness, or major personal crises. The therapist faces challenges keeping the client in the emotions and thoughts she brings to therapy, and the contact form between them can often seem like of a mixture of deflection, in which the client avoids dealing with what is unpleasant (Chapter 17), and confluence, where the client agrees with everything the therapist suggests and has few opinions of her own (Chapter 12). The therapist and client are easily stuck in self-monitoring's opposing pole, and it can be difficult for the therapist to make the client aware of other needs they may have in the situation. The best way may be for the therapist to repeat and reinforce what the client says or try to contradict the client and see if she reacts.

Summary

In this chapter, we have described what we mean by the concept of self-monitoring, how this contact form is useful in important processes where choices are made, and that it is about slowing down the pace and taking the time to weigh the options; taking time for self-reflection and self-assessment. We have described the contact form's polarity—to give oneself impulsively over to others and to be spontaneous—and challenges that clients may experience when there is too much or too little of one of these aspects of the contact form.

References

Frankl, V. (1947/1966). *Kjempende livstro* [The struggle for meaning]. Oslo: Gyldendals Fakkelbok.
Gilbert, M., & Evans, K. (2000). *Psychotherapy supervision: An integrative relational approach to psychotherapy supervision*. Buckingham: Open University Press.
Jørstad, S. (2002/2008). Oversikt over kontaktformer [Overview of contact forms]. In S. Jørstad & Å. Krüger (Eds.), *Den flyvende hollender* [The flying Dutchman] (pp. 128–139). Oslo: NGI.
Joyce, P., & Sills, C. (2014). *Skills in gestalt counselling & psychotherapy* (3rd ed.). London: Sage.
Mann, D. (2010). *Gestalt therapy: 100 key points and techniques*. New York: Routledge.

Mjelve, L. H. (2016). Parallel processes in counseling for schools. In J. Roubal (Ed.), *Towards a research tradition in gestalt therapy* (pp. 271–289). Newcastle upon Tyne: Cambridge Scholars.

Parlett, M. (2015). *Future sense*. Leicestershire, UK: Matador.

Perls, F. S., Hefferline, R. F., & Goodman, P. (1951). *Gestalt therapy: Excitement and growth in the human personality*. London: Souvenir Press.

Spagnuolo Lobb, S. M. (2005). Classical gestalt therapy theory. In A. L. Woldt & S. M. Toman (Eds.), *Gestalt therapy: History, theory, and practice* (pp. 21–39). London: Sage.

Spagnuolo Lobb, S. M. (2013). *The now-for-next in psychotherapy: Gestalt therapy recounted in post-modern society*. Siracusa: Istituto di Gestalt HCC Italy.

Wheeler, G. (1998). *Gestalt reconsidered* (2nd ed.). Cambridge, MA: CIGPress.

Chapter 17

Deflection

In many situations we avoid dealing with what others say. This can cause irritation, but it can also have advantages. When the pressure of work becomes too great, it is both good and necessary to be able to deflect thoughts and feelings by doing things such as losing ourselves in a good book, surfing the web, or watching television. In some cases, it can be a good survival strategy to think about something else. Many of us cover our eyes or look away when we watch frightening scenes in films. We comfort children when they fall down and assure them that it is going to be all right. When a loved one falls ill, we sometimes make light of the situation, assuring them that they will soon recover, even when we know that that is not the case. In addition, it is important to be able to stay level headed in crises or challenging situations (Hostrup, 2010).

In this chapter, we describe different forms of deflection, how they affect contact between us, and how they are expressed in everyday life. We show how we work to recognise and explore these forms of deflection in different situations in therapy, coaching, and supervision.

Definition of deflection

The word 'deflection' comes from the Latin *dēflexiōn-*, and can be translated as 'bending away from something'. The contact form deflection is defined as diverting attention away from something in a given situation and 'a way of taking the heat off the actual contact' (Polster & Polster, 1974, p. 89).

Deflection is a mental process in which we ignore what others say or do. It can feel like there is considerable distance between us, and contact becomes superficial. In some cases, deflection can stand in our way, such as in situations where we sense inner turmoil or are uncertain, or where we make light of something in order to escape discomfort. We can also divert attention with the words we choose, for example, when we say 'you' in a general sense when the word 'I' would be more relevant. The statement 'you have to pull yourself together' generalises an experience, and is often an expression of a need to create distance between ourselves and our feelings, when in fact saying 'I need to pull myself together' accurately describes the phenomenon we experience. This is a form of

DOI: 10.4324/9781003153856-20

deflection that can help us when a situation involves more discomfort than we can handle. For example, when we witness a car accident, we can experience a need to avoid feeling the emotions that come up. In that case we might say 'you really think about your mortality when you see an accident' instead of 'it made me think about my own mortality', which is more direct speech. In these cases, deflection becomes an unconscious avoidance strategy that keeps unpleasant or overwhelming emotions at bay.

The use of 'you' instead of 'I' can also be a way to avoid personal feelings or getting too close to something or someone. In some situations, however, it can also be of great help. A participant in an Arctic expedition who was interviewed described his emotional walk across the ice with the pronoun 'you': 'You just have to take it one step at a time and you'll get through it'. This formulation helped him to safeguard his personal experience and thus allowed him to create distance in the situation there and then. Deflection became an important part of the way he safeguarded his own experience.

In conflict-ridden situations it can often be useful to be able to 'beat around the bush', as is often done in diplomacy and in politics (Polster & Polster, 1974). Escaping from the situation in crises or acute situations physically or emotionally is a known survival strategy. How appropriate this escape is depends on how aware we are of our strategy and whether there are other, more appropriate ways of handling the situation.

Deflection and its opposing polarity

Because deflection is about avoiding something, it naturally follows that the opposite polarity is to accept and be present in a situation or sensation (Joyce & Sills, 2014). Just as a photographer adjusts focus before taking an image, we sharpen our attention to make things clear in the situation.

We have seen that the span of the contact form's polarity describes how our needs in the field are different and often contradictory. Sometimes the contact is characterised by the need to think about something other than what is figural or otherwise avoid getting to the point. Perhaps we can all identify with trying to avoid something that is staring us in the face by pushing it into the background. Other times contact moves towards the opposite end of the polarity, where the need to accept something and be present in what is going on around us comes to the foreground. The contact in these cases is characterised by having a clear focus on the subject at hand, such as working with others to solve a task or training for an athletic event. Here, the challenge is that we can blindly focus on one issue or task and exclude the possibilities inherent in allowing events to unfold and seeing what emerges.

The tension between the poles can be illustrated as follows:

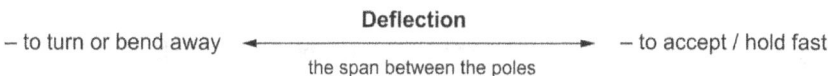

Deflection

– to turn or bend away ◄─────────────────► – to accept / hold fast

the span between the poles

One example that shows the challenge we can face in this tension between polarities can be seen in the case of Mohammad, who is struggling to write a project assignment at work. He has a short deadline and sits at his desk in deep concentration writing for several hours when he suddenly discovers that his thoughts are elsewhere. The temptation to get up from his desk is great, and he chooses to go for a walk instead of forcing himself to stay where he is. On his walk he gets new ideas, and what he struggled with while at his desk falls into place. He feels himself becoming more creative as he moves his body and lets his thoughts flow freely away from the task at hand, and that the urge to get up was not a deflection, as he first thought, but rather an inspiration to move forward in his process.

He faces a new challenge when he returns to work: sitting down at his desk again to work with the new ideas rather than turning away, by for example reading the newspaper, checking emails, or organising files on his computer.

The struggle and tension between the desire to write and the desire to do something else can become very clear in such situations. Two conflicting needs are expressed (see Chapter 6 on field theory). The next example shows a situation in which conflicting needs appear between Laura and her colleagues.

Free-flowing thoughts versus focus

Laura is in middle management in an institution and has been asked to lead a task force that will create a proposal for an education program for employees. There are three members in the working group, and Laura is in the first meeting with the other two, Barbara and Bob.

Even though the three all know each other, they have never worked on a project together. It is therefore natural that they spend some time warming up with small talk. Laura is pleased that they can talk freely, and waits to interrupt the small talk because she experiences that they are having a good time together. She tells herself that this is a good start for their future cooperation.

Bob suddenly interrupts and says: 'Shouldn't we get to work?' He looks at Laura with a frustrated expression.

Laura becomes more focused. It is time to stop the small talk. She straightens up in her chair, clears her throat, and starts talking about what they need to do. Bob's intervention helps her to focus.

Laura joins in the pleasant social chat when the three initially meet, and she avoids taking responsibility for holding the focus on the task at hand. She is not aware that she has two conflicting needs as the group leader, and that this means that, up to the point of Bob's intervention, all three avoid embarking on a task that is demanding and uncomfortable. As group leader, Laura becomes aware of the tension between the need to think about something else and to stay present in what is happening around her. In other words, she notices how good it can be to be social, but at the same time how important it is to focus on the task they need to finish.

Figure-ground and deflection

Deflection is not originally one of Perls' contact disturbances (as he referred to them), but comes from Miriam and Erving Polster (1974). Perls had intended to call his new form of therapy 'concentration therapy' or 'focus therapy', because he claimed that people often spoke in clichés, thus avoiding unpleasant feelings and situations (Perls, 1947/1969). He believed that by increased attention, people would become more conscious and concentrated so that the focus of their interest could become apparent. In figure-ground thinking (see Chapter 2), the object of attention—that which is figural—becomes clear or unclear depending on the degree of attention the individual has in the situation, and how important the figure (need) is to the individual. We see the same polarities in Zen Buddhism, which Perls was influenced by (Clarkson & Mackewn, 1993). The aim is to pay attention and be present in the moment, while at the same time letting thoughts and feelings pass by without being affected by them. Strangely, Perls did not refer to this as a contact disturbance.

Deflection and focusing alone or together

In the example of Laura and her colleagues, it is the nature and importance of the task that helps influence whether the group members chose to do something other than their work ('turning away') or focus on their task. If you are alone and have tasks to be performed, as the example with Mohammad shows, it is your own thoughts and feelings that affect how you handle the situation you are in—whether you are focused in front of your computer working or whether you constantly interrupt yourself by checking Facebook, reading messages on your phone, or starting to tidy up around you.

If you perform tasks together with others, the relationships between all participants will affect how the situation is handled and the task is resolved. A team at work that has a deadline to deliver on a project can run into difficulties if one or more of its members does not follow up, as the example above with Laura shows. This can create quite a bit of tension between those who feel the need to finish on time and those who do not seem to be taking it seriously. The result can be that the quality of the group's work is poor or that they do not finish their tasks on time.

Couples or families can also experience challenges in sorting priorities, such as when important tasks need to be carried out at home or at work. A couple that disagrees on whether to spend the money they earn on vacations and recreation or save to buy a new apartment lack a common goal. Both risk dissatisfaction if they are not able to reach an agreement. In the same way, conflict can arise in families with children if the parents do not agree on how to raise their children and lack awareness of which disagreements need to be dealt with and which are better left alone. It is important to be conscious of when deflection is appropriate, such as putting aside irritation that can arise due to clutter and noise, in contrast for example to pointing out when agreements are broken and tolerating the discomfort that the confrontation entails.

Working with deflection in therapy

In many situations, the need to avoid addressing unpleasant or difficult situations conflicts with the need to stay the course and do what needs to be done. In therapy, these conflicting needs often appear in themes the client brings in as well as in the contact between therapist and client. Often the client herself is not aware of this and needs support from the therapist to become aware of how she avoids that which is unpleasant.

In therapy, we try to hold the client in the situation that arises so that she can experience how she constantly avoids what she senses and interrupts herself. For example, we can say: 'I hear that you have started to talk about something other than the accident you were in. Can you instead repeat how you experienced driving off the road?' We can also hold the client in the situation by repeating the client's own words: 'I heard you say that you were scared when the car drove off the road. Is that right?' Another way the therapist can hold the client in the situation is by pointing out particular body movements, laughter, or a smile when there is no correlation with what the client says. For example: 'I notice that you start laughing when you tell me about your sick husband. What's it really like for you that he's sick?' This allows the client to feel the discomfort that the deflection helps her keep at bay and thus become aware of her other needs. Holding the client firmly in that which is uncomfortable can in fact be a way to support the client.

Being sent to therapy

For many of us it can be challenging to seek out therapy, especially when we are not aware that we need it or how a therapist can help us. We can also deny that we have problems or delay dealing with challenges until someone gives us reason to do so, as the example with Robert shows.

Robert seeks out a gestalt therapist because one of his friends thinks it will be good for him. In the first session he tells the therapist that this friend was with him when he booked the appointment. Robert does not know whether or not he has problems. He explains that he has a part-time job in addition to his studies. His studies aren't going well, which he says is due to the fact that he has to work so much because he spends a lot of money. When the therapist asks what he spends money on, Robert replies evasively with 'hobbies and stuff like that'. When the therapist asks again, he admits that he spends a lot of money going out in the evenings. He says that he drinks a lot but does not feel that it is a problem.

When the therapist talks to Robert, she becomes aware that he looks around and is restless when he speaks. It appears as if he is uncomfortable answering the therapist's questions, and she wonders if he is trying to hide something from her. She thinks about the friend who encouraged Robert to seek therapy and decides to ask more about her client's life and thus hold him in this feeling of being uncomfortable.

After half an hour in which the therapist has explored how Robert is doing, he gradually becomes more uneasy and shows signs that he feels uncomfortable. Hesitantly and softly he says that life is really very difficult. He is constantly trying to push difficulties away, and thinks it is shameful that he cannot handle his studies, that he drinks too much, and lacks control over his life. As Robert speaks, he looks at the therapist who has tears in her eyes and sees that she is touched by his openness.

Robert came to therapy at the urging of his friend. The therapist's questions and exploration of how Robert is doing is a way to hold him firmly in his uncomfortable state, which is expressed in bodily unrest and his voice. When Robert first acknowledges to himself and to the therapist that he is having a hard time, it becomes easier to address his problems. Robert has avoided seeing the seriousness of his life situation. It is only when this realisation comes to him that the contact between them changes and Robert can truly take responsibility for the choices he makes.

Using 'you' instead of 'I'

Examples of difficulties for which clients seek therapy can be a lack of feeling that they are able to cope at work, that they lose motivation for things they previously enjoyed, or that they struggle in their relationships with partners or friends without understanding why. Susanne contacts a gestalt supervisor because she struggles in her job as a teacher, and the principal has recommended that she do so.

Susanne tells the supervisor that she continually comes unprepared to teach. She is not able to keep order in her classes and feels she has to do something about it. The principal is concerned about the situation. He has recommended that she go to supervision and will pay for it.

While speaking with the supervisor, Susanne sits uneasily, seems restless, and has little eye contact with the supervisor. She talks quickly in a loud voice about her work as a teacher and about how she feels at home. Some time into the conversation, she says: 'You get so frustrated with these students. You'd think that when they're fourteen they'd have learned to sit still'. She continues: 'It's hard to prepare at home because there are so many things that need to be done. And my husband's pretty fed up at this point'.

SUPERVISOR: 'Susanne, I notice that you say "you" sometimes when you're talking about yourself. I wonder: can you repeat the sentence and notice what it's like to say "I" instead of "you"?'
SUSANNE smiles a little at the therapist's question, and says: 'Yes, I'm sure I can, if I can remember what I said!'
THE SUPERVISOR says: 'Just now, you said "I" and not "you".'

After the supervisor repeats the sentence, Susanne replaces 'you' with 'I', and says: 'I'm so frustrated with these students. I would think that they would've learned to sit still at age fourteen'. She pauses for a moment and then says: 'This was different, I can really feel how frustrated I am. I don't know what to do with them, it's just terrible'. Susanne has tears in her eyes and looks directly at the supervisor. The supervisor can feel that she is both sad and happy about Susanne's new insight, which she shares with Susanne.

This situation is another example of a client not seeking therapy (or supervision) on her own initiative. In this case, it was the principal who was concerned about Susanne and how she does her job, and therefore suggested she seek help. The supervisor holds Susanne firmly in her experience by repeating Susanne's sentence and asking her to replace 'you' with 'I'. Susanne becomes aware of the feelings she has tried to distance herself from, which in turn allows her to become aware of the seriousness of the classroom situation. The contact between Susanne and the supervisor changes. When Susanne acknowledges that she is responsible for the unrest in class and that she does not know what to do, the motivation to change the way she is towards her students and the supervisor can come from within herself and not from the principal or supervisor. Susanne's experience of being held firmly in her own experience and taken seriously by the supervisor can be important for her and help her to take both herself and her students more seriously than she has done thus far.

Deflection and bodily unrest

As therapists, we often take our point of departure in the words our clients use, as the example with Susanne shows, or in the content of clients' words, as the therapist does with Robert. However, when deflection is figural, it may be equally helpful in many situations to comment on the bodily unrest we become aware of in the client or ourselves.

In the example of Susanne, the therapist could say: 'I see you are restless and don't look at me when you talk. Is there anything that's hard to talk about?' The conversation might then develop as follows.

> Susanne denies that there is anything that is difficult to talk about, but her body language becomes more troubled, which the supervisor points out by saying: 'I hear you deny that it's hard, at the same time I see you sitting even more uneasily, so what you're saying doesn't match what you show me. I think there's something bothering you'. Susanne starts crying and nods to the therapist and says: 'Oh . . . it's so hard at work, I don't know what to do . . . '
>
> The supervisor leans forward and says with a gentle voice: 'I understand that. Let's first spend some time on what it's like to be you in this difficult situation, before we explore what you can do next . . . '

This approach is a confrontational way of holding Susanne firmly in her own experience, and the supervisor will consider carefully the point in the conversation at which she makes such direct observations. It can be a relief for Susanne that the supervisor takes her seriously and shows interest in how she is doing by pointing out what she sees and hears.

Turning away instead of standing firm

Some clients are in life situations where they feel unable to change things, describing how worries and bad feelings paralyse them in everyday life. Learning to turn away rather than standing firm on can occasionally be helpful in such situations. Look at the following example with Diane.

> Diane has sought out a therapist because she is having a hard time while her twenty-year-old son is on a three-month overseas trip. She thinks about him all the time and is very worried. Diane uses the first therapy sessions to talk about how she worries, lies awake at night, and struggles to eat. Diane speaks intensely at her sessions as she looks right at the therapist. The therapist feels she needs a break. After thinking about it for a minute, the therapist suggests that they stand up and walk around the room together

a bit. Diane accepts the therapist's invitation, but continues to talk as if she is not aware that they are walking together. The therapist asks Diane to stop talking for a moment and instead look around the room as she walks. Diane looks around and at the therapist. The therapist asks Diane to describe what she sees around her. Diane does so while turning her body towards what she sees. The therapist notices that Diane breathes more deeply, and she herself feels that her muscles are less tense, which she tells Diane. When asked by the therapist if she is aware of her body, Diane says that she feels that she is breathing more easily and that she is aware of her body, which was not the case when she was sitting on her chair talking. When they return to their chairs, Diane feels that she has had a break from her worries.

Here, the therapist distracted Diane for a period of time from being focused on her son, based on the need she herself felt to have a break from how she was feeling. This increased Diane's attention to her surroundings and enabled her to see more than her own worry. Diane and the therapist did this experiment after they had first focused on Diane's worry and feelings. They then examined the opposite polarity: to turn away from the worry. Diane experiences how she can turn her attention elsewhere when she feels she is being engulfed by worry. She also becomes aware that she noticed her body only after walking around the room.

Diane is immersed in her worries about her son and her attention to her surroundings goes to the background. Our surroundings are out of focus when we are in the opposite pole and keep going from one thought to another. Because deflection is often a mental activity, it can be useful for both client and therapist to turn their attention outwards to their surroundings or inward to their breathing and bodily sensations in order to become more aware of the quality of the contact between them.

Summary

Diverting attention can sometimes provide a good break from the stress and bustle of everyday life. Deflection from intrusive demands and obligations or shying away when something becomes too challenging can provide calmness and be a good coping strategy. After some time has passed, we are again challenged to sharpen our focus without shying away from what is unpleasant, and realise that things are what they are, that the task must be done. We continually move between the extremes of the polarity—between the need to stand firm and be focused and the need to distract ourselves and avoid what is unpleasant.

In this chapter, we have described situations in which people have sought therapy or supervision when they have felt they were locked into one of the poles and have not been conscious of their conflicting needs. Once they have become more aware of the conflicting needs to turn away and to stand firm and of the span between them, they can more easily grasp challenges they face, take responsibility for the choices they make, and be aware of the contact between themselves and their surroundings.

References

Clarkson, P., & Mackewn, J. (1993). *Fritz Perls*. London: Sage Publications.

Hostrup, H. (2010). *Gestalt therapy: An introduction to the basic concepts of gestalt therapy* (D. H. Silver, Trans.). Copenhagen: Hans Reitzlers Forlag. (Original work published 1999)

Joyce, P., & Sills, C. (2014). *Skills in gestalt counselling & psychotherapy* (3rd ed.). London: Sage.

Perls, F. S. (1947/1969). *Ego, hunger and aggression*. New York: Vintage Books.

Polster, E., & Polster, M. (1974). *Gestalt therapy integrated*. New York: Vintage Books.

Part 4

Process models

In gestalt theory, there are several models that are used to describe the processes people go through in their attempts to creatively adjust to the challenges they meet in a world that is continually changing. These models are simplified images of reality; their purpose is to make it easier for us to understand how people experience and are in contact with their surroundings over time and how they seek to satisfy their needs at any given time (see Chapters 4 and 6). We show an example of this with Tom, who has several needs he tries to meet one early morning on his way to work.

> Tom is on his way to the bus. He is running late for an important meeting at work that is happening in half an hour. Suddenly he discovers that he forgot his cell phone at home. He turns and runs back home as he thinks about the fact that he will be even later for the meeting. He struggles to unlock the door and frantically looks for his mobile phone, which he finds under the newspaper on the breakfast table. He sees that the lunch he had packed for himself is also on the table, so he takes that with him as well. As he locks the door, he looks at his watch to check the time. He realises that he will not catch the bus he had planned to take. As he walks to the bus stop, he texts his boss to say he will be fifteen minutes late.

Many diverse needs to be met

Tom's situation is likely something many can identify with. Many of us have experienced running late in the morning. There are often many things to remember and many expectations to be met, both from ourselves and others.

In this example, we saw that Tom needs to get to a meeting on time. This means that he has to catch the bus at the right time. He also needs to bring his cell phone. By choosing to go back to get his phone, he also chooses a situation in which he will not be able to get to the meeting on time. We can speculate that he is running

DOI: 10.4324/9781003153856-21

late because he read the newspaper at the breakfast table and forgot the phone and lunch underneath it. Tom has several needs; we see that his needs to go to work and get to the bus coincide. However, his need to read the newspaper before he leaves and to go back for his phone when he forgets it are to some degree conflicting needs in terms of going to work. On the other hand, he may need his phone at work and have a job where it is important to stay informed about the news, so these needs might actually coincide with the need to be at work. It may therefore be that what creates unrest for Tom this morning is that he went to bed too late the night before and overslept in the morning.

The purpose of the example is to show how different needs with varying degrees of importance provide different choices and create different processes. We see that Tom realises he has forgotten his phone and chooses to turn back to get it. The process of 'going to work' changes to 'going home'. Once he found his cell phone, he was again in the 'going to work' process. Here we see an example of how a process can change when a new need is expressed. In his field theory, Lewin described how the different needs of the field affect and help organise the field, and that this helps create movement in the field. This is illustrated in the example with Tom (Chapters 1 and 7).

Process and change

'Process' comes from the Latin word *processus* and means 'advance' or 'progress'. The term is related to the verb *procedere*, which means 'to advance, appear, or proceed'. When we use the term 'process' in gestalt therapy, we sometimes mean the way in which something moves forward and other times that something has moved, evolved, and changed. The close connection between the concepts of process and change becomes clear here. In any process there is a change, and in any change there has been a process. In the second part of this book we described the theoretical basis from which gestalt therapy views change, with reference to Beisser's theory of paradoxical change (Chapter 4).

Perls was interested in the idea that all life is process and flow, and that nothing is static (Clarkson & Mackewn, 1993), which he showed in his therapeutic work. In therapy it is also relevant for clients to become aware of how they are in contact with their surroundings, such as exploring the themes they bring in. As therapists, we see that there is often a connection between the topics that clients bring in and the process, in other words *how* the topic is brought into the therapy room. In many cases, clients are not aware of how they contact others. They can act automatically, creating challenges in their lives and in the therapy room. Therefore, gestalt therapists are interested in the client's life story and how the relationship develops between therapist and client (Yontef, 1993; Joyce & Sills, 2014). The therapist works to increase the client's attention to the topic brought in, to how the two of them experience being together in the therapy room, and to the process that evolves between them.

Three process models

This section describes three theoretical models that map how processes and change occur over time. We show how a process can constantly change shape and direction, how it can sometimes become static or fixated, and how in therapy we can support the process so that it can flow in a more meaningful way. These theoretical process models are associated with previously described concepts and models such as field theory, formation of figure-ground, regulation of needs, creative adjustment, the paradox of change, and contact (Part 2). We briefly reflect on what is meant by process and change and justify our choice of concepts and process models. The three models described are: the process of contact, the process of experience, and the process of change.

All three models are built on the original version of Fritz Perls's 'disturbance cycle' or 'cycle of inter-dependency of organism and environment' described in *Ego, Hunger and Aggression* (Perls, 1947/1969). He took the terms he used in his earlier version of the model, such as 'sensation', 'feelings', and 'action', from Smut's (1927/1987) description of experiences and Sullivan's (1953) belief that life is process and flow, ideas that Perls was well acquainted with from his initial period in New York. This cyclical model takes its point of departure in the idea that life is itself a cycle that can be seen in nature and the seasons, and coincides with his theory of how individuals self-regulate and the principle of homeostasis (see Chapters 1 and 3). He claimed that the individual has a need (an urge) for homeostasis as well as a need for disturbance and excitement, and that these are complementary needs that are the foundation of our existence. Perls, influenced by Friedlaender (Frambach, 2003), was especially interested in the moment in the cycle that an individual is in balance, which he called the 'zero point' or the 'creative void' (Clarkson & Mackewn, 1993; see also Chapter 20).

We describe these three theories or process models because they each emphasise different aspects of a process and because they are all useful in clinical practice and coaching. Our main reason for including these particular models is that they can be considered educational aids when a therapeutic process stagnates, when a therapist or coach and client experience that they are not able to finish work they begin, find themselves in a struggle with conflicting needs, or discover that they lack awareness of and attention to their needs in the situation.

Adapting to the environment

The processes of contact and experience are based on Fritz Perls' first model. He developed this model together with Goodman into what we today call *creative adjustment*, a process in which humans creatively adapt to their surroundings (Perls et al., 1951; see Chapter 5). The example with Tom presented earlier shows such creative adjustment.

Later gestalt theorists developed their own process models based on Perls' original model, in which they combined and focused on the various elements of a therapeutic process (Clarkson & Mackewn, 1993). The most well-known of these models has several names, among others, the 'awareness-excitement-contact cycle' (Zinker, 1977), the 'gestalt experience cycle' (Zinker, 1994), or the 'continuum of experience' (Melnick & Nevis, 2000). The models are often described as circles or arcs (Zinker, 1977; Clarkson & Mackewn, 1993), and show a cyclical movement in a process over time. Perls was inspired by the repeating and cyclical changes of seasons in nature, and therefore applied the term 'cycle' to his model (Clarkson & Mackewn, 1993). In the following chapters, we return to the discussion of whether process models should be described as sequences, arcs, or circles, and justify our choice in this book.

Staemmler called his theoretical model a process theory of change. This model is based on Fritz Perls' 'neurosis model' and is described in Chapter 20.

References

Clarkson, P., & Mackewn, J. (1993). *Fritz Perls*. London: Sage Publications.

Frambach, L. (2003). The weighty world of nothingness: Salomo Friedlaender's "Creative indifference". In M. Spagnuolo Lobb & N. Amendt-Lyon (Eds.), *Creative license: The art of gestalt therapy*. Wien: Springer Verlag.

Joyce, P., & Sills, C. (2014). *Skills in gestalt counselling & psychotherapy* (3rd ed.). London: Sage.

Melnick, J., & Nevis, S. (2000). Diagnosis: The struggle for a meaningful paradigm. In E. C. Nevis (Ed.), *Gestalt therapy* (pp. 57–78). US: Gestalt Press.

Perls, F. S. (1947/1969). *Ego, hunger and aggression*. New York: Vintage Books.

Perls, F. S., Hefferline, R. F., & Goodman, P. (1951). *Gestalt therapy: Excitement and growth in the human personality*. London: Souvenir Press.

Smuts, J. C. (1927/1987). *Holism and evolution*. Cape Town, SA: N & S Press.

Sullivan, H. S. (1953). *Interpersonal theory of psychiatry*. New York: Norton.

Yontef, G. M. (1993). *Awareness, dialogue & process*. New York: The Gestalt Journal Press.

Zinker, J. (1977). *Creative process in gestalt therapy*. New York: Random House.

Zinker, J. (1994). *In search of good form*. San Francisco: Jossey-Bass Publishers.

Chapter 18

The process of contact

In this chapter, we describe the creative adjustment and phases of a process in which people connect with people, situations, or things in the environment in order to meet their needs (Perls et al., 1951). This is called the 'contact process'. Its focus is on how the contact between people or between people and things they connect with in their surroundings develops, and on the contact people have with their experience of satisfying their needs at any given time.

Perls et al. (1951) describe such a contact process with the example of a person who knows that she is thirsty and needs to drink. In the following example, Edward becomes aware that he is thirsty. He makes contact with a physiological need in his body, and that need becomes figural for him. Edward connects with his surroundings by looking around. He uses his contact functions (p. 127) by looking for water, and contacts it by going to the water and drinking it. When drinking, he senses the water in his mouth, oesophagus, and stomach; he has contact with the water's taste and temperature, and senses that he is no longer thirsty. The need goes to the background, the figure can change, and Edward can become focused on new figures.

Phases in a contact process

The way contact changes—from the point at which Edward becomes aware of a need and something becomes figural, until the need is met and goes to the background—is perceived differently at the beginning, during, and end of the contact process. Fritz Perls therefore categorised this process into four phases (Perls et al., 1951, p. 403):

1   *Fore-contact*: The person has a beginning sense that something new is about to emerge. Attention is given to the surroundings and one's own body, without clear needs or figures. In this phase, Edward is not aware that he is thirsty, but has a sense of unease in his body.

2   *Contacting*: This is a phase in which the person:

    a   becomes aware of something or someone as possible figures in the environment or in the body that engage him emotionally.

DOI: 10.4324/9781003153856-22

b   chooses or discards possible figures. He actively connects with and explores obstacles, and deliberately processes various figures to find direction for his wishes. Edward feels uneasy and becomes aware that his mouth is dry and that he is thirsty, and he begins to look for water.

3   *Final-contact*: At this point, the person is not worried about the surroundings or his body; now it is the experience of the need being satisfied that becomes is clear. There is a spontaneous alignment between action and experience, movement and emotion. In this phase, the person is aware of the surroundings, which can provide a new experience of the other and who they become together. Edward drinks the water and notices that he is calmer. It is good to feel that his thirst has been quenched and to be content. He may feel happiness when he tastes the cold, refreshing water and smiles at those around him.

4   *Post-contact*: The need has been met and there is fluid interaction between the person and his surroundings, without a distinction between figure and ground. Edward relaxes in his chair.

The phases of the contact process can be drawn as an open circle, which illustrates that the process can continue on into a new circle (Figure 18.1).

An example of a contact process

The various phases of a contact process can often be difficult to recognise and are usually more complex than in the example with Edward. We therefore show an example with Therese, where the environment changes and she must deal with different people within a few hours.

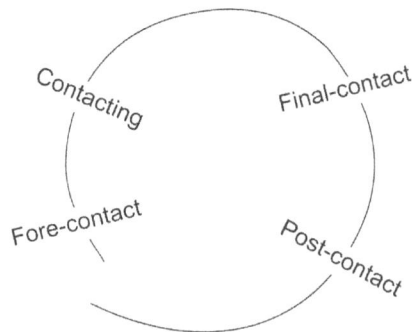

Figure 18.1 The contact process as a circle.

Therese is invited to a party where she knows only a few people. As she enters the party, she hesitates a little just inside the door and looks around. There are a lot of people talking to each other, but she does not know any of them. No one comes over to welcome her, and she feels both vulnerable and excited.

Therese is in fore-contact; she is in a situation where she first feels insecure and spends some time figuring out who the guests are and what she wants to do, since no one welcomes her. She has been looking forward to the party, but at the same time dreading it. She hopes to see some friends she has not seen in a long time.

She is not sure whom to approach. Her need is unclear and there is not a clear figure. The fore-contact phase is characterised by a situation that is not yet organised clearly into figure-ground. In this phase it can be difficult to know what is important; this can be experienced as unpleasant, confusing, and chaotic (Latner, 2000). There can be a lot of excitement and unrest about the unknown possibilities that are in the situation, as we see in the example.

The fore-contact phase often goes unnoticed when we meet others because the process flows into the next phase. For example, when we have clearly defined tasks at work, the figure (task) is clear, and we often perform it without thinking about it. However, we can notice tension or unrest when tasks are finished and we are waiting for the next assignment or looking for new tasks. We can become aware that we are in a fore-contact phase in the beginnings of new situations when we are unsure how to behave, unsure what is expected of us, or do not know what we want.

Therefore, the length of a fore-contact phase varies, depending on how quickly we choose to contact (make contact with) that which we need or interests us in the situation. If we have defined goals in advance and know what we want, fore-contact can be almost non-existent. However, in a new situation it can be good to take the time to explore the opportunities that are there. In this way, we do not opt out of anything that is in line with what we really want.

Contacting phase

Therese eventually helps herself to a glass of wine. She tastes the wine before she greets any of the other guests. After a few moments of small talk, she sees her friend Mona, who invited her to the party, approach her. Therese is glad and relieved.

Nothing captures Therese's interest (no clear figure) until she sees the wine. She then chooses to help herself to a glass, despite the fact that no one has invited her to do so. When she drinks the wine, she has contact with the taste and might feel the effect of the alcohol. It might be good for her to hold the glass as she prepares to follow her next need, which is to greet (contact) some of the other guests. Theoretically, we can say that she is in a transition between the fore-contact and contacting phases, where there is no strong interest in anything in particular. The figures she contacts are unclear. It is only when she sees her friend that Therese expresses happiness and a clear figure becomes apparent. There is now an interest and movement in the situation.

The contacting phase is characterised by the fact that something captures our attention (becomes figural) in a situation, as we see in the example with Therese. It is in the contact phase that we consider and choose or opt out of various possibilities and needs in the situation. There is a greater degree of distinction between figure and ground. If others in the situation respond to us, we can experience that the process is evolving. We build on each other's statements and actions.

It is in the contacting phase that we try out different possibilities. We contact different figures to see which is most consistent with the wishes and needs in the situation, as Therese does before Mona contacts her. It might be that there were several interesting people at Mona's party, but Therese excludes them when she chooses Mona. We can continue to observe Therese after the point at which her friend contacts her.

Final-contact

Mona gives Therese a hug, and they start talking to each other with engaged and eager voices. Mona takes Therese over to some of the other guests who are standing talking together. They greet each other, and soon Therese is included in their conversation. They laugh and enjoy themselves. The conversation flows; Therese is happy and at ease. The excitement she initially experienced is gone. She also sees some friends she had been looking forward to seeing again, and who she would like to get to know better. They eat and are engaged in a discussion about immigration and migration, something Therese is interested in. The sound level and tempo of the discussion increase, they speak at the same time and gesticulate.

Here, Therese is included by Mona, and she becomes part of the conversation that flows easily. The contact Therese experiences is different at this point. She is in the full contact phase; hesitation and uncertainty are gone. During this phase, she and the others have a common understanding of what is important to them and the activity they are engaged in, as well as a common experience of fluidity between them. The figure is clear. Everything else goes to the background, and together they have developed a meaningful situation.

In the final-contact phase, the choice between different needs is made and we can be completely immersed in what we do. We experience a meaningful contact with the situation or the others that are in the situation with us. We have now fully contacted what we longed for or wanted. We can have moments of happiness or an 'aha' experience where we gain an extended or new understanding of something we were previously stuck in or lacked answers to. We are very much aware of the situation we are in and can experience bodily reactions, such as Therese had in the form of lightness in the body, or in the form of palpitations, tremors, or tears (Latner, 2000).

Post-contact

Post-contact is used to describe the phase that comes at the end of a contact process, when we are satisfied and finished. Post-contact is often expressed by ending the situation. We retreat and reflect on what has happened, what we have experienced, new insights we have gained, and occasionally what we regret. It is a time for contemplation and rest and is sometimes accompanied by sensations of bodily calmness and quiet. The former figure goes to the background; the field is again undifferentiated, and remains so until we become aware of new, possible figures.

We can illustrate what Therese experiences as the party draws to a close.

Therese has enjoyed food and drink with her friends at Mona's party. She feels that the evening has flown. Several guests are starting to leave, and she feels it is time for her to leave as well. She is tired, calm, and very happy. She finds Mona and thanks her. She tells her how happy she is that she was invited, how nice she thinks it has been, that she has felt that the others enjoyed her company, and that she has made some new friends. Back home she stays up for a while, reflecting over and enjoying the memories of the evening before she goes to bed.

Here, we show how Therese becomes aware of when she has 'had enough' and feels finished and satisfied with the evening. Her interest in the others is becoming less and she is no longer hungry or thirsty. This also applies to many of the others at the party. Therese becomes quieter and more withdrawn; the need for rest comes naturally. It is time to leave and give feedback to Mona about how she experienced the party.

Transitions between phases

It is often in the transitions between phases that we become aware of the process is and where we are in it. We illustrate this with an example taken from Martina's aerobics class.

Martina attends a weekly aerobics class together with several people she knows. She has been going to class for a while now and feels that she is becoming stronger and more flexible. What she is becoming increasingly aware of, however, is how difficult it is for her every time the woman who leads the class gives them new exercises.

Class has begun one day; they have started up with music and the choreography they usually do. Martina thinks to herself that she can follow the rhythm and manage to do the movements by listening and looking at the leader. Suddenly, she becomes aware that she is doing something different than the person next to her. She sees that the leader has begun to move her legs back and forth in a new way and that her arms are moving at the same rate. Martina stops, listens to the music, and starts copying what the leader does. Her body moves again in time with the music, and she is back in the flow of the choreography. Then it happens again: the leader again changes the way she moves her arms and legs. Now Martina is more focused, and after stopping again for a moment she manages to move in the way the leader does. Her legs go back and forth, her arms up and around. Again, she manages to follow the new movements, and the flow returns. The transitions between the different exercises cause her to stop, but she notices that the more her attention is on the leader, the less amount of time she needs to stop and the more she cuts out all her thoughts. Every time she starts thinking about something else, she comes out of the flow of the movements and does not notice that the leader switches exercises. Sometimes she experiences that she flows with the music and all the others who are doing the same exercises and moving at the same pace together with her.

In this example, we see that every time Martina stops moving, she is in fore-contact for a moment before she again makes contact by following the music and copying the leader's movements. When she flows with the music and movements, she is in final-contact until the movements change and she returns to fore-contact.

This example also shows how bodily movements are affected by the mind, vision, and hearing. It is not possible for Martina to think her way to how to move her body, but she can think that she needs to concentrate on copying the leader's movements and following the music. When she 'surrenders' her body to try out new movements and bodily impulses, she experiences either flow in her movements or a need to stop and start over. Previously, we described how we eventually can become conscious of what we initially sense and become aware of without words, and how this increased awareness and consciousness leads to new gestalting processes (Part 3, Chapter 8). In other words, there is a close correlation between our level of consciousness and attentiveness, and how the process we are a part of is shaped and developed, as the example with Martina shows.

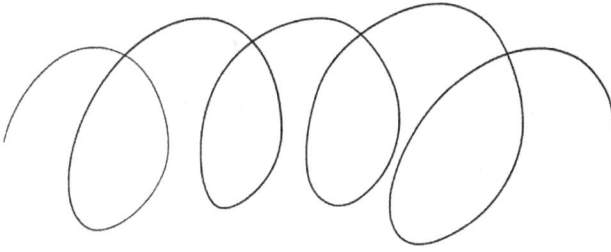

Figure 18.2 The contact process illustrated as spiral.

In the preceding example, we describe several contact processes that follow each other, where Martina's first discovery of a transition between two exercises can be perceived as a transition to a new contact process. She goes from fore-contact to contacting, but no further. The transitions become easier when Martina is conscious of them and uses her experience of how her thoughts affect the rhythm of the process. When several contact processes follow each other, we can use a model of circles that follow each other in the form of a spiral, rather than using the model of a circle, as on p. 258. This is illustrated in Figure 18.2. Experience in life and in the therapy room shows that contact processes follow each other, and that we can sometimes see that there are many small processes within a larger process. We often see this first in retrospect.

We can see from Figure 18.2 that the circles in the spiral have different forms. This illustrates that processes are always different in length and intensity.

Interruptions in the contact process

Earlier theorists (Perls, 1947/1969; Polster & Polster, 1974; Zinker, 1977) have described what they call 'interruptions' in a cycle. We disagree with this. A process can never stop. It may feel as if we stop, that we are not moving forward, but that indicates that the process changes direction, character, or shape. It is possible that earlier theorists used the term 'interruption' more in terms of changing direction, but this was not clarified. We prefer to avoid the word 'interruption' so as not to create unfortunate associations. Instead, we describe how the process can *change direction, stagnate,* or *become automatic.*

Contact processes in the therapy room

The therapist is aware of the contact process and transitions she experiences between the client and herself during the therapy, as well as how the client describes contact in her close relationships. As therapists, we often experience that it can feel as if the process between us and our clients stops or stagnates. It is as if we continually need to start over, there is no sense of flow. We can feel dissatisfied with ourselves as therapists and the processes we are a part of (Selmer, 2016). We show an example of this with Brian, who is in a life crisis when he seeks out therapy.

Brian has come to therapy because his wife left him. He is in despair and does not know how to handle the situation alone. He talks the entire first session about what has happened and tries to find explanations as to why his wife left him. The therapist listens with great warmth and empathy. She thinks it is important for Brian to tell his story.

In this situation, Brian and the therapist are in the contacting phase most of the time. The only figure the therapist is interested in is Brian's despair over the fact that his wife left him. There is little fore-contact, because Brian's despair captures the therapist's attention right away. There are small moments of final-contact as the therapist listens to Brian's story, but when Brian again starts to wonder why his wife left him, the engagement is less, and they are again in the contacting phase. There is no time for them to talk about what this conversation was like for Brian, since he is unable to stop telling his story. There is no post-contact. The therapist is aware of where they are in the process, something she will remember and take into account in future sessions.

Brian continues to share his despair over his wife having left him for several consecutive sessions. The therapist eventually becomes aware that Brian does not show much emotion or look at her when he speaks. She herself feels a vague sense of sadness and notices that she is less engaged in Brian's narrative. She has heard the same story several times. She thinks that Brian holds back his feelings and that it can be useful for him to become aware of how he does this.

At one point during the fourth session, the therapist intervenes on the basis of what she observes: 'Brian, I see that you look down a little bit when you talk. Can you keep doing it while you continue to talk?' Brian looks at the therapist for a moment, then looks down and talks about his wife. After a while he stops talking and again looks at the therapist. The corners of his mouth tremble and he has tears in his eyes. The therapist notices that she is sad and that her eyes are moist. 'I see there are tears in your eyes, and I notice that I'm sad. What is happening to you right now?' Brian starts crying quietly; neither of them says anything for a while.

Here, the process moves into the final-contact phase as the therapist asks Brian to keep looking down when he speaks, and he then looks at her and starts crying. By making him aware of where he looks when he speaks, the therapist leads his attention to his eyes and body and away from his mind. Brian becomes aware of where he looks. He experiences how different it is to look away from and to look directly at the therapist. This change in attention leads to a spontaneous, bodily reaction, first in Brian in the form of movement in the muscles around his mouth and tears in the eyes, and then in the therapist in the form of sadness. They are more together in the moment instead of being focused on Brian's story. They connect with their own feelings and a different type of emotional contact with each other.

Brian continues to cry while the therapist sits quietly and breathes calmly. He looks at her and says, 'I'm becoming aware of how sad I am, it's like I have a lot of tears inside me that I've held back. It's actually good to cry . . . even though I'm not used to crying . . . and even though I'm sad, I feel a little better'.

THERAPIST: 'Yes, it was a relief for me, too. I kind of felt like I was on the outside when you were talking. It was completely different for me when you looked at me. I knew I could be with you and at the same time be aware of my own feelings. It was like we were flowing more together'.

BRIAN: 'It's weird that there was such a big difference between talking without looking at you and when I looked at you. I was kind of more inside myself in a way when I didn't look at you. Maybe I felt alone and tried to connect with you, make you understand me. Yes, I think I was trying to explain to you how I was doing. That's why I talked and talked. I didn't know any other way to do it'.

THERAPIST: 'I understand that. And now you have experienced a new way to connect with your feelings and me. This might be an experience you can take with you in other situations as well'.

BRIAN: 'Yes, I've never thought about where I have my eyes when I talk to someone. At least I want to pay more attention to what I do with my eyes in the future. Maybe I haven't been aware of this in my relationship'.

Here, Brian and the therapist sit and reflect on the conversation and the contact process between them. They are in the post-contact phase. Brian tells the therapist what he has become aware of and how he feels after crying. The therapist tells Brian how she experienced the change in contact between them in the various sequences of the sessions. At the end of the session, the therapist highlights Brian's new experience and how he can take it with him to other situations. He has gained a new awareness of how he uses his eyes and where he looks, and that this can affect contact between him and his wife. This is a topic he needs more time to explore further in therapy.

In this session, the therapist uses her attention to how the relationship between them changes, how the process takes shape, and what phases in the contact process they are in at any given time. Brian continually told his story because he did not feel that the therapist understood him. He did not experience having contact with himself or the therapist, even if this was not something that he was aware of. The therapist's hypothesis was that by increasing Brian's attention to how they looked at each other, something new could happen between them. Here she relied on the paradoxical theory of change: 'change occurs when one becomes what he is, not when he tries to become what he is not' (see Chapter 5). First, it is as if Brian sensed that there was a change in the therapist when she made him aware of where he directed his gaze and asked him to keep talking without looking at her. He looked at her, and the therapist sensed a wonder in him over the experiment she suggested. He continued to talk with a new awareness of his eyes and where he directs his gaze. The change came spontaneously when he looked right at the therapist and stopped talking. The contact between them changed; they have experienced something new together and are in the final-contact phase. Here it is clear how their increased attention lead to this movement in the field between them.

When there has been a clear final-contact in a therapy session, as in this example, there is more 'to harvest' in the post-contact phase. Brian and the therapist have a shared experience that is integrated when they talk about it. In therapy, it is often easy to forget the significance of this particular stage because the situation has ended and what was unpleasant and unfinished goes to the background. When her client leaves the therapy room, however, she meets everyday life and the new experiences can be quickly forgotten. The therapist is therefore interested in raising Brian's awareness of the work they did together, of Brian's bodily sensations, and how he experienced the contact with himself and between them differently after the experiment. She also shares what happened to her, which she thinks can create fewer projections and a stronger feeling of safety between them. When the therapist asks Brian if he notices that he does not look at others when he speaks, she wants to put the new experience into a larger context in his life. Here it is as if the therapist contacts something new, and had it not been for the fact that the session was over, they could have begun a new contact process. Brian, however, takes the therapist's question with him and can reflect on it alone if he needs to, or can bring it up in the next session.

The contact process described as circle, spiral, or sequences

The purpose of describing the contact process as a circle and spiral is to show how an ideal contact process can unfold. This type of description makes it easier for the therapist to become aware of where in the process she and her client have challenges and what she needs to explore further with her client in order to support the flow and contact between them. In the example with Brian, he and the therapist move from fore-contact to the contacting phase and then to a new fore-contact. This is repeated several times before they come to final-contact and post-contact. The process is not completed and does not create satisfaction for either of them until after a long period of time. Some theorists (Bloom, 2010; Gaffney, 2009) argue that it is better to describe the process in sequences, in which the therapist can be aware of which sequence of the process she is in at all times. It can be easier to show how she and her client move from one sequence to another in the process without thinking that they move backwards, which is easy to do when the model is in the form of a circle or a spiral. It is at all times the therapist who chooses how she uses the model and whether she envisions the process in a circle, spiral, or in sequences. In the next example, we show how the process is often in the fore-contact phase, and that it takes time for the process to move into the next phases.

Silence in a therapy group

This example is taken from a therapy group with six people who are meeting for the third time.

> The group leader, Mark, sits in his chair waiting for the participants to enter the room. They greet each other and Mark as they enter and sit in a circle chatting with each other until Mark says it is time to start. He begins by saying that he is happy to see them all again. He wonders how they are and if there is something in particular they want to share with the others. It is quiet for a while until Ingrid says that she feels unwell and that she had considered not coming, but that she is happy to be there now. Again, it is quiet. Some look around, others look down. After some time, Mark says: 'It's fine to sit in silence. Pay attention to what it's like for you, and feel free to tell us as you become aware of what you notice'.

Here we see how the group is in fore-contact after Mark welcomed them and as they wait for someone to say something. Ingrid brings in a possible figure when she says she is unwell and was unsure if she would come. No one contacts that figure, and they continue in fore-contact until Mark brings in a new possible figure when he makes the participants aware of the silence and asks how it is perceived.

> Sara spontaneously says that she finds it very uncomfortable to sit still, that she is worried, and that it makes her want to run out of the room. Kathrine follows up and says she does not like it either. She struggles to breathe while saying that she does not know what to say. Clyde says he

does not care whether anyone says anything. He is concerned with how his youngest son is doing because he is alone at home; he is worried about whether or not his son is okay. He had also wondered if he would come to group today, because of his son. Morten interrupts him and says that Clyde can call his son to check on how he is, a suggestion that causes Clyde to shake his head.

Here we see how different group members react to the theme Mark brings in. The group is now in the contacting phase, where they talk about how they experience silence in the group. This changes when Morten brings in a new theme or possible new figure by following up what Clyde says.

'It's nice that you suggest that Clyde can call his son, Morten. I see that you, Clyde, shook your head when Morten made the suggestion. Maybe you have the sound on, on your phone, so he can call you if necessary?' Clyde confirms this, and Mark continues: 'Can those of you who haven't said anything about silence in the group say something about it?' Sally responds and says she finds it uncomfortable and that she needs the conversation to move on. Morten disagrees and says that he very much likes the silence. He thinks it gives them a sense of calm that makes it possible to notice what is going on with each of them as individuals, something Lisbeth agrees with. She says that she struggles many times to keep up with the conversation when the others talk. She has so much stress and pressure in her life and comes to this group because she needs something else.

Mark leads members back to the topic of silence in the group after first clarifying this with Clyde. They are still in the contacting phase when the other three participants express their experiences of and needs on the subject of silence.

The group members continue to talk about how differently they experience silence, that it was good to hear what it is like for the others, and that they become more aware of how they experience silence. Sara says it is easier to be quiet when they agree to do so than it is when there are expectations that someone should say something. Kathrine spontaneously says that she has never thought about the fact that she is constantly waiting for someone to say something, and that she worries about saying the right thing, what the others think of what she says, when to say something, and so on. The other group members respond one by one to say how they recognise themselves in what Kathrine says. One word leads to another, they speak faster with louder voices, and some smile and laugh.

Mark breaks in after a while and says he understands that they have made some new discoveries. He asks them to say something about what it has been like to exchange these experiences on the subject of silence in the group. Clyde responds by saying that he has become aware of how he has pushed away his discomfort when there is silence by thinking about something else, which he also did today. Lisbeth goes on to say that she has discovered that she has given herself permission to be quiet and Sally has become even more aware of her own impatience and that she has many expectations of Mark and the others. Sara recognises herself in what Sally says, while Morten has become aware of how he places his chair a little outside the others in the group and is mostly paying attention to himself and his own breathing. Finally, Katherine says how happy she is that she dared to say how difficult the silence has been for her, and that she now believes that she will manage to handle silence and waiting in a different way.

In these two paragraphs, we see how group members say more about how the topic affects them. A change occurs in how they talk together after Katherine says how she experiences the silence. The volume of their voices increases, and the contact takes a different form. It is as if they are flowing together and are in final-contact. The post-contact starts when Mark asks them to share what it is been like for them to talk about the topic. Together they reflect on their new experiences about themselves and as a group.

In this example, the process (the silence of the group), is also the theme or figure that the leader chooses to explore. Through the process, the participants have gained new awareness of themselves, how they were in contact with the others and with themselves, and creatively adapted to the situation in the group. This experience can lead to new themes to explore, either in the group or individually, such as whether participants recognise the way they adapted in the group from other situations in life. They can also experiment in the group by being silent for a long period of time or by doing the opposite and talking all the time, to raise awareness of the phenomenon of silence and expectations.

Creative adjustment

When Perls and Goodman presented the concept of creative adjustment in their book *Gestalt Therapy* (Perls et al., 1951), they described both a theory of self and a theory about the course of contact in a process. In this book, the two theories, or models, are presented in different chapters (Chapters 7 and 18). Both models describe how we creatively adjust to a situation, and in addition we have devoted Chapter 6 to the concept of creative adjustment. Our desire to present the theories separately is based in a wish to give the reader an understanding of how the individual models can be used as support in therapeutic practice, where the self model focuses on who the therapist and client become together in the therapy room and the process models focus on where the therapist and the client are together in the process. It can, however, also be useful to use both models of creative adjustment in one and the same therapy session, which we show briefly at the end of this chapter.

In the description of the process of creative adjustment, Perls and Goodman envisioned that various aspects or functions of the self are active in the various phases of the contact process (Perls et al., 1951). As previously described, the self is divided into three functions (Chapter 7): the impulse function is what is expressed in the fore-contact phase, which includes sensations and impulses. The I-function leads us to think, consider, and act, and signals the contacting phase. The personality function, who we become in a situation and with others, is expressed in both the contacting and final-contact phases.

For example, in a therapy session, the therapist may feel frustrated and confused when nothing becomes apparent between her and her client. In these cases, it can be useful to think that there is no clear figure here. No need is expressed; we are in fore-contact. At this point the therapist may be especially aware of sensations and impulses in herself and in the client, and thus become aware of the possible needs of the situation. The therapist might also become aware that she is being especially careful and worried about her client, and may think: 'Now I'm almost like an overprotective mother', which is an expression of the personality function. The therapist can then wonder who the client becomes with her. She has increased attention to the possible figure she can contact and is in in the contacting phase.

In the example with the therapy group, the group is in fore-contact until Sara spontaneously says that she finds the silence uncomfortable. She has an impulse to speak (impulse function) on the basis of bodily sensations of unrest and excitement in the group. Sara's statement prompts more people in the group to share how the silence affects them. The process in the group has changed. Some speak, and some are quiet; they are in the contacting phase. We can imagine that the group leader is interested in who the members of the group become together (personality function) when he later asks those who have not spoken to tell how they feel in the group. He supports them in talking (I-function) and at the same time follows up the figure of silence. This leads to members talking and sharing more and to a change in the process. The group is in final-contact when members become engaged and personal (personality function). Near the end of the session, Mark supports participants in reflecting on who they felt they were during the process, so that they can become aware of the possibility of different ways of being and how they influence and are influenced by others.

Summary

In this chapter, we have described a process consisting of four phases in which contact changes in and between people over a period of time. The model is based on how needs arise and become clear, where something figures against a background, and how needs are contacted and satisfied and then go to the background so that new needs or figures can be formed. The contact process is based on what Fritz Perls originally called creative adjustment, which describes a process in which people creatively adapt to their surroundings (Perls et al., 1951). The needs a person becomes aware of and attempts to satisfy, and how that person adapts, depends on the person and her surroundings. The four phases of the contact process are fore-contact, contacting, final-contact, and post-contact.

It is the therapist's awareness of the phase in which she and her client are at any given time that makes this theoretical model useful in therapeutic work. This is what we show in the example of Brian, where the therapist eventually becomes aware that they are mostly only in the contacting phase. In the example of the therapy group, Mark becomes aware that the silence in the fore-contact phase is a recurring theme in the group. It occupies him so much that it becomes a figure he chooses to contact. He also feels a growing unease when the group becomes quiet. Although he is conscious that this unrest is natural in the fore-contact phase, he experiences it more strongly in the third meeting than he did in previous meetings. He is also conscious of the time when he stops the discussion and asks how the session was for the participants. He also ensures that there is time for post-contact.

In some situations, the challenge is to choose a figure when the client does not have a theme to bring into session, and at other times the therapist is unable to stop the client's narrative for fear of rejecting the client. During sessions the therapist asks herself what she becomes aware of in order to understand where she and the client are in the therapy process. She is interested in whether the topic the client brings in interests her. The therapist herself is part of the process, and it is therefore important that she can observe herself, the client, and the relationship between them, and be aware of the contact and process in order to choose what she says and does with her client (Yontef, 1993).

References

Bloom, D. (2010). Commentary 1: Let's go round again: Cycle of experience or sequence of contact? Dan Bloom has another go with Seàn Gaffney. In S. Gaffney (Ed.), *Gestalt at work*, vol. 2 (pp. 126–139). Los Angeles: The Gestalt Institute Press.

Gaffney, S. (2009). The cycle of experience re-cycled: Then, now . . . next? *Gestalt Review*, *13*(1), 7–23.

Latner, J. (2000). The theory of gestalt therapy. In E. C. Nevis (Ed.), *Gestalt therapy: Perspectives and applications* (pp. 13–56). Cambridge, MA: Gestalt Press.

Perls, F. S. (1947/1969). *Ego, hunger and aggression*. New York: Vintage Books.

Perls, F. S., Hefferline, R. F., & Goodman, P. (1951). *Gestalt therapy: Excitement and growth in the human personality*. London: Souvenir Press.

Polster, E., & Polster, M. (1974). *Gestalt therapy integrated*. New York: Vintage Books.

Selmer, J. W. (2016). Nøkkelen til oppdagelse er din. Hvordan skape bevegelse i låste situasjoner? [The key to discovery is yours: How can movement be created in fixed situations?]. *Norsk Gestalttidsskrift*, *2*(13), 72–83.

Yontef, G. M. (1993). *Awareness, dialogue & process*. New York: The Gestalt Journal Press.

Zinker, J. (1977). *Creative process in gestalt therapy*. New York: Random House.

Chapter 19

The process of experience

The process model discussed in this chapter is the process of experience. Here, instead of describing how contact develops, as we do in Chapter 18, we describe the experience a person acquires through a process of becoming aware and conscious of a need—how energy is mobilised based on an increased awareness of acting and satisfying the need—until the person feels satisfied and can rest. The model was developed by Fritz Perls' successors from the Cleveland Institute in the United States, Ed Nevis and Joseph Zinker (Clarkson & Mackewn, 1993). Our presentation of the model is taken from Zinker's 1977 book *Creative Process in Gestalt Therapy*.

Zinker explains his interest in developing a theoretical model of how people can become aware of their needs and satisfy them:

> If I know what I want, I will not look to other people to tell me what I want, nor will I project my own needs on to others. Existentially, my awareness will make it possible for me to take responsibility for actions I take to get what satisfies me.
>
> (p. 94)

As an example of how we do not take responsibility for our own wishes and needs, Zinker mentions a married couple where one fails to tell the other how upset she is about what the other has said, and indirectly punishes her by being silent and shutting her out emotionally. This can happen either because the person is not aware that she is angry, or that telling the other that she is angry is too frightening. Zinker argues that sharing feelings is better than not expressing them at all, and that dealing with emotional expression is difficult because both parties have already forgotten or have become tired of the original experience.

By becoming aware and conscious of our feelings here and now, we can take responsibility for how we express them and how we act and are in the world with others. A student expresses this in the chapter on awareness (Chapter 8). Zinker (1977) formulates it thus: 'Gestalt therapy emphasizes not that we live for the moment, but that we live *in* the moment; not that we meet our needs immediately, but that we are present for ourselves in the environment' (p. 95).

DOI: 10.4324/9781003153856-23

The process of experience is a model that therapists can use in collaboration with clients so that clients can learn to take care of their own processes from the point at which they become aware that they have a need until the point at which they can act on that need, and can ultimately rest. The model can help clients become familiar with where in the process they are, at which stage they tend to react automatically, where they have their strengths, and where they have challenges and opportunities for development. They can discover and experience that the process is different, depending on the situation. With some people the process flows, at times they might discover that they act too quickly, while others can become paralysed, struggle, and stop and remain dissatisfied.

Phases in the process of experience

The process of experience is divided into six phases: sensation, awareness and attention, mobilisation of energy, action, contact, and withdrawal. This process and its associated phases can be drawn as a wave or an arc to illustrate how the energy in an experience process is built up before we act and how the energy goes down when the need is satisfied (see Figure 19.1).

The experience process can also be drawn as several successive waves, to show how a process never stops and is constantly changing. The waves in such a process will have varying degrees of length, intensity, and shape, as shown in Figure 19.2.

The model shows how emotions, actions, and moments of contact are constantly moving and occur in waves, and that these waves are a metaphor for life as it is experienced. We show this in an example with Emily.

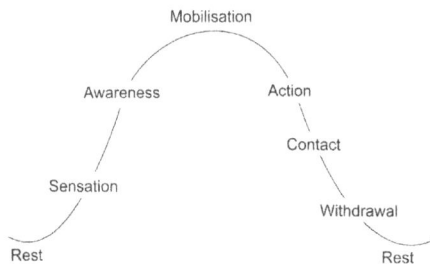

Figure 19.1 The process of experience as a wave or an arc.

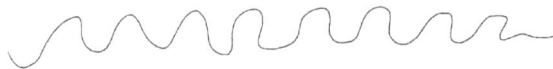

Figure 19.2 The process of experience as multiple waves.

Emily has just ended a phone call with a friend, and wonders what to do. She is a little worried and thinks it might be good to go for a walk to get some fresh air. She realises that she has been sitting all morning, even though she has the day off. As she sits and tries to decide whether to go out, she notices that her bodily turmoil is increasing. She gets up, puts on a jacket, and leaves her apartment. As she walks, she feels how good it is to move her body and breathe in the warm air. She walks faster and farther than she had planned to because it is so nice to be outside. When she returns home she sits down, satisfied, and rests.

The first phase of the process is when Emily becomes aware of her bodily unease. She notices and becomes aware of a feeling without knowing what it is. This awareness leads to thoughts of walking and fresh air; she becomes conscious of a need. This need becomes clearer when she becomes conscious of the fact that she has not been out all day and that her bodily turmoil is increasing. This is what we call the mobilisation of energy for an action. Emily's action was to put on her jacket and go for a walk. While on her walk, she is aware of how good it feels to walk and breathe the air. At that point she is in contact with her action: walking and breathing outside in the fresh air. When she returns home she sits down, withdraws, and rests.

We will describe each phase of the process of experience and how it can be expressed in more detail.

Sensation

In the first phase, we can recognise what we described in Chapter 8 in relation to awareness and the process of awareness: we feel that there is something in the environment or ourselves that is troubling or influencing us. It might be that we sense a tingling in the body or a movement or change in people around us, which arouses our curiosity.

Awareness

The transition to the next phase is almost imperceptible. The process changes; we become aware of signals from the body or environment and begin to become aware that we have impulses, without realising what these impulses are. We experience a beginning consciousness before we are able to put our experience into words and understand the form our experience takes. We gradually become aware that our impulses have a direction, and our needs and desires begin to take form.

Mobilisation

Now we are aware that there is something we want or do not want to do. We explore how we can meet the need that arises and how we can respond to our surroundings. We consider various possibilities and weigh the pros and cons of these possibilities when the needs are in conflict with each other. As we explore and contemplate, the body mobilises energy that we can experience as an increased heart rate, faster breathing, and more physical and mental activity, and we become engaged, excited, and eager; we are ready for action.

Action

The action we take might be to follow the impulses we have in a situation. The action can come spontaneously and quickly, or we can carry out projects that have long been planned. We can have a conversation with a good friend, listen to a piece of music, find solutions to challenges we face, or perform tasks at home or at work. Actions can be something we do with others or perform alone. This phase can go quickly or continue for a longer period.

Contact

This phase corresponds to what we call final-contact in the process of contact and is closely related to the action phase. Here we are in contact with and aware of the action we take. We can be completely engrossed in and be committed to our action, and we can gain new insight and feel satisfaction as we act. We can be sensitive to emotions and be engulfed by joy or sorrow.

We near the end of this phase gradually when we become aware that we are satisfied and that our need has been met.

Withdrawal

When we are conscious of being satisfied, have done enough and feel done, we end the action and go to the next phase, in which we gradually withdraw. In this phase we reflect on the action and integrate new experience before letting go of what we have done. We do nothing and rest until a new need arises.

Challenges in the various phases

The description of the process of experience and its phases has thus far been focused on conducting a course of action where the process flows from sensing something to becoming aware of a need, satisfying it, and withdrawing. There are, however, many situations in which the process does not lead to satisfaction.

In the example with Emily, there is progress in each phase because she becomes aware of what she feels, thinks, wants, and does. The challenge for many of us is situations where we are not satisfied or do not meet our needs, where we struggle, are dissatisfied, and ask ourselves how we can move forward and what we can do differently in life. In this type of situation, we may be unaware of how we adapt and deal with the challenges we face. It may be that we act automatically, by reflex and habit, rather than with a conscious attention to our surroundings and ourselves. Many seek therapy or coaching when they face challenges and the realities of life feel insurmountable. In clinical work, the therapist can rely on the model of the process of experience in order to see where in the process the client can become more aware and the phase in which she struggles.

From the therapy room: becoming aware of the body

Stuart has been undergoing therapy for a while because he feels burned out and is on sick leave. He has a responsible position in his company and works a lot, is married and has two young children. The therapist notices that Stuart becomes eager quite quickly when they converse, though he can be both moody and sad when he arrives. The therapist is often fascinated by Stuart's eagerness when they talk, and she wonders if he is aware of how quickly he mobilises energy and becomes eager. When she mentions this to him, he recognises what she says and responds very quickly that he thinks that this is one of his problems. He engages quickly both at home and at work. He is good at finding solutions, which is one of the reasons that he has a job that entails so much responsibility. As they continue to talk about the topic, Stuart offers several suggestions of ways to solve the problem of becoming so eager so quickly.

THERAPIST: 'Do you realise that you're doing it now too, trying to find solutions very quickly?'

STUART: 'Yes, you're right, it happens automatically. But what should I do about it? I'm tired of constantly thinking that I'm going to solve everything for everyone at home or at work'.

THERAPIST: 'It seems as if you're almost out of breath, and I notice that I'm tightening my body'.

STUART: 'I breathe, but it's like I'm not aware of my body or myself, I'm just concerned with my thoughts and the problems'.

THERAPIST: 'It's great that you're aware that you're thinking and trying to find solutions. I know I started to breathe a little more easily when you said that. Becoming aware of what you're doing is what's important; that's how change starts'.

STUART: 'But I don't know what I'm doing, I'm just concerned about finding solutions to my problems and the problems of everyone around me'.

THERAPIST: 'And that's exactly what you're doing—trying to find solutions. It's not wrong, you're aware of something that makes you tired and burns you out. You're not going to fix it right now. You can just continue to sit here with me and be aware that you're mobilising and moving quickly to action without being conscious of it when you do. Right now you are aware of this, and that's enough for now'.

STUART: 'I feel like I'm getting restless and impatient when you say what you say, I want to get up and do something'.

THERAPIST: 'Sure, let's get up and walk around the room a little bit'.

They walk around for a while Stuart continues to talk enthusiastically and eagerly. The therapist asks him to walk faster and speak even more eagerly, which he does.

After a while, he stops and looks at the therapist and says: 'I'm getting so tired, I want to sit down. I thought it would be better to walk around talking instead of sitting and just thinking about how I feel. This is how I burn out. I just do things on autopilot instead of being aware of what I want. I don't want to walk around in this room with you and be eager, I want to sit and notice what I'm feeling, even though it's uncomfortable'.

Here, Stuart has spontaneous insight into what makes him so tired. The therapist first tries to help him become aware of this by telling him that he knows what he is doing. That does not make sense to Stuart, so the therapist experiments with increasing his pace by walking and talking more quickly. This reinforcement gives Stuart an experience of how his physical unease is a signal of how uncomfortable it is for him not to have a solution. In the past, he has not been aware of how this unease affects him. He also experiences that by mobilising and acting automatically in response to the therapist's suggestions, without awareness of how he is feeling, he becomes tired. The therapist is working here to help Stuart become more aware and conscious in the first three phases of the process of experience: sensation, awareness, and mobilisation of energy. Stuart's challenge is that he acts automatically, without being aware of any contradictions or resistance that may be inherent in his actions.

In later sessions, Stuart and the therapist explore the bodily sensations he becomes aware of as he begins to mobilise energy before taking action. In this way he becomes more familiar with and aware of signals from his body. These signals can help him to act less automatically and give him information about the pace he has when he speaks.

Eventually, Stuart no longer needs to be on sick leave and goes to therapy less often. One day at a session he tells the therapist that he has been offered a new position at work. It entails a lot of travel, something he enjoys. He is, however, unsure whether to accept the position, because it means he will be away from his family quite a bit. As he talks, the therapist notices that he leans forward and faces her as he speaks eagerly, something she remembers well from their previous conversations. She asks him to pay attention to how he sits and talks. He responds right away that he feels the eagerness throughout his body but is also aware of unease or tension in his diaphragm. This is the first time Stuart describes tension in his diaphragm, something that piques the therapist's interest.

THERAPIST: 'Can you describe the tension you feel?'
STUART: 'Yes, it's tight all the way up to my sternum'.
THERAPIST: 'How tight is it?'
STUART: 'Not very much, but it's still uncomfortable'.
THERAPIST: 'How big is the area that's tight?'
STUART: 'It's pretty big'. He uses his hands to indicate how much of the area is tight. The therapist notices that she is also tightening her body and breathing more shallowly.
THERAPIST: 'I notice that I'm only inhaling to the point where the tightness in my body starts. How deeply are you breathing?'
STUART: 'Down to my diaphragm. It's not a problem to breathe'.
THERAPIST: 'Can you hold your hand on your diaphragm and *be* the tension, talk as if you are the tension?'
STUART: 'Yes. I'm tense, I'm tightening my muscles. I'm being careful—no, I want to say that I'm a little scared, I'm worried'. Stuart straightens up a little in his chair, and with both feet on the floor he looks at the therapist and says: 'Yes, I'm actually scared, I'm tight because I'm scared. This doesn't feel good. Maybe I'm more afraid of this job than I realised. Maybe it's too much for me now, right after I've been burned out. I think I'll talk to my boss again and ask more about what it actually involves'.

Here, Stuart becomes aware that he is afraid of the new job by exploring the sensations in his diaphragm. He realises that the tension signals fear when he gives it a voice and speaks as if he were the tension. The therapist wants Stuart to become aware that he is the one who tightens his muscles, that these muscles are part of him, and that he should take signals from his body seriously. When Stuart gains new insight about the fact that he is scared, he immediately associates it with the offer of a new job. He realises that he also contains contradictions, and he begins to consider whether to say yes or no, which is new to him. Now he uses past experience of being burned out as part of this consideration.

Many clients who come to therapy are not used to sensing their own bodily reactions and signals from their surroundings. They have not learned to use their senses, and often act on impulse or on the basis of ideas and thoughts about what they should do or what they think their surroundings think they should do. In therapy, they can become aware of this and learn to sense both inward and outward. The therapist can teach them how to be aware of how they breathe, how they sit in their chairs, how they use their eyes and voices (see Chapter 8 on awareness and Chapter 11 on experiments). In the example, we show how useful and necessary it is for Stuart to take time to explore bodily sensations—to be in the first two stages. With increased awareness, the choices can become less automatic, and the client can see new and unknown possibilities for action. We saw that Stuart acted on impulse when it came to what he wanted, without being aware of fear or resistance. He needed to develop awareness of his sensations before he could become aware of the polarity of desire (see Chapter 10 on polarities).

Challenges in mobilisation

In the chapter on polarities (Chapter 10), we provided an example where Therese has challenges when mobilising energy in order to make choices and act. Together with the therapist she explores how she tends to choose what is safe, and as she explores the polarity—her desire—she experiences that she becomes engaged and mobilises. It is possible to mobilise energy by clarifying and working with a single unknown pole or by exploring both polarities.

In therapy, a certain amount of excitement and energy is needed to get to the action phase. Important signals for the therapist are when she feels little interest or engagement or perhaps becomes bored while simultaneously observing a lack of mobilisation in the client. When the therapist becomes aware of a lack of energy in the room, she can alert the client to this by for example sharing what she observes in the client or feelings in her own body. Together they can reinforce how they sit and speak in order to clarify and mobilise, or the therapist can suggest that they get up and walk around the room as they talk. They can stop and 'observe' the client and therapist chairs together and describe what they see and hear. They mobilise by walking, observing their energy while sitting, and reflecting together. They can compare how their bodies feel when standing, and how it is unlike when they sat. These are different ways the client can become aware of signals from the body when energy is low, allowing her to mobilise, become engaged, and want to act.

Clients who come to therapy when they are scared and experience anxiety are often easily able to mobilise thoughts and feelings, and can sometimes be frightened by how these thoughts and feelings can lead to actions. In therapy, it can be necessary to dampen the tension by helping clients become aware of how they can limit sensory stimuli. These clients should not be stimulated in the therapy room (Melnick & Nevis, 2000). In the example of Diane in Chapter 17 on deflection, you see how the therapist helps her turn attention away from the concerns she has for her son by looking around the room (using the contact features, Chapter 9) together with the therapist.

When clients are feeling low, they might need help mobilising energy. The therapist can do this by exploring injunctions and expectations that the client feels are difficult, as Tanya does in the example in Chapter 13 on introjection. Tanya received support from the therapist to mobilise energy by working with conflicting needs she felt in relation to her parents, her boyfriend, and herself.

The action phase

There are many people who are good at planning and mobilising, but who do not act due to a fear that they might make the wrong choice or that their plan is not good enough. They think that they need to plan better or weigh the pros and cons one more time, or perhaps they do not know enough about their options. In therapy and coaching it can be helpful for the therapist or coach to be part of this selection process and to make the client aware of how movement and progress stops. Often, we must explore the desire to make a perfect choice and the fear of failure. We recognise the contact form introjection: the client needs to do so much and needs control (Chapter 13). Together, the therapist and client can explore what it is to be perfect and when something is good enough.

We can see conflicting needs in therapy and coaching when there is a high degree of mobilised energy, such as when the client wants to quit smoking, lose weight, or refurbish her house, but never moves beyond the planning stage. In those cases, clients often tell us what they think they should do without being aware of whether they actually *want* to do these things. They are not aware of what is stopping them from acting, and that they have rules for what they should or must do (a high degree of introjection). In these cases, it can be helpful to explore whether or not they example want to stop smoking and make them aware of what is stopping them from doing so. They can then become aware of how challenging it is to change old habits and do something new. The choice and how to implement it become more realistic, and the process of becoming conscious is also a meaningful act.

Contact and challenges in the withdrawal phase

Difficulty in the withdrawal phase is not infrequent. We can be critical of ourselves and the environment and have an idea that our action or choice was not good enough. It can be difficult to enjoy work we have done well and withdraw and rest (Zinker, 1977). We can recognise this in situations where we are unable to finish tasks, as the example of Eve shows.

Eve is conscientious and wants everything she does to be done well. She is rarely completely satisfied with what she does and does not believe positive feedback she receives from others. She has spent several months in therapy and talked a lot about how difficult she thinks it is to finish tasks. It is as if she will never be satisfied. Her boss is constantly complaining that she has to finish what she is working on so that she can begin new tasks. She can stay at work long into the evenings to rewrite documents to make them even better. She feels she goes in circles in her mind, is tired and sleepy, and struggles more and more with confidence. In their sessions, Eve and the therapist have explored what happens when Eve is at work, what it is like to stay at her desk and write, and what kind of feedback she gets at work. Eve realises that she often enjoys staying at work to write, to form thoughts and sentences, but that she finds it difficult to hand the completed document over to her boss. When she does so, she becomes very insecure, especially when her boss does not comment on the material Eve sends her.

In chair work between Eve and her boss, Eve explores her ideas that her boss is not happy with how she does her tasks at work. Eve eventually realises that it is not her boss, but rather she herself who is critical of whether or not the work was done well enough, and that she has projected this onto her boss (see Chapter 14 on projection).

Through the chair work, Eve mobilises energy. She takes action and becomes aware (contacts) that her boss is not the one who can satisfy her need to finish her tasks, but that she herself must resolve her own inner conflict in order to be satisfied and feel ready.

The therapist invites her to do a new chair work where she lets the critical Eve who wants to be perfect talk to the Eve who would like to finish the task she is working on. Eve changes what the chairs represent, and speaks as both sides of herself. The therapist asks Eve to stand up, move back from the chairs, and formulate a sentence that includes the content of what she has said in both chairs.

While standing back a bit with one chair on either side, she says: 'I want to be perfect and I want to finish. And that's me right now . . . hmmm, yes, that's the situation right now at any rate. Now I want to finish . . . it was a relief to say that . . . and maybe I don't have to be perfect . . . ' She sits down again and reflects on this new realisation with the therapist.

Here we see how important it is for Eve to experience that it is her inner conflict that causes her not to finish her tasks at work. Through this experience, she comes into a deeper contact with the need to be perfect and the conflicting need to finish, and she realises for a moment that what she does might be good enough. This paradoxical change comes as an expression of the contact she has known with her needs and with the support she has experienced from the therapist. The theme Eve brought into therapy is existential and important to her. It is related to her need to be perfect and can be linked to what we have previously written about existential pressure (Chapter 2).

Reduction of excitement, withdrawal, and rest

Eve's involvement in her inner conflict diminishes as she becomes aware of and acknowledges her conflicting needs, making it possible for them to go to the background. She becomes able to reflect on these needs and can integrate and learn from the experience and gain wisdom (Melnick & Nevis, 2000). When her engagement declines, Eve becomes calmer, which means she can relax more.

In the next example, we show how the therapist supports Eve in the latter part of their therapy work in relation to reducing tension and ending the therapy session.

Eve tells the therapist how difficult it has been for her to accept that something is good enough, and says that it is wonderful that she now feels she is somewhat able to relax her demands on herself at work. She smiles and is happy when she speaks, and is about to continue when the therapist interrupts, pointing out that she sees that Eve's breathing is deep and relaxed as she speaks. Eve nods, breathes more easily, and sits further back on her chair. The therapist says that she notices that she also breathes more easily and feels calm. Eve nods and says that it is good to know that she is breathing and that her body is heavy and relaxed. The therapist encourages her to spend some time sitting and feeling her breathing and body, which Eve does. After a while she begins to yawn, her face and body relax even more, and the therapist waits a few minutes before pointing out that it seems a natural place to end the session.

By pointing out what she notices about Eve's breathing and body, the therapist supports Eve's awareness of how she breathes and helps her to keep from re-mobilising by rethinking her experiences. Eve is supported to reduce the excitement and energy she gained through her new realisation and rather to stay in the moment with her new insight. By becoming aware of her breathing and body, she can feel satisfaction and a reduction of excitement, and is able to be present in her own experience and feel rest. Eve can later reflect on and experience how the new insight affects her at work and at home. Giving time to attention in moments of completion, withdrawal, and rest is important and necessary in a busy everyday life. It is important for therapists to pay attention to this when working with clients who place high demands on themselves and have an existential pressure to be perfect (see Chapter 13 on introjection).

Completion and unfinished situations

Unfortunately, there are experiences that can feel too overwhelming and difficult, where engagement and excitement do not subside by themselves. These can be existential experiences such as death, illness, divorce, and loss, but can also be associated with a positive process such as falling asleep, dreaming, fantasising, and celebrating. In such situations, the client may need support to reduce and remove the energy she has mobilised. If this is not done, the experience cannot be integrated and completed and can have a repetitive and disruptive effect on current and future experiences for the client (Melnick & Nevis, 2000).

In the chapter on creative adjustment (Chapter 6), we describe Fritz Perls' understanding of how unfinished situations tend to affect people later in life, the challenges this can create, and how therapists can work with these unfinished situations in therapy. Painful and unfinished situations tend to be mobilised when people encounter new endings, especially when these endings are difficult and important such as sudden death, illness, or accidents. It is also the case that endings themselves can be experienced existentially, as a reminder of the fear that the end is nearing, that something is over (p. 27).

If the client brings in life situations that have to do with challenges with finishing, whether it be work tasks, relationships, relocation, or other changes in life, it is important that the therapist is aware of how previous endings can come up. It is also natural for the therapist to pay extra attention to how she and the client conclude their work, whether it is an individual therapy session, the last session before a vacation, or the end of the therapeutic relationship.

The experience process: a model of waves, arcs, or sequences?

Initially we described how the process of change can be viewed as a wave, an arc, or as multiple waves or arcs. In the examples, however, we have shown how the undulating movement can stagnate; there is a lack of progress in the process and the therapist and client work in one of the phases in order to raise awareness and create new movement. It is difficult to imagine how a wavelike movement could include stagnation and repetition of earlier phases. In such situations, it can in many cases be easier for the therapist to envision a model of sequences in which the movement is from one sequence to another, for example from becoming aware of a new sequence in which the client acts automatically and without awareness, and then into a new sequence of increased duration, leading to mobilisation, and so on. This coincides with the criticism that has been raised towards seeing the process of contact as circles (Chapter 18), and we recommend here that therapists themselves choose how to use the model, either sequentially or undulating.

Summary

Being aware of needs and taking responsibility for choices and actions is fundamental in gestalt therapy. In this chapter, we have described a theoretical model that shows the process through which a person has a sense of a need until she becomes aware of the need, mobilises energy to make choices and act to meet the need, contacts the action, and ultimately becomes satisfied and can withdraw. This process is usually painless and fluid, and the client has an experience having her needs met. There are, however, situations in which this does not happen. The flow is gone; we become frustrated with ourselves or our surroundings and experience discomfort and misunderstandings. Clients often come to therapy when they feel the process is stagnating and they are unsatisfied. The therapist works to help the client become aware of where in the process she is struggling, to become aware of bodily sensations, understand how she can mobilise energy and use that energy to make good choices, and how she can feel that she has met her needs, is satisfied, and can withdraw.

In the examples from the therapy and coaching room, we have shown that Therese is good at noticing sensations and bodily reactions but struggles to mobilise and act. Stuart can mobilise and act, but is not aware of bodily signals, while Eve can produce and persevere, but struggles to achieve completion. Therese's challenge is that she is cautious and avoids difficulties, unlike Stuart, who throws himself into new challenges without exploring them well enough first. Eve is focused and does not let go. She needs help to see that everything does not have to be perfect and that it is possible to be in a situation that is unknown and new. These are examples of how people can act and experience being in various ways in various situations. They have different opportunities for development, which they experience when the therapist or coach helps them become conscious and aware of the process.

References

Clarkson, P., & Mackewn, J. (1993). *Fritz Perls*. London: Sage Publications.
Melnick, J., & Nevis, S. (1992/2000). Diagnosis: The struggle for a meaningful paradigm. In E. C. Nevis (Ed.), *Gestalt therapy* (pp. 57–78). Cleveland: Gestalt Press.
Zinker, J. (1977). *Creative process in gestalt therapy*. New York: Random House.

Chapter 20

The process of change

Changing ourselves—our actions and behaviour—is one of the most difficult things we do. At the same time, we are always changing; we are never the same. In this chapter, we use a clinical example to illustrate the phases in the model and show how the process can develop over time. This change model is based on therapists' experiences of having clients over time who are unhappy, frustrated, and whose change process has stagnated. The purpose is to show what therapists can do in each phase to create movement to the next phase.

Staemmler and Bock's process theory of change (1998), which we refer to in this book as the change model, is based on Fritz Perls' neurosis model. Perls explained his model in the course of four lectures he gave in 1966 (the transcribed lectures are described, among other places, in Fagan and Shepherd, 1970/2006).

Staemmler and Bock developed a phase model where time is an axis, based on their own experiences from clinical practice. They described each phase on the basis of long-term data collected from their own and others' therapy practices, which they compared to Perls' description of client behaviour. They analysed and categorised this data and compiled an overview of common and characteristic elements in each phase (Staemmler, 1994).

Fritz Perls' neurosis model

Perls developed his process of change model based on his experience with clients. In this model he described clients' behaviour as neurotic. He reworked his original model many times. We summarise Perls' model here because it forms the basis for Staemmler and Boch's process of change model.

Perls' point of departure for the model was that he believed that humans created inappropriate strategies to avoid being aware of challenges, pain, and fear. People were not aware of these strategies, and much of Perls' therapeutic work shows how he worked with clients in different sequences of therapy to raise awareness of their behaviour.

DOI: 10.4324/9781003153856-24

Perls divided a change process into layers, which he named according to his experiences from therapeutic work with clients. He changed the name and significance of the layers throughout his years as a gestalt therapist, which has caused great confusion for later gestalt therapists. Here we present a summary of his theory based on Staemmler and Boch (Staemmler, 1994):

1   Neuroses are the opposite of authentic life. Being authentic means being finished with neuroses and is one of the goals of therapy.
2   Neuroses are considered to be structures with four or five layers.
3   These layers can be described independent of the specific psychological content the client brings to therapy.
4   The term 'layers' describes a form of behaviour that is related to the content of therapy at any given time.
5   Therapy often begins with the client playing different social roles and games. The first layer is usually the 'phony layer' or 'cliché layer'.
6   At the end of therapy, after going through all the layers, the client experiences authentic feelings such as sadness, anger, orgasm, or joy.

The layers of neurosis Perls describes are:

1   The phony layer
2   The phobic layer
3   Impasse
4   Implosion
5   Explosion

The phony layer was described earlier. In the phobic layer, the client is mobilised and often frightened, and her avoidance strategies are often reinforced as she begins to become aware and understand that actions do not lead to change. Impasse is described as a dead end, where the client sees no way out of her desperate situation. At the impasse the client experiences that she does not know who she is, that past ways of being do not allow her to move forward and that she is losing control of her life and her situation at the moment. A spontaneous contraction (implosion) occurs when the client has been at an impasse for long enough, followed by an explosion of emotions leading to what Perls called an authentic way of being, where roles and games are over.

Perls had great faith in what was later formulated by Beisser as a paradoxical change (Chapter 5). He therefore challenged and provoked clients with the intention of getting them to the next layer of neurosis so that a spontaneous change could occur.

The change model is based on three assumptions:

1 The therapist works dialogically.
2 The therapist's main task is to increase the client's awareness and help her to be conscious of her life situation.
3 The therapist adheres to the principle of the paradoxical change theory (Chapter 5).

The change model describes five phases: stagnation, polarisation, diffusion, contraction, and expansion. These five phases follow one another in time, although in many cases clients move back and forth between phases.

First phase: stagnation

At the beginning of a change process, we can see the various phenomena that can correspond to what Perls called the phony layer. At this stage, the client is unaware of how she really is and pretends that everything is fine. There is a lack of congruence between what she says and what she shows, and it may seem that she is superficial and plays roles. She can be frustrated by the conditions in which she lives. She feels depressed and functions poorly at home or at work and has chronic headaches or other physical symptoms that make life difficult. She wants to get rid of her symptoms, but nothing has helped. She may feel helpless and that she is a victim of her symptoms, and she does not know how to live with them. In this situation, the client tries to satisfy her needs in many ways and hopes to get outside help.

Clients who come into therapy in the first phase have in common that they do not experience progress in their personal development. They feel trapped and stuck; they do not see that they can influence their situations and take no responsibility for them. This does not, however, mean that clients are passive—on the contrary. They talk about their problems, often seek help from a therapist, and try to find solutions by switching jobs, moving, or other practical measures without bringing about the desired changes (Eie, 2005).

During the stagnation phase, the therapist is interested in recognising avoidance strategies the client uses to avoid becoming aware of the fear and uncertainty that arises when an unknown and challenging situation is not dealt with. In such situations, clients may feel threatened and become extremely rigid, which can affect their relationships with others. The therapist explores and works with among other things the forms of contact that emerge. Because the client usually blames the environment at this stage, various forms of projection work, such as role-play and the projection chair, are helpful (Chapters 11 and 14). The therapist can also work on how she and the client are together in the therapy room. For example, the therapist may point out that the client smiles as she complains as she shares what is going on with her by saying something like: 'When you say that everything is fine, I feel turmoil in my body and am not sure if I believe what you

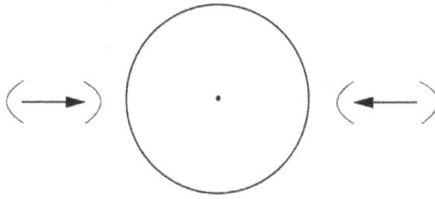

Figure 20.1 Stagnation: it can seem as if the client is only affected by external forces.

say'. The therapist can also explore the impulses and bodily sensations she or the client has, in order to raise awareness of how the client currently feels, as opposed to how the client thinks she should feel.

As shown in the illustration of this phase in Figure 20.1, there are arrows coming from outside, pointing towards the client. The arrows symbolise forces that either come from the environment or are outside the client's area of responsibility.

In this phase, the therapist works to raise the client's awareness of the situation she is in so that she can become aware of the suffering that has been placed on her by outside sources on the one hand, and what she can take responsibility for and do something about on the other. The therapist explores underlying unsatisfied needs and what the client does to maintain stagnation, which we illustrate in the following example with Miriam.

Miriam comes to therapy because she feels that she is in an untenable life situation. Her husband, Steven, was in a car accident two years ago and is partially disabled as a result of the injuries he sustained. He lives at home and they have relatively good support arrangements, but the situation involves a lot of work for Miriam. She has had to reduce her work hours as a result. When she comes to therapy, she is pale, tired, and speaks softly, often choking up. The therapist notices that she is moved by the story Miriam tells, and has great sympathy for her in her new life situation.

In their first few sessions the therapist lets her talk and complain about the difficulties, without doing or saying much. Gradually, the therapist notices that Miriam constantly complains about how difficult her husband is, how little the children involve themselves in what needs to be done, and that there are constantly new caregivers coming and going. She talks about how much she has to do and says she feels exhausted and helpless. When she speaks, she sinks into her body and speaks in a low, complaining voice. It is as if she is trying to show the therapist how hurt she is, but the therapist is not completely convinced because the client's words and body language do not seem to be congruent—it is almost as if she exaggerates. The therapist notices that she listens to Miriam with less interest and sympathy.

In the following sequence, Miriam complains about what the changed life situation has resulted in for her, and how she feels that the responsibility rests on people and events outside herself. There is a lack of congruence between what she says and what she shows the therapist, and she seems to be self-pitying rather than suffering. She feels that she has stagnated, that life as she knew it is over. She is in the stagnation phase. The first step in a change process is to acknowledge that she has stagnated. The therapist is interested in how they can bring Miriam's situation at home into the therapy room here and now.

> THERAPIST: 'I can understand that you feel that life as you know it is over, and it must have been a big shock to you when your husband was in the accident'.
>
> MIRIAM: 'Yes, it was just awful to see Steven afterwards. He was in so much pain, and I coped so badly. I think I should've handled it better than I did'.
>
> THERAPIST: 'You did the best you could. I don't know how I would handle what you've experienced'.
>
> MIRIAM: 'Do you think so?'
>
> THERAPIST: 'Yes, I don't think you've fully understood what kind of stress you and your husband have been subjected to and the pressure you're living under. No one can prepare for an accident like this and the way it changes your life'.
>
> MIRIAM: 'That's true, it's just so awful'. The muscles around her mouth tremble and there are tears in her eyes. 'I never imagined this could happen to us'. There is a change in her body; she straightens up a little and looks right at the therapist.
>
> THE THERAPIST feels warmth and sadness, looks directly at Miriam and says in a low voice: 'And it happened to you and your husband. Your lives are completely changed. Life is sometimes terribly brutal'.
>
> MIRIAM cries quietly, but breathes a little more deeply than she did earlier in the session, and says: 'Yes, it's just terrible and so incredibly painful, and I can't handle it anymore. Everything is different'.
>
> Miriam continues to cry for a while and says that she feels calmer. It is as if she has realised that this is the way her life is right now. They talk about this insight together before they finish the session.

The therapist brings Miriam's situation into the room by saying that she cannot imagine how she herself would cope with such an accident. She expresses her thoughts about Miriam and her life situation with much respect and warmth, without being sentimental or being circumspect about what she thinks. She thinks that it is necessary to confront Miriam with what cannot be changed. Her husband was in an accident and they both experience suffering that was caused by external forces. This confrontation causes Miriam to become aware of the grief she is holding back, and, for the first time, she feels pain and helplessness. This insight is the first step towards the transition between the stagnation and polarisation phases, and comes spontaneously. It entails a paradoxical change. By complaining about how difficult life is and what everyone else is doing wrong, Miriam has thus far avoided feeling the pain. Her underlying need to grieve is expressed, and the resistance, the fear of feeling the pain that has had a stagnant effect, is in the background. In the first phase it is necessary to help the client to become aware of what she has been exposed to from the outside, an aspect of her situation for which she is not responsible and cannot change.

The process of change model places great emphasis on the transition between the phases as well as what can prevent and create movement to the next phase.

When Miriam arrives next at her next session, she again complains about her husband, children, and helpers. It is as if the insight she gained at the last session is forgotten. The therapist points this out. Miriam nods and agrees that it was an important session for her, but that she still has to deal with the consequences of the accident along with all the problems and worries the situation brings to everyday life. The therapist emphasises that she understands that there is a big difference between recognising that the accident has happened and living with the consequences. However, it is unclear if Miriam hears what the therapist says. She does not look at her and continues to talk. She seems rushed and frustrated, and her voice is sharper than the therapist is accustomed to hearing her. Miriam's disappointment with those around her reveals that she has high expectations of her surroundings, which the therapist thinks is important to explore. She also thinks that her disappointment extends to her as a therapist.

Miriam still feels that she has stagnated. Therapy has not solved her practical everyday problems, although she has been helped to recognise the pain and grief she feels about the accident. The therapist now concentrates on raising Miriam's awareness of how she complains to others, to see if she can eventually become aware of her own experience and what her underlying needs are.

Exploration here and now

The therapist chooses to continue the session by exploring the client's expectations of her and the therapy, since she has a hypothesis that Miriam is critical.

THERAPIST: 'It sounds like you're not happy with me and what we've done together so far'.

MIRIAM: 'It's been good to talk to you and it felt surprisingly good to cry last time. But it's like you don't understand how I feel and don't want to help me'. She talks in a low voice and looks down. It is unclear if she is annoyed or upset.

The therapist says with a calm and gentle voice: 'You are right that I don't understand exactly how you feel, probably no one can. Maybe you're hoping that I can do more for you than I'm able to'.

Miriam looks at her beseechingly, as if expressing expectations without even being aware of it, and says: 'I need your help. I don't know how to handle everything on my own'.

The therapist repeats her question. Miriam looks a little surprised, as if she is taking in what the therapist says for the first time, and answers: 'Maybe I expect too much from you. Maybe I'm hoping that you can get rid of my problems, but you can't. It's good to talk to you anyway. I feel like you listen to me, but that doesn't solve my problems'.

THERAPIST: 'I'm glad it's good for you to talk to me, and I also wish I could help you more in your everyday life. And it sounds like you have high expectations for me and others around you'.

MIRIAM: I think we should help each other. I've always thought that I have to help others, not only Steven. And I think that's why I expect that others will help me. I've never thought about it like that before. I kind of expect everyone to be like me'.

Here, the therapist keeps Miriam in the moment by repeating her question about expectations. She thinks it is important that Miriam be aware of all the expectations she has, both of herself and the outside world. Expectations are often a mixture of introjection and projection (Chapters 13 and 14), and it is only when Miriam realises that her automatic belief that others are the same as she is, is not a truth, that change can happen (Chapter 5). She begins to become conscious of and take responsibility for how she assumes things about others that actually are about her.

In this and the next sessions, they further explore what Miriam expects from her family and helpers. Miriam reflects on what she thinks those around her 'should' help her with, and what she is disappointed and annoyed with them about. Gradually, Miriam realises that there are differences in her expectations and that it is unreasonable for her to expect her children to take responsibility for their father, but that she can expect them to help her when she occasionally asks them to.

She also realises that the therapist cannot solve her home situation, that it is her responsibility, but that the therapist can help her sort and reflect as they have done in their sessions so far.

The therapist continues to explore introjects and projections together with Miriam because she sees how Miriam is still locked into unrealistic expectations of her surroundings. This is one of the things that prevents her from taking responsibility for what she can do.

Eventually it becomes clear that Miriam's greatest challenges are in relation to her husband. She feels he is difficult and unreasonable, and she does not know how long she can stand to be his caregiver. The therapist suggests an experiment in which Miriam can alternately pretend to be Steven and herself in chair work (see Part 2, Chapter 8). Miriam agrees, and the therapist asks Miriam to start off by being Steve. It is hard for Miriam to find a way to sit, because Steve often sits on a couch or special chair. The therapist finds some pillows and an extra chair, and Miriam tries out different combinations until she finds a comfortable position. The therapist asks what it is like for her to sit as Steven, and Miriam replies that it is okay, but very strange. She feels stiff and uncomfortable and finds it difficult to be her husband.

The therapist asks her to go to her own chair, which Miriam does right away.

MIRIAM says spontaneously: 'Oh, it's much better to sit as myself in this chair, I'm not as tense here. But I feel like lying down, not sitting up like I am now'.

THERAPIST: 'Can you look at the other chair with all the cushions and imagine Steven sitting there? See if there's anything you want to say to him'.

MIRIAM turns slightly, looks at the chair, and says in a weak voice: 'You don't understand how difficult this is for me. I really want to help you, but I'm so tired. I just want to sleep'.

MIRIAM, as her husband: 'Yes, but I'm completely dependent on you. I can't manage by myself. I'm in so much pain and feel like everything is meaningless. I'm so scared'. When she talks as if she is Steven, she moves her body as if she's in pain and looks sadly at Miriam.

MIRIAM: 'It's so hard for me to listen to you and it's hard that you're so dependent on me'.

The therapist asks Miriam to get up and stand with her to look at the two empty chairs that represent her and her husband.

MIRIAM: 'It was difficult to be my husband. It's as if I forget how hard it is to be in pain and to be so helpless. I feel guilty and that I shouldn't complain so much'.

THERAPIST: 'Yes, it's hard for both of you. You're tired and need help, and he is helpless'.

MIRIAM: 'Yes, it's a bad situation to be in'.

THERAPIST: 'What can you say to your husband now? Can you continue the conversation?'

> MIRIAM sits in her own chair and says to the other chair: 'Steven, I forget so easily what it's like to be you when I'm in the middle of everything I have to do. I just don't know what we can do'. She has tears in her eyes and sits bent forward.
> MIRIAM, as her husband: 'Don't cry, I can't stand to see you crying and feeling sorry for me'.
> MIRIAM: 'I don't feel sorry for you. I'm crying for us and for the situation we're in together'.

By reflecting on her projections and expectations of others, Miriam takes more responsibility for her own situation. In the chair work with her husband, she realises that she attributes being difficult to him, rather than seeing how difficult it is for her to be with him. This projection of difficulty is likely true. Steven is likely having a hard time in reality. She also becomes aware of the underlying introjects she sends to her husband: that he should not pester her and be difficult.

As the therapist works with introjection and projection, they explore what is in Miriam's way, keeping her from moving on. Her ideas about her future fell apart when her husband was in the accident. She adapts to this new situation by approaching her surroundings with the notion that they can save her from the consequences of the accident, and thus she becomes more helpless than she really is. She needs to see herself and her life situation with new eyes and to understand how the situation with a disabled husband actually is. The world is not as she thought and expected; it is therefore important to work with the notions she has about herself and others. The stagnation phase has a lot to do with how she imagines that others should be towards her. In the next phase, she begins to understand that it is really about herself—about how she wants to be with herself and her own conflicting needs.

Different needs and conditions during the stagnation phase

Needs can be different. Some are related to people's daily lives, such as the need to shop for food, get to work on time, pick up children from day care, and so on (Chapter 5). Other needs may feel more important and be more existential, such as the need to have someone to love, be safe with, or live meaningfully with (see Chapter 2 on existential pressures). The first are referred to as everyday needs and the second as underlying needs. Underlying needs are often implicit and more difficult to become aware of. As previously mentioned, it is important to make the client aware of the expectations and needs she has, so that she becomes aware of what she assigns to others and what she herself can take responsibility for and do something about. The client is directly responsible for the subjective conditions she creates along the way, but she is not responsible for external conditions, which are also not the reason for therapy. It is important that the therapist does not confuse subjective obstacles to change with objective obstacles that are part of external conditions. In Miriam's case, an external obstacle might be a lack of home helpers or carers. It is important that the therapist does not see it as her job to get more help for Miriam. However, she can explore what it is like for Miriam to have little help, if there is something Miriam does that prevents home helpers from coming to them or if there is something she can do to get more help.

During the stagnation phase, the therapist is interested in how the client relates to subjective conditions that she can influence in the situation. She notices whether the client avoids doing something that hinders her satisfaction or is passive and does not do what is necessary in order to be satisfied. The therapist might ask herself: 'What does the client do or fail to do that makes her unhappy?'

There are also situations in which the client herself is unable to do what is necessary to improve her situation. One reason might be that she lacks the capacity or ability to do what is necessary to be satisfied. In these situations, the therapist might ask herself: 'Does the client lack some capacity that would make it possible for her to do what she needs to be happy?' The therapist can detect if the client lacks such a capacity by observing and being aware of the client's response to her interventions. She can then see if the client avoids tolerating difficulty and discomfort and does not meet her need for that reason, or if the client does not have the necessary ability needed to move forward.

We return to the therapy session with Miriam.

During one session, the therapist hears Miriam complain that she does not have enough help getting her husband to and from his appointments for treatment. Miriam sits uneasily in her chair and feels like giving up. The therapist wonders about Miriam's unease and asks her what is stopping her from driving her husband herself. Miriam shamefully tells the therapist that she does not know how to drive. She is so afraid of driving that she has never dared to take a single driving lesson. The therapist says she understands that that makes her more dependent on help from others.

THERAPIST: 'What's it like for you that you don't drive?'
MIRIAM, with a resigned voice: 'Right now it's very inconvenient'.
THERAPIST: 'And you're still just as scared to drive?'
MIRIAM: 'Yes, I've actually become even more scared and find it difficult to be a passenger when I'm in a car that's driving over bridges and through tunnels'.
THERAPIST: 'So you'd rather be dependent on finding someone else to drive when it's necessary?'
MIRIAM shakes her head and says: 'I have to, even if I don't want to'.
THERAPIST: 'And I hear that you choose not to explore how you can start driving. I respect that choice, especially because it has consequences for you'.
MIRIAM: 'It's good to hear you say that. I don't see how I can handle it'.

It is important that the therapist make Miriam aware that she chooses not to explore the possibility of learning to drive a car. When Miriam confirms that it is her choice, she accepts the disadvantages of her choice. It is an acknowledged part of her, and she can move on to exploring the conflicting needs that the therapist has noticed and made clear to her.

In the transition to the second phase, the therapist must work to increase Miriam's awareness of her conflicting needs and of the avoidance strategies she uses hinder her development. Many clients end therapy when they become aware that they have been in a victim position and have not taken responsibility for the situation in which they find themselves. They have the resources and knowledge to deal with challenges on their own, and end therapy.

The transition to the polarisation phase

The transition to the polarisation phase is gradual, and manifests as the client becomes aware of how she hurts herself by complaining and blaming others, being helpless, and playing roles. She acknowledges that she has underlying needs that have not been met by this way of being. The new insight brings her into a new and unknown situation where emotions such as fear, uncertainty, indecision, distrust, and doubt can arise. These emotions can correspond to what Perls called the phobic layer, which causes a lot of inner tension and struggle.

The client can express such tension bodily by moving one part of the body while another part is at rest. For example, she sits and moves her legs while her upper body is still. It can be expressed verbally by the client with statements such as 'I want to . . . but I don't dare to' or 'On the one hand I feel like . . . on the other hand I'm happy the way things are'.

Miriam is at a new therapy session. This time she tells the therapist that she would like to go on vacation with a friend, but she is so afraid that Steven will not manage at home without her and of what he will think about her going on vacation. She feels that she needs to get away—it will help her to be more patient. She sits uneasily on her chair, her eyes are fixed on the therapist, and she speaks in a calm voice. She says it's hard to know what to do and that she thinks about it all the time. The therapist explores these conflicting needs by using two chairs. One chair represents the Miriam who wants to 'get away', and the other represents the Miriam who is 'afraid that Steven will not manage without her'. The therapist lets the two sides of Miriam talk together and makes sure Miriam moves between the chairs when appropriate.

'Get away': 'I'd love to travel. I need a vacation and it's so important to me to do something just for me'.

'Afraid that Steven will not manage': 'But what if Steven can't handle my not being there? I feel so guilty just leaving him, he's so dependent on me'.

'Get away' to 'Afraid that Steven will not manage': 'Yes, it's not easy to be him, but it only gets worse if you get worn out and break up. I long for a little sun and warmth and to feel like I'm alive'.

'Afraid that Steven will not manage': 'But can I just leave him? Isn't that selfish? He's the one who needs to get away, not me'.

'Get away' to 'Afraid that Steven will not manage': 'Typical you—you only think about others and never about yourself'. At this point, 'Afraid that Steven will not manage' leans forward and raises her voice.

'Afraid that Steven will not manage': 'No, that's not true, I just feel really bad for Steven and can't stand that he's in pain. I don't think I can talk to him about this trip. It will make him so unhappy'. Here, Miriam speaks in an unsteady voice, and it seems like she is about to start crying.

The therapist ends the chair work and asks Miriam what it was like. Miriam replies that it was just awful. It becomes clear to her how scared she is that Steven might feel abandoned by her, and how difficult it is for her to do something for herself because she fears that he will be hurt and unhappy with her.

THERAPIST: 'It sounds like you recognised that you have two conflicting needs: one that wants to go on vacation, and one that doesn't want to hurt Steven. And I heard you say that you recognise a part that only thinks about others, and that doing something for yourself is selfish'.

MIRIAM squirms: 'Yes, I always think more about others than myself. I think I've already said that I think we should help each other'.

THERAPIST: 'I notice that you move around on your chair when you say you have to help others. Can you exaggerate how you twist?'

Miriam moves her upper body one way and her legs another. The therapist asks Miriam to get up and continue to twist her body. It becomes clear how the upper body tries to move in one direction while the legs go in another direction. The therapist asks Miriam to pay attention to what is happening to her and what she feels in her body. After a while, Miriam stops the movements and sits down again.

THERAPIST: 'So now you really got to feel the conflict in your body. You want to help and be kind to Steven and at the same time you want to think about yourself and go on vacation'.

MIRIAM: 'Yes, I really felt it. It was like I was being pulled in two directions. It was as if my upper body was holding back while my legs wanted to move'.

THERAPIST: 'So the legs wanted to move . . . ' The therapist repeats what Miriam says.

MIRIAM: 'Yes, my legs want to go on vacation, but my upper body is holding me back. That was weird. I haven't ever really thought about it, but it's true that when I want to do something without Steven, I get uneasy in my body. Then my heart starts beating fast, and I get worried about whether he thinks I don't care about him, since I want to do something without him'.

THERAPIST: 'That makes sense. And now it looks like your body is calmer, am I right?'

MIRIAM: 'It's as if I see how I stop myself by constantly thinking about what other people need and how I don't know what's going on with me and what I need. It's a relief to see it, because I understand more about myself and what I've been doing in my life, not only with Steven, but with my friends, too. And even with my own family. I always helped my little brother and I couldn't stand it when our mother was mad at him and hit him. I felt so sorry for him and felt that I had to take care of him when my mother didn't'.

THERAPIST: 'I'm touched when I listen to you. It warms me to hear the insight you have about yourself now, and how you took care of your little brother when you were young. I think it was wonderful for him that you were there then'.

During this session, Miriam becomes aware that by thinking about others and always being the one who helps, she has prevented herself from getting in touch with what she really wants and needs. Taking care of others has been her creative adjustment since she was a child. It was easier for her to take care of her little brother than to see him hurt when her mother was angry and hit him. This insight comes when the therapist asks Miriam to exaggerate the movements she has in her body, and she becomes aware of how her body moves in two different directions and between two different needs. Miriam sees how she has been the helper all her life, and that she has not been aware that she has more choices today than she did as a child.

This insight leads to a paradoxical change for Miriam. She has no longer stagnated, but rather has moved on to the polarisation phase. Miriam has become aware that she is divided between two conflicting poles. One pole, the need to get away and go on vacation, represents an impulse that is moving forward or is expanding. This is called expansion. The effect of the second pole, her concern for her husband and her need to help, inhibits her in the form of a backward or inward movement, which is called contraction. Psychologically, the expansive pole represents the client's predominantly unsatisfied needs at the moment, while the contractive pole is what she does, thinks, and feels that prevents her from satisfying that need, that is, her avoidance or resistance.

Theme and underlying needs

The two elements, the dominant unsatisfied need and avoidance, shape what is called the theme of Miriam's process of change.

There is a difference between ordinary, everyday needs and underlying needs, as we discuss on p. 294. For Miriam, an everyday need is how she can get help to care for her husband. The need is expressed through her suffering and is the reason she seeks therapy. An underlying need often makes itself apparent in the exploration between therapist and client, and is more existential. In this process, the underlying theme the client brings in will be expressed. This underlying theme is not necessarily the reason the client says she has come to therapy; Miriam says that she has come to therapy to get help to manage her daily life. When the underlying need emerges and the therapist and client begin to understand what the client's theme is, they have moved to the next phase. Miriam's theme is her inner conflict between her need to get away and do something for herself and her need to take care of her husband. Her underlying developmental needs are closely related to the theme she is now becoming aware of.

Second phase: polarisation

In Figure 20.2, two arrows point inward and represent the contractive pole, and two arrows point outward and represent the expansive pole. In Miriam's case, the contractive pole is the force triggered by her having to help others, and the expansive pole is the force triggered by the fact that she wants to do more for herself. Miriam's change came when she acknowledged that she was getting in her own way by being concerned with what others needed and not paying attention to what she herself wanted to do. She sees herself in a new way. She is aware that she is responsible for her own actions and that her idea that others would help her

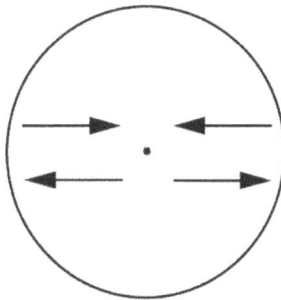

Figure 20.2 Polarisation: the client experiences conflicting inner forces.

did not match reality. On one hand, this insight makes her more ready to work on herself in therapy, and on the other, she is confronted with the fear and discomfort of being responsible for her own situation.

In this phase, it is useful for the therapist to rely on the theoretical models of polarity work described in Chapter 10. It is important to pay particular attention to the contractive pole and help the client become aware of how she prevents herself from satisfying her actual needs. In this phase, the internal struggle between conflicting needs can be almost unbearable for the client. The tension between holding on to previous solutions and the discomfort of following the new and underlying developmental needs can create a lot of fear and discomfort. We described this tension in what we called the desire/fear model (Chapter 10). We take a closer look at how the therapist explores this with Miriam at a later session.

Miriam is at a new session where she is again discussing how she can tell Steven about the vacation she is planning. She understands that it is up to her to talk to him, and that unless she does there will be no vacation.

THERAPIST: 'What is it that you are afraid your husband will say when you tell him that you're going away?'

MIRIAM: 'Maybe I'm mostly afraid he'll think I'm selfish'.

THERAPIST: 'Are you selfish?'

MIRIAM: 'No, the opposite, I never think about myself. I'm not allowed to be selfish. It's amazing how strict I am with myself'.

THERAPIST: 'Yes, that's how it sounds. And now you don't dare to tell your husband that you want to go on vacation because you don't want to be selfish'.

MIRIAM: 'I want to think about myself, and I get so scared when I think about talking to my husband about my plans'.

The therapist suggests that Miriam explore the side of her who is afraid of being selfish. When she is the scared Miriam, she feels chest contractions and struggles to breathe. The therapist stands next to her and encourages Miriam to breathe with her. She thinks it is important for Miriam to feel her presence when she is scared, so she rests her hand lightly on Miriam's shoulder. After the experiment, Miriam says that she became aware of how severe her fear was and that she had not realised that she was so scared. It becomes a little easier for her to accept that she finds it difficult to talk to Steven. She recognises that she has been scared previously, before Steven got sick, and that that fear has now been strengthened. The therapist says that she felt calm and at the same time very touched when Miriam was scared, and that she realises that it is difficult for Miriam to have such a strong internal conflict.

Here, the therapist works with Miriam to help her experience how the contractive pole feels in her body and to gain insight into how the underlying fear affects and prevents her from talking to Steven. The goal of the therapist is not that Miriam be able to talk to Steven; that is the ground. The figure is that Miriam must take ownership of her own avoidance strategy. Here, Miriam is in transition to the diffusion phase.

Not all clients need to move on to the next phase; many are happy to be aware of their inner conflicts and the insight this gives them. It is important that the therapist be aware of the extent to which the client can move on in her life without further exploration of conflicting needs and whether it is perhaps time to end the therapy.

The transition to the diffusion phase

The transition to the next phase means that the client has become aware of how she prevents herself from meeting her underlying needs and is conscious of her own responsibility for the situation she is in. The responsibility can feel daunting; it is challenging to recognise the fear and discomfort of being in the contractive pole. It is important that the therapist understand the client and can be with her in her stuck state. The situation is be reminiscent of what Fritz Perls called the impasse, but it does not fully encompass the chaos and confusion the client can experience when she is on her way into the diffusion phase. Now, the internal, unbearable conflict gradually ends, and there are no longer clear conflicting needs. Now the client has many confused thoughts and associations, and memories and images from the past might emerge and go to the background in quick succession, but it does not appear that this flow of thought leads to a solution for the client.

At this point it might be that the client no longer knows what the problem was. She can be forgetful, confused, and disoriented, and she can feel empty. Physically she might feel dizzy or nauseous and her movements might be poorly coordinated and lack direction. The growing confusion might be at least as unpleasant and frightening as the inner conflict she was in. There is no visible way out of the chaotic situation, and the more the client tries to find a way out, the more chaotic it becomes.

Third phase: diffusion

The third phase, diffusion (Figure 20.3), marks a turning point in the process of change. The inner war is over, and a new situation begins, where absolutely everything is moving. The movement has no order; it is scattered in all directions. We see how Miriam and the therapist experience and work in this phase.

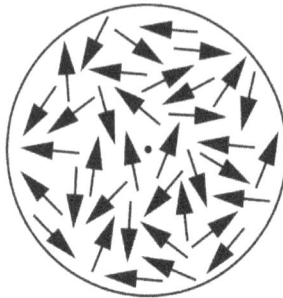

Figure 20.3 Diffusion: the arrows in all directions inside the circle show how everything feels chaotic and confusing.

At the next session Miriam arrives a little late, which has never happened before. She says she does not know what is going on with her. She is forgetful, angry, and confused, and does not know if there will be a vacation. The days just go by and she is not able to do as much as she usually does. When she talks, she seems dejected. Her eyes wander around the room and her voice is less energetic than usual. The therapist is confused about the change in Miriam but chooses not to say anything about what she thinks.

MIRIAM: 'I don't recognise myself, it's like everything is chaos. It feels so pointless to get up in the morning. It's as if nothing matters anymore. Steven is mad at me for not being there when he expects me to be, and it's almost like I don't care that he gets annoyed. I try to help him of course and to do what I usually do, but it's as if he's no longer important'.

The therapist does not know what to say or do, but moves little closer in order to show Miriam that she is there with her. After a little while she says: 'Mmm. This sounds very uncomfortable. I notice that I'm feeling very serious, and at the same time I think that you feel that you're changing, that everything is moving now, everything is flowing'.

MIRIAM starts to tremble a little and complains of a headache: 'I never have headaches. Maybe I'm sick? Maybe I'm getting the flu?'
THE THERAPIST says with a warm voice: 'I don't know. Maybe you feel sick, maybe you're very tired and sad. I see you're shaking—do you feel that?'
MIRIAM: 'Yes, it's really uncomfortable, I don't understand anything. I had decided to go on vacation and started getting ready to tell Steven. I'm

shaking because I'm freezing, maybe I'm going crazy. Maybe this is too much for me'.

THERAPIST: 'I can put a blanket around you and be with you. I don't think you're crazy even if you feel this way. I think you're reacting quite normally even if you don't experience it that way'. The therapist puts a blanket around Miriam's shoulders, and she breathes a little more deeply. Her body calms down a little. The therapist is aware that she has become calmer now that she understands that Miriam is in the diffusion phase.

The therapist leans toward Miriam and says: 'I understand that this is really difficult and that you feel everything is chaos. In the kind of process that you're in now it's very common to enter a phase where you don't know who you are. It's like a transition between the Miriam you know and a new and unknown version of yourself'.

Miriam cries a little and says nothing.

Here, the therapist is with Miriam in her confusion and unease. She is not trying to find a solution for Miriam in the midst of her chaos; she thinks the most important thing is that Miriam has some sort of understanding of the situation she is in that makes it possible to deal with and that she hears that the therapist has hope for her. At the beginning of the diffusion phase it is important for the client to become aware of bodily sensations without the therapist doing anything with those sensations. Her job is to be with the client and tolerate that the client does not know what she wants.

In this phase, clients can often feel that they are in an existential crisis where life feels meaningless. They feel stuck and that life can almost not be borne. The lack of meaning can in some cases make the client want to escape from the whole situation, either by thinking about taking her own life or quitting therapy. It is important that the therapist can be with the client in her chaos and let her know that the process she is going through is meaningful. It is unknown and frightening, but not meaningless, even if the client does not see meaning in the moment (see Chapter 2 on existential pressure).

After a while the therapist says: 'I recognise your reaction from my own life when I was in a crisis and didn't know which way was up. I got through it, but I remember how awful it was to be in the middle of it and to not know what was ahead of me'.

MIRIAM: 'It's really good to hear you say that. I didn't think anyone could understand. And you thought everything was hopeless?'

> THERAPIST: 'Yes, I did, and I know that some of my clients have experienced the same, and that they have always been able to move on when they dared to be in the unknown'.
>
> MIRIAM. 'I can barely stand it. The worst thing is that I can't see any meaning. It's like there isn't a light at the end of the tunnel'.
>
> THERAPIST: 'I get that. And you will see the light. If I didn't believe so, I wouldn't be sitting here with you today'.

In this new and unknown situation Miriam is in, the therapist chooses to share from her own experience, both from her personal life and as a therapist. It is important that the therapist share her own experience and use her knowledge when she is with Miriam in this phase. Miriam can then rely on the therapist's words and borrow her hope when she herself has none.

The transition to the contraction phase

The contraction phase can be compared to what Fritz Perls called the 'death layer'. The name does not have its origin in the client feeling metaphorically 'dead', but rather refers to the fact that she has an awareness that she is afraid to die or disappear. She no longer knows who she is and is afraid to give up control and all her ideas of who she is. She might face feelings such as total helplessness, desperation, panic, or disgust, and might have considerable bodily pain or discomfort as well as thoughts that revolve around what she is experiencing.

> After a few weeks of turmoil and chaos, Miriam is back in therapy. She seems desperate and says that it is getting harder and harder to be her. She sees no end to this uncontrollable and chaotic state. She is moody and feels empty. The therapist asks her to describe where she feels empty, and Miriam points to her chest. The therapist asks her to describe the emptiness, which Miriam does with a few words. Her face is expressionless, she is silent and continues to hold her hand on her chest. The therapist asks her to be empty. Miriam begins to breathe heavily and becomes more restless in her body. It is as if her body is contracting, and she starts shaking.
>
> MIRIAM: 'I don't know what's going on with me. It's like my body is moving by itself. I get so scared, it's awful. I want to cry and just give up'.

Fourth phase: contraction

At this point Miriam is in the contraction phase (Figure 20.4). Here, all the forces in her body are directed inward. She becomes very frightened and feels

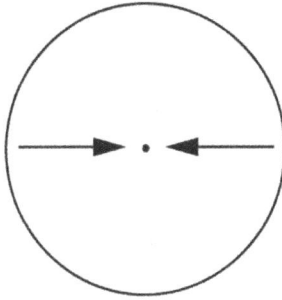

Figure 20.4 Contraction: the arrows point inwards and show the direction of the forces.

the need to surrender to the new and unknown. The therapist knows how to be vigilant and present with Miriam; it is as if she is preparing to join her fight. She knows from past experiences with other clients that if Miriam dares to surrender to the unknown and the fear it entails, the expansion phase will come spontaneously.

> THERAPIST: 'I'm here, it's not dangerous. Your body does exactly what you need. You can let it take over for you and your thoughts'.
>
> Miriam trembles and breathes. The therapist sits next to her and rests her hand lightly on her knee. She repeats that she is there and that all is well. She asks Miriam to breathe. Miriam breathes and bends forward in her chair. Her body twitches; now and then she sobs. The therapist rests her other hand on Miriam's shoulder so that Miriam knows that she is there beside her. At the same time, she breathes and says 'Mmm'.

Fifth phase: expansion

> Miriam shakes in her chair and suddenly sobs loudly. She cries and cries. Her nose runs and her tears flow without her noticing; it is as if her whole body is crying. The therapist is still sitting next to her without saying anything. Gradually Miriam's crying ceases and her sobs are fewer and farther between. She shops shaking. Miriam looks at the therapist with tears in her eyes, takes a tissue and dries her eyes and nose. Then the crying starts again, and Miriam surrenders to it again. After crying for a while, the periods of silence become longer. Finally, Miriam straightens up in her chair, looks at the therapist, and smiles a little.

MIRIAM: 'I'm completely worn out. It's as if everything inside me was pushing to get out. I just couldn't hold back. It's strange—and sort of nice,
too, as if I'm lighter now in a way. It almost feels like a purification
process. I never cried like that or let myself just surrender to despair. It
actually feels better now, and it was so good that you were here'.

THE THERAPIST has tears in her eyes, and says: 'And it was so good to be
the one sitting next to you. I'm so touched that you dared to surrender
with me'.

MIRIAM also has tears in her eyes, and says: 'I still don't know who I am
or what to do, but right now it's like I'm not worried about it. It's as if
I see you better, my body is calmer and I'm actually very happy'. She
is almost a little euphoric. 'What am I worried about? I can just talk to
Steven about this vacation. He's a reasonable man'.

Now Miriam is in the expansion phase. She has surrendered and followed her
body's contraction, which spontaneously led to change and expansion. The therapist has been with her, physically taking care of her and supporting her in the way
she felt Miriam needed. She has also participated in Miriam's struggle and been
aware of Miriam's and her own impulses.

During the expansion phase (Figure 20.5), the client is often happy and relieved
and can feel great peace and satisfaction. The fight is over, a solution for the original conflict has made itself apparent, and the path to meeting her needs becomes
visible and possible to navigate.

Change and time

The example of Miriam shows how a client can be in a process of change for a
long time. We rarely see clients go through all phases in one session—it is usual

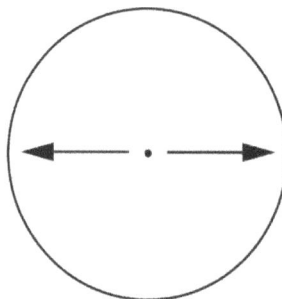

Figure 20.5 Expansion: the arrows point outwards to show that the direction of the forces
is now the opposite of the contraction phase.

that clients spend a long time in the first two phases and often move back and forth between phases. Some clients return to the polarisation phase after being in the diffusion phase for a while. This may be because the therapist does not recognise that the client's confusion and chaos is a sign of movement, but on the contrary interprets it to mean that they are getting worse and tries to create structure and experiment with conflicting needs she sees in the client's chaos. Sometimes the client cannot stand to be in the diffusion phase. It can be so upsetting and filled with so much anxiety that she chooses to maintain control and stay in the polarisation phase or return all the way back to the stagnation phase. Some clients are satisfied with awareness of internal conflicts and remain in the polarisation phase. Perhaps their need is satisfied when they realise that they are responsible for dealing with their own challenges; this might be enough to enable them to find satisfactory solutions.

The therapist's role and function

It is important that the therapist is aware of the client's process throughout and understands that the different phases require different approaches. In the first two stages it is useful and necessary for the therapist to bring the client's situation into the therapy room, either by working on the relationship between them or by bringing people and situations from the client's life into the therapy room by means of experiments such as role-play and chair work. It is important to note that the client can sabotage herself and her development, and that there is a difference between the underlying developmental needs and the need to maintain the status quo. In the diffusion phase experiments are ended, and the dialogue with and presence of the therapist are crucial. The therapist draws attention to the relationship between herself and the client, where she can use her own experiences and must tolerate the process in order to hold the client in unpleasantness and discomfort. During the contraction phase the therapist holds and supports the client so that she dares to feel the fear and discomfort and to believe in the change. When expansion comes, the therapist shares in the client's joy and relief and reflects on the new experience.

If the therapist becomes frightened or uncertain in the process, it is important that she takes that uncertainty and fear seriously. There may be signals that the client is not ready to be in the unpleasantness of this process of change, that she is going too fast, or that they are in a different phase than the therapist thinks. It may also be that the therapist herself is not ready to be with the client in such a process, or that she lacks knowledge or experience. In such a situation it is important that she seek supervision to further explore the sensations and unrest she experiences.

When the process of change is too demanding

Being in this type of change process can be too demanding for some clients. This is especially true of the diffusion phase, where a lack of meaning and direction in the process can be too daunting and challenging. This may apply to clients who do not have a level of self-support, network, or structure that enables them to be in this type of challenging process. Having regular routines, such as a job to go to, friends and family who care, and past experiences of handling difficult situations are factors that together make it more likely that clients can tolerate a process that can at times feel completely unbearable.

If the therapist doubts the client's capacity and life situation in a change process, it is important that she change her therapeutic approach. She can, for example, keep the client in the polarisation phase by constantly exploring difficult individual situations from the client's everyday life. She can also explore the client's life situation further and see if it is possible for her to create more structure where it is lacking. If the client is on sick leave or unemployed, the therapist and client can explore ways to create daily routines. The therapist can also support the client to contact former friends or groups, or to go on walks or involve herself in activities. If the client is in a major crisis and at the same time has a small network, the therapist may contact the client's physician, mental health carer, or other institutions that may be relevant to the client. The therapist's ability to be present with care and empathy while being aware of the limitations and possibilities of the therapy situation is fundamental in all work with people, and its importance is illustrated especially well in this model.

Summary

The change model can be used in all change work but is especially suitable when working with clients who are in crisis or have been exposed to traumatic experiences. The model provides a structure for therapists that can be useful in practice but is not a recipe for what therapists should do; rather, it is a guideline or map that can be used to navigate the process. It is especially important that the therapist is aware of which phase she is in with the client and is aware of the choices she makes in the different phases.

The steps in a therapeutic process of change are described in the example of Miriam, and the characteristic conditions of each phase are highlighted. In the examples, you can recognise therapy work described elsewhere in this book, including the work on polarities and various forms of contact. We have also shown how the therapist can use chair work through the example of Miriam's conflicting needs in relation to her husband, and how the therapist uses chair work in internal conflicts. In all phases in the example, it is important for the therapist to hold Miriam in what she describes as difficult, while at the same time supporting and challenging her to explore different needs and opportunities. In this way, the therapist helps her to gain new experiences. In such a challenging process, the therapist relies on the theory of paradoxical change and does not push for a change to occur but is instead with the client with a great deal of awareness and attention to her and the process between them.

References

Eie, E. (2005). Fra full stopp til vekst og utvikling [From a complete stop to growth and development]. *Norsk Gestalttidsskrift*, 2(2), 21–34.

Perls, F. S. (1970/2006). Four Lectures. In Fagan, J., & Shepherd, E. L. (Eds.), *Gestalt therapy now: Theory, techniques, applications*. (pp. 14-38). Gouldsboro, ME: The Gestalt Journal Press.

Staemmler, F. M. (1994). On layers and phases. *The Gestalt Journal, 17*(1), 5–30.

Staemmler, F. M., & Bock, W. (1998). *Ganzheitliche Veränderung in der Gestalttherapie* [Holistic change in gestalt therapy]. Wupperthal: Peter Hammer Verlag.

Index

Page numbers in *italic* indicate a figure on the corresponding page.